THE WAY OF THE FIVE SEASONS

by the same author

The Way of the Five Elements
52 weeks of powerful acupoints for physical, emotional, and spiritual health
John Kirkwood
ISBN 978 1 84819 270 6
eISBN 978 0 85701 216 6

of related interest

Qigong Through the Seasons
How to Stay Healthy All Year with Qigong, Meditation, Diet, and Herbs
Ronald H. Davis
Foreword by Kenneth Cohen
ISBN 978 1 84819 238 6
eISBN 978 0 85701 185 5

The 12 Chinese Animals
Create Harmony in Your Daily Life through Ancient Chinese Wisdom
Master Zhongxian Wu
ISBN 978 1 84819 031 3
eISBN 978 0 85701 015 5

Principles of Chinese Medicine
What it is, how it works, and what it can do for you
Second Edition
Angela Hicks
ISBN 978 1 84819 130 3
eISBN 978 0 85701 107 7
Discovering Holistic Health series

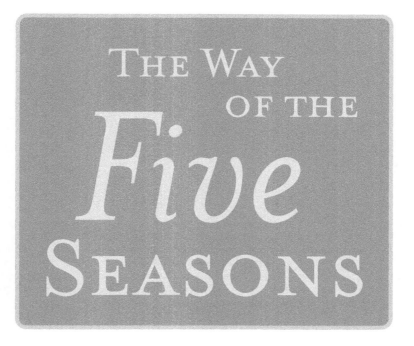

THE WAY OF THE
Five
SEASONS

Living with the Five Elements
for Physical, Emotional
and Spiritual Harmony

JOHN KIRKWOOD

SINGING
DRAGON

LONDON AND PHILADELPHIA

The 12 meridian pathways are illustrated by Lyndall Bryden.

First published in 2016
by Singing Dragon
an imprint of Jessica Kingsley Publishers
73 Collier Street
London N1 9BE, UK
and
400 Market Street, Suite 400
Philadelphia, PA 19106, USA

www.singingdragon.com

Library of Congress Cataloging in Publication Data
Names: Kirkwood, John (Professor of Chinese medicine)
Title: The way of the five seasons / John Kirkwood.
Description: Philadelphia : Singing Dragon, 2016. | Includes bibliographical
 references and index.
Identifiers: LCCN 2015038698 | ISBN 9781848193017 (alk. paper)
Subjects: LCSH: Five agents (Chinese philosophy)
Classification: LCC B127.F58 K57 2016 | DDC 610.951--dc23 LC record available at http://lccn.loc.
gov/2015038698

British Library Cataloguing in Publication Data
A CIP catalogue record for this book is available from the British Library.

ISBN 978 1 84819 301 7
eISBN 978 0 85701 252 4

Printed and bound in Great Britain

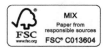

Contents

Acknowledgements

They say that all fiction is autobiographical. This work of non-fiction is no less so, distilled through my every experience over six decades. The list of people to acknowledge is therefore extensive. Rather than attempt to compile such a catalogue, I have chosen to describe the kinds of people who have influenced, taught, helped, loved, supported and guided me to the place from which this book emerges. Thus, with great gratitude, I thank: my family who have given me life, love, connection and belonging; all the teachers who have shared their knowledge and shown me a path through life; all the loves of my life who have haped and grown my heart; all the many friends all over the world who have been good and supportive companions; all the spiritual guides and teachers who have nudged me along the path of realisation; True Nature, the true author of this book, that which is the nature of me, you and everything.

Notes on the Text

- Throughout this book I have capitalised Element, Five Elements, Constitutional Element, Extraordinary Vessel, Official and the substances of Qi, Blood and Essence in order to distinguish the context-specific usage herein from the more common usages of these words.

- In Chinese medicine each internal organ is only one aspect of a much wider energetic system. For example, capitalisation of 'Large Intestine' signals this referencing, while lowercase 'large intestine' refers only to the organ from a Western perspective.

- 'Essence' is used in two senses: from the perspective of Chinese medicine, 'Essence' is the substance known as *jing*; from the perspective of the Diamond Approach, 'Essence' is the true nature of who we are.

- I have italicised Chinese words such as *shen* and *jing* but not 'Qi', 'yin' or 'yang', which have more fully entered modern usage.

Preface

My Journey with the Five Elements

One day in February 1991, I was working with a client in my office in Palo Alto, California. It was a normal day, a normal session of massage and acupressure, nothing remarkable. There was nothing to indicate that something was about to happen that would chart the trajectory of my life.

As my hands were gliding up and down my client's back, a thought suddenly sprang into my mind. I remembered that months before, my friend Michael had recommended a workshop on the Five Elements of Chinese medicine. *About time I looked into that*, the thought said. Soon after that, I heard the mail delivery drop through the slot of the front door.

After my client had left, I looked through the mail. The usual clutch of business offers went straight into the recycling. But among them was a brochure from the Traditional Acupuncture Institute of Maryland offering a workshop entitled 'Redefining Health'. As I read beyond the rather bland title, I realised that it was the workshop on the Five Elements that I had just been thinking about.

The coincidence, the synchronicity of this, was too great to ignore. It became very clear that I had to go to this workshop. Two months later I travelled to the Lone Mountain Center in San Francisco along with 50 or so others to check out what these acupuncturists from the East Coast were on about. There I met my new teachers: Bob Duggan, Diane Connelly and Julia Measures. That weekend was a whirlwind of new ideas and possibilities. What happens, they asked, if we take down the treatment room walls, throw away the needles and take the core principles of Five Element acupuncture out into the world? How can we use the Five Element model to move energy in ordinary life situations – at the office, in our personal relationships, at the supermarket? How can we become practitioners to life?

I was very excited about these ideas. I was already a practitioner in the treatment room. But to take this practice into the whole of my life and into all my relationships? This was revolutionary. I don't normally embrace new methods so quickly, but straight away I took to this like a duck to Water, and to Wood, Fire, Earth and Metal. My journey with the Five Elements had begun.

In November 1991 I began my deeper studies with Bob, Diane, Julia and also John Sullivan. These four teachers made regular trips to San Francisco over the course of the next year to instruct our group of 20 in what they called the SOPHIA Program.[1] We came from all walks of life. Some were health practitioners like myself, others were people from business and commerce, artists and freelancers. We studied each of the Five Elements in its own season, beginning with Metal in the autumn of 1991, then Water in the winter, Wood in the spring of 1992, Fire in the summer and Earth in the late summer. Through a range of teachings, activities and practices, we immersed ourselves in each Element and learned its gifts for us as well as its challenges.

In November 1992 our group met for the final time and our year-long training was over. Bob, Diane, Julia and John went back to Maryland and we graduates were left feeling more than a little cut adrift. The work had become so important, so meaningful in our lives, that we were not ready to stop there. So we began to meet as a group on our own to explore how we might continue this work with the Elements. We met socially with an eye to seeing what might come next. At our first meeting there were 14 of us; at subsequent meetings the numbers dwindled until just five of us remained: Jenny Josephian, Tom Balles, Susan Leahy, Devi Brown and myself. Two acupuncturists, a landscape gardener, an accountant and a massage therapist. Later we were joined by freelance adman Daniel Meyerovich and acupuncturist Keith Stetson.

What arose was the notion to offer experiential classes in the Five Elements to introduce this remarkable wisdom to others. We dubbed ourselves Five Hands Clapping, a rather whimsical allusion to the Five Elements and Zen mystery. We began our workshops in 1993. Each of us would prepare a presentation, exercise or activity to bring out one or more of the qualities of the Element of the season. Our aim was to create a pool of Water, of Wood, of Fire, of Earth, of Metal for people to immerse themselves in. What we discovered was that each class became like a treatment. The acupuncturists found that their patients who attended the classes responded as if to treatment with needles. Some people would feel like a million bucks afterwards. Others would feel awful as if having a treatment reaction. One person even stormed out of a class and was never seen again. Almost everyone was strongly affected in some way.

One of the things we discovered was that many people would feel a great resistance to coming to one particular Element workshop and would find 15 good reasons not to attend. I myself had the experience of getting sick just before a Wood class and could not go. When the very same thing happened the next year, I realised I had a great resistance to exploring the Wood Element and forced myself to attend anyway.

After three years of offering classes, there were only four instructors left. We decided to take a break from teaching and began holding workshops for ourselves. These became retreats and we would meet in a location that suited the season. We prepared activities for ourselves. We cooked for each other in accord with the Elements. And we explored keeping silence.

These retreats were very fruitful and provided the support for much deeper exploration of the Elements within ourselves. For me they established a rhythm of living with the Elements that has never diminished, but rather strengthened with the passing years.

The final year of Five Hands Clapping was 1999. Our numbers had dwindled to three and so we disbanded the group.

This period of Five Hands was a rich and seminal one for me. Many of the ideas, inspirations, exercises and activities that were generated by this amazing group were later to find their way into my own teaching of the Five Elements and into this book.

In December 2006 I returned to live in Australia after almost 19 years in California. I settled in the Adelaide Hills and began to focus on the practice of Five Element acupressure that had been my work in Palo Alto. Also I began to teach the acupressure course at Adelaide's Natural Health Academy. I took over the diploma classes there and also began a series of advanced acupressure classes that owed much to the Five Hands model.

The next thing to arise was a newsletter. In the southern autumn of 2009, the idea just popped into my head, just like that thought back in 1991. I began to write an E-zine that I called 'Bubbling Spring' after the first point of the Kidney meridian. This publication explored the attributes, associations, resonances and Gifts of the Five Elements while at the same time offering a forum for practitioners and others interested in the Five Elements to contribute, comment and advertise.

This proved of great value to many readers, yet I feel that I was the greatest beneficiary. By imposing deadlines on myself, over the course of four years and 19 issues, I forced myself to dig deep, deeper and then deeper still into myself, my understanding, my knowledge and experience to craft newsletters of value. This process required large amounts of reading and research which greatly deepened my understanding of this ancient wisdom. And, not least, it was a training ground for writing. Writing seems such a simple thing, until you go to publish.

More recently a new series of workshops has arisen which I call *Seasons of Life*. They draw upon the model of the SOPHIA course, Five Hands Clapping workshops and my own 25 years of living with the Elements. These seasonal workshops offer an immersion in the Element of each season as well as a supportive group setting to explore at depth the resonances of the Elements in oneself. Now in its third year, Seasons of Life has been profoundly transformative for many people. There has been physical healing, psychological understanding, emotional balance and spiritual development. I include myself in this.

These workshops have provided a place where the material of this book has been trialled and out of which new ideas for the book have sprung. I want to acknowledge the contribution that all of the attendees of this group have made to the development of this work.

Most recent of all in my exploration of the Five Elements has been the writing of a fortnightly blog. This focuses on the acupoints, exploring the nature and uses of each point at physical, psycho-emotional and spiritual levels. Intended as a practical guide to the uses of the points in modern life, the blogs have been well received by practitioners, students and clients alike. In fact, it was this blog that led to the creation of my first book, *The Way of the Five Elements*.

When I originally submitted to Singing Dragon publishers the manuscript of the book you now hold in your hands, it was politely declined. However, Jessica Kingsley herself saw the value of the blog and invited me to write a book based on it. As this spin-off book neared completion, Singing Dragon reconsidered my original magnum opus and offered to publish it as this current title.

Those who have already read *The Way of the Five Elements* may therefore notice some overlap in the material. While there is some repetition, I hope readers will appreciate the fuller, expanded treatment that this volume offers.

Which brings me to the present. As Steve Jobs put it in his famous 2005 address to Stanford University graduates, you can only connect the dots in retrospect. By writing this little history, I see how the dots have led to the publication of this book. What began with a thought popping into my head during a massage session in 1991 has led me through 25 spirals of the Elements cycle. I use the word 'spiral' because we don't return to the same place each year. We return changed, with more wisdom, more depth and more consciousness.

This book is the condensation of this score and more of cycles. I hope that readers can find some of the excitement, the understanding and the wow of living life through the guidance of the Five Elements. As I have.

The Diamond Approach

In the year 2000 I began to study with a teacher of the Diamond Approach, a path of realisation whose fundamental practice is ongoing inquiry into the truth of one's present experience. While it is a modern teaching, it contains much that is familiar from Eastern traditions such as Buddhism, Taoism, Sufism and Vedanta. One of the things that sets it apart from these other traditions is its use of modern psychological understanding to support spiritual unfolding. The teaching developed through A.H. Almaas who describes the work this way:

> The Diamond Approach is a contemporary teaching that developed within the context of awareness of both ancient spiritual teachings and modern depth psychological theories; hence, the perspective of this teaching recognises the inherent synthesis between the spiritual and the psychological domains of experience. The spiritual and the psychological can be separated only in theory, for in experience they are two dimensions of the same human consciousness. Recognizing this truth makes it possible to approach the path to inner realization informed with modern psychological knowledge, and thus allows the process of understanding one's psychological experience to open one's consciousness to the deeper truths of our spiritual nature.[2]

When I was 13 years old and began to conceptualise, I rejected the Christian teachings to which I had been exposed as a child and became a committed and vociferous atheist. Not realising then that I'd thrown the baby out with the bathwater, I spent the next three decades finding my way back to a spirituality that was meaningful to me. The way back led me through humanistic astrology, spiritualism, Tibetan Buddhism, Zen Buddhism and shamanism. Following a gross betrayal by a Mexican shaman, I felt spiritually adrift. It was in this place at the turn of the millennium that I discovered the Diamond Approach.

I signed up for a series of ten sessions with a teacher in this school and was openly curious. About the fourth or fifth session I found something subtle but significant was changing in me, as if something was awakening. I have now been working with my teacher for 15 years and he has been a wise and loving guide through many dark passages and blissful states.

In 2002 A.H. Almaas, who to me will always be Hameed, began to teach a group again for the first time in about 20 years. I just happened to be in the right place at the right time to join the Diamond Heart 6 group which has been taught by Hameed and Karen Johnson for the past 13 years. This group of seekers has become a kind of spiritual family for me. Its field is palpable to me wherever I go.

It is said that our work in the world is a blend of all we have met. So it is natural that my work with the Five Elements should be influenced by this spiritual path. My work has become a blending of the ancient Taoist model of the world and the modern spiritual path of the Diamond Approach. It is a natural blending. Many of the fundamental tenets of Taoism are shared by the Diamond Approach. Sometimes I find passages written by the Taoist sages over 2000 years ago and I feel like I'm reading one of Hameed's books.

It seems to me that the Diamond Approach is articulating many of the understandings of the ancients but using modern language and drawing upon modern psychological knowledge, mapping this world view in a way that is both detailed and appropriate for the modern world.

Throughout this book I have tried to present the views and perspectives of classical Chinese medicine. At the same time I have included other perspectives. The Western medical view is included as is that of Western naturopathy. So too are the ideas of Western and Eastern philosophers of two millennia. The understandings of over a century of psychological understanding also form a large part of the text. In the sections on the spiritual realm of the Elements, the Taoist and Confucian views appear side by side with those of the Buddhist, Hindu, Sufi and Diamond Approach traditions.

What holds all of these ideas together, what anchors the whole structure of the book, is the Five Element model. It is a model that is ancient yet perfectly applicable to the contemporary world. Simple. Sophisticated. Elegant. Timeless.

John Kirkwood
Adelaide Hills
September 2015

Part 1

Preparing for a Journey

———————————————

Chapter 1

How to Use This Book

Living the Book

It is amazing how many people, when I mention the Five Elements, say, 'I've always wanted to know more about that.' Well, this book tells you more.

But it is more than just a collection of information that satisfies the mind's curiosity. It certainly does contain a lot that is interesting, but it is much more than that. What this book offers is a practical guide to using the Five Element model in your daily life in ways that can improve your physical health, foster mental ease and clarity, create more emotional balance and bring you closer to spirit which is the True Nature of who you are.

The way these changes can come about for you is by evoking each Element in turn, immersing yourself in all the manifestations of that Element and engaging with its qualities in all areas of your life and your being. The more you actively call the Element into your life, the more the gifts of that Element will be revealed within you.

When you have this kind of access to an Element, you are able to experience the world and interact with it through the strengths and gifts of that Element. If you have access to all five, then you are living a full life. You are able to live fully from all possible phases, all possible perspectives. The corollary of this is that if you are closed down or stuck in an Element, you are unable to perceive and experience the capacities and gifts of that Element. It closes you down to one area of human life.

The way to get the most out of this book is to 'live the book' over the course of a year. This is how I wrote the book, by living each Element chapter in its own season as thoroughly as possible. While the material may be *read* at any time, the chapters are best *lived* in their own seasons. This is because nature provides us with five seasons that are perfectly aligned with the vibrations of their corresponding Elements. For example, the Water Element is most prominent in winter. Winter provides us with cold days and long dark nights, the better to rest, sleep more and gather our resources. It supports us to stay home and do less. And it gives us the opportunity to find our still places, to go inward and explore the depth of ourselves. If we do spend the winter immersed in the Water Element, we are much better prepared to take advantage of everything that the Wood Element has to offer in spring. Rested and restored as we are, we can leap up and move forward with a spring in our step, put plans into operation with vigour and purpose, fully supported by the energy in nature that is doing exactly the same thing.

If you choose to accept this mission of living the book, start by reading Part 1 of the book. Then choose the Element chapter that corresponds to the season you are currently in and begin there. If you are part way through a season and don't have time to fully explore all the exercises and activities, that's okay, the season will come round again next year and you can finish then. I know from long experience that when you immerse yourself in an Element in its own season, you are inviting its wisdom in. This begins an alchemical process that is as magical as it is mysterious.

The focus of this book is on actively engaging with the Elements. It offers a range of methods of doing this. There are several categories of activities which are described in more detail in Chapter 5. These activities include movement, cooking, gardening, journaling, visualisation, meditation, dialogue and self-acupressure. All of these activities I have used myself and many have been used with groups, so I know they can work. Since we are all very different people with unique backgrounds and experiences, some of these activities will resonate more than others. Some of them might feel awkward at first, but I encourage you to give them all a try. You never know if you'll find some new way into yourself by trying something unfamiliar.

Each Element chapter is divided into three sections, each of which focuses on one level or expression of human life. The first of these levels is the physical body, its structures, organs, tissues and systems. The second is the psycho-emotional body, made up of thoughts, beliefs, self-images, emotions and reactions. The third level is that of the spirit, that part that is neither body, personality nor history, and which is both eternal and non-dual. I will explain more about these three levels in Chapter 4.

If you have got this far into the book, then you are probably a person who has an interest in self-awareness and self-exploration. What the book offers is a simple yet elegant model of the world that is perfectly suited to this endeavour. The Five Element model arose out of the philosophy of Taoism which sees everything in our world as arising out of the void or the Great Mystery. Moreover, we and everything else in the world are being continually recreated moment by moment out of this void. Thus, we are both separate and indivisible at the same time, like waves arising out of the same ocean.

The philosophy that underpins the work of this book presupposes that we are both wave and ocean. There is a particular wave of you which eats, sleeps, thinks, feels, goes to work, has relationships and hobbies, and eventually dies. And there is the ocean of you that is also the ocean of everyone and everything, an ocean which never dies and is indestructible.

The activities in the book encourage you to explore yourself at all levels of your human existence. By so doing, you are allowing the Great Mystery to express itself more completely in this strange and wonderful world of ours.

Becoming a Practitioner to Yourself

In our quest for good physical, mental, emotional and spiritual health, we all need the help and guidance of specialists. When we have a physical illness, we seek a practitioner such as a doctor, an acupuncturist, a naturopath or a chiropractor. When we feel our mental and emotional state is interfering with our functioning in the world, we seek psychological help from a counsellor, therapist or psychologist. And when our spirit is suffering, we seek guidance from spiritual individuals or groups who can support the unfolding of that part of us which is eternal.

All of these sources of assistance are invaluable to us as we move through the many changes and phases of our lives. But we may overlook the inherent wisdom within ourselves. Some have called this place the inner doctor, the part of us that truly knows what is best for us. Others have referred to it as our inner guidance or inner self. But it is often not an easy thing to contact that place within us, that part of us that knows the best way we can heal ourselves and support ourselves to grow into our greatest potential.

Just as we seek out practitioners to help and guide us to greater health, we can look for and discover the practitioner inside us. This is the practitioner who is closest to us, most attuned to us and most interested in our health and development. It is our inner doctor, our quiet voice, our kind guide.

How do we find this amazing person? Well, she is right there all the time. The way we find her is to discover what gets in the way of hearing her voice. What lies in the way are things like fears, judgements, beliefs, self-criticism and negative patterns that run our thinking.

There are many ways to explore these impediments to finding our inner practitioner. Psychotherapy offers tools to understand the way our mind functions, and through that understanding, brings more of ourselves into conscious awareness so that our behaviour changes. There are spiritual practices like Buddhism, mindfulness practices and energetic practices like yoga and tai chi. All of these practices offer methods of uncovering the stillness within.

What this book offers is a model for self-understanding which has its origins in China several thousand years ago and which has been moulded to our Western perspective of the world since the 1960s by several generations of Five Element practitioners. This model provides us with a framework that organises the whole of existence into five categories, each with its own vibration. These five meta-vibrations provide the template for everything.

As we begin to understand how these five vibrations operate within us, we get to see to what extent they are expressed in healthy and balanced ways, and also to discover what is out of balance, stuck and not working well.

This book will guide you through this Five Element landscape and train you to become practitioner to yourself. While you won't abandon all those other practitioners who have helped you and will continue to help you in your journey to health, you will learn to find the most important practitioner in your life: *you*.

Chapter 2 ————————————————————

The Five Element Model

Origins and History of the Five Elements

Throughout this book I use the term 'Element' to refer to the five different vibrations of all things. Some scholars and practitioners do not use the term 'Elements' but refer to them as the five phases. This more accurately describes the cycle as a series of stages and avoids confusion with the concept of an Element as a component part. While I agree that *phase* is a more accurate description of what is occurring, I have stayed with the word 'Element' because it has so thoroughly taken root in common usage. As long as it is clear that we are referring to a phase of a cycle and not to a constituent like hydrogen, then I see no problem using the word 'Element'.[1]

Naturalists

The earliest developments of the Five Element perspective are lost in the mists of prehistory, since writing did not develop in China until about 1200 BCE. But it is clear that this way of viewing the world was based on a close observation of nature. Because of its monolithic land mass, China is much less connected to the sea than is Western Europe and so the ties of its people to the land were deeper.[2] Whereas in Europe proximity to the seas led to prolific trade, in China the dependence on the produce of the land was profound. This shaped the very social structure of society and deeply influenced the philosophy of the Chinese people for millennia. The perspective of the simple farmer who was in close contact with the rhythm of the seasons informed the development of the Five Element model.

The first articulation of this nature-based perspective was in the third century BCE by the School of Naturalists, or the Yin-Yang school, which attempted to explain the universe in terms of the forces of nature: the polarity of yin (dark, cold, female, receptive) and yang (light, hot, male, assertive); and the Five Elements of Water, Wood, Fire, Earth and Metal. The perspectives of this early philosophical school became absorbed into the later development of Taoism.

Taoism

Taoism is named after that pillar of Chinese philosophical writing the *Tao Te Ching* whose authorship is ascribed to Lao Tzu. Whether Lao Tzu (literally Old Master) was a historical personage has been a matter of scholarly debate. Be that as it may, the text itself is real and the earliest extant version dates to about 300 BCE. It is a short work of great influence. In fact, its impact cannot be overstated since its philosophy shaped the thinking of many other philosophical schools to follow. Moreover, its cosmological perspective became inextricably interwoven into Chinese medicine. Literally translated as the *Classic of the Way of Virtue*, this book has more than 250 English translations. Its meaning is often as mysterious as the Great Mystery of the Tao itself. But what is clear is that it is based on the principles of yin and yang, and living in accord with the harmony of nature.

The other great pillar of Taoist literature is the *Neijing Su Wen* or *The Yellow Emperor's Classic of Medicine*. The *Neijing* purports to be a series of conversations between the mythical Yellow Emperor Huang Di and his ministers. Huang Di ruled China around 2500 BCE. However, the text of the *Neijing* we have today was believed to have been written around the second century BCE. It has become the foundational source of Chinese medicine for over 2000 years. It comprises two books each of 81 chapters. The first book, *Suwen* or *Basic Questions*, is the most commonly cited. It covers theory and diagnosis in Chinese medicine. The second part is known as the *Lingshu* or *Spiritual Pivot* and contains details of acupuncture practice.

The principles of the Naturalist school now became clearly articulated. The Neijing explains how the natural forces of yin and yang, Qi and the Five Elements can be understood and used to bring balance and harmony to life. Thus, the Neijing does not only give details of a system of medicine but is in fact a model of holistic living in all realms of human life. It does not separate external changes such as geographic, climatic and seasonal, from internal changes such as emotions and reactions.[3] In this sense it is the first book of holistic medicine.

A reading of this 2500-year-old text seems surprisingly apt for our modern world:

These days people have changed their way of life. They drink wine as though it were water, indulge excessively in destructive activities, drain their *jing*

(Essence) and deplete their Qi. They do not know the secret of conserving their energy and vitality. Seeking excitement and momentary pleasures, people disregard the natural rhythm and order of the universe. They fail to regulate their lifestyle and diet, and sleep improperly. So it is not surprising that they look old at fifty and die soon after.[4]

The influence of this text on Chinese medicine and Chinese thought in general cannot be overstated. Not only did it influence the theory and practice of acupuncture, massage, diet, herbs and lifestyle in China over the next two millennia, its teachings also found their way into other Asian cultures, particularly Japan, Korea and Vietnam.

Decline of Acupuncture and the Five Elements

During the Qing dynasty of the Manchus (1644–1911) acupuncture began a long decline in favour of herbalism. It has been suggested that the Manchus, invaders from the north, were afraid that their physicians were going to murder them with needles and ordered acupuncture not to be used.[5] What is more, the system utilised by herbalism was not related to the Five Element system, but to one known as Eight Principles for Differentiating Syndromes. So not only did acupuncture suffer a decline, but also one of the fundamental principles on which it had been founded, namely the Five Elements, lost its influence.

Another historical development contributed to the overall decline in all kinds of traditional medicine, namely that of rapid Westernisation in the latter part of the nineteenth century. Once Western allopathic medicine was introduced into China, it quickly supplanted the traditional medicine. This process was further accelerated by the collapse of the dynastic system in 1912. A law was passed in 1929 prohibiting the practice of the old medicine. The period that followed saw China descend into the chaos of civil war, invasion by Japan and further civil war, culminating in the eventual takeover by the Communists in 1949.

Taking over a ravaged country, Mao Tse-Tung was eager to find a system of health care that would support China's vast, growing and impoverished population, and so turned to the traditional methods. In 1958 he famously declared that 'Chinese medicine is a great treasure house. We must make all efforts to uncover it and raise its standards.'[6] With that encouragement, a new system of medicine was created that was based on traditional methods but which was in alignment with the Communist principles of rationalism and atheism. What emerged was a system that became known as Traditional Chinese Medicine

(TCM), a system that became codified and taught in colleges rather than by the old way of learning from a master.

This is the system that was in place when US president Richard Nixon made his historic visit to China in 1972, an event which radically opened China to Western contact and trade. The form of acupuncture and herbalism that was subsequently exported to the West was a system that had been carefully culled of anything of a spiritual nature and which contained little of Five Element theory.

The Five Elements Move West

While this great leap forward into TCM was developing in China, European practitioners had already become interested in Chinese medicine. The first European to become skilled in acupuncture was the sinologist George Soulié de Morant who was publishing works on acupuncture in French as early as 1929. What he brought to Europe predated the development of TCM and so was more aligned with the ancient methods. Indeed, his writings contain much that was to find its way into Five Element acupuncture but which was omitted from TCM. His influence on the development of acupuncture in Europe has earned him the title of grandfather of traditional acupuncture in the West.

Another Frenchman, Jacques Lavier, was responsible for the spread of these ideas throughout Western Europe through his writings and the conferences he organised. Lavier exerted a particularly strong influence upon the early English acupuncturists and could be said to have been the principal cause of the early elevation of the Five Element method in England. English acupuncturists Denis Lawson-Wood (1959),[7] Felix Mann (1962)[8] and Mary Austin (1972)[9] all published books on acupuncture which focused on this method.

J.R. Worsley and Five Element Acupuncture

It was in this climate that J.R. Worsley, a practising osteopath, began to study acupuncture. He was a graduate of Lavier's historic 1963 seminar in London and later made trips to China, Taiwan and Japan to study with masters whose techniques were largely in alignment with the methods he had already learned through Lavier.

By the time Worsley began teaching in about 1966[10] his method of treatment, focusing on the Five Element model, was already established. This was before the codification of TCM and the Eight Principles method by the Chinese authorities. What had happened was that the ancient methods that were abandoned by the

Chinese in the 1970s took root and flourished in a most unlikely environment: England.

Meanwhile, in the USA, the American journalist James Reston brought the attention of his country and the world to the wonders of acupuncture as a result of his own emergency surgery in China in 1971.[11] His appendectomy was performed using acupuncture needles in lieu of anaesthetic. The news sparked interest among Americans wanting to study acupuncture. Two years later, a group of American students, most notably Bob Duggan and Diane Connelly, went to England to study with Worsley. They returned to the USA to establish their own college of acupuncture in 1974. This Traditional Acupuncture Institute (TAI) began teaching its first class in 1981.

In 1987, at the request of patients, TAI began a program they called School of Philosophy and Healing in Action (SOPHIA) to teach laypeople the ancient wisdom, rooted in nature, that underpinned its master's program in acupuncture. The SOPHIA program is now an integral part of the acupuncture degree, signalling that the practice of acupuncture comes from the depth of the practitioner and is not simply an analytical exercise. This is the program that I had the great fortune to attend at its only incarnation in San Francisco, California. The influence of my teachers, Bob Duggan, Diane Connelly, Julia Measures and John Sullivan, has been immense.

Since TAI began breaking down the acupuncture treatment room walls and taking the underlying principles out into the world, the Five Element perspective has penetrated into many areas. There are Five Element exercise programs, Five Element music and movement styles, Five Element life coaching, Five Element diets and cookbooks. There has been an upsurge of interest in Five Element feng shui. There are various kinds of Five Element bodywork including acupressure, shiatsu and Chi Nei Tsang. There is Five Element Chi Kung, Five Element yoga and the Five Element dance movement style of Wu Tao. There seems no limit to the application of these ancient principles to modern life.

Five Element Theory

What follows is a brief overview of the theoretical principles underpinning the Five Element model. Knowledge of these foundations is important in order to understand the ways in which the energies of the Elements operate and interact with one another and therefore impact our lives. We begin at the place where these five energies originate.

One Becomes Five

One

Let us take a look at the cosmological view from which this Five Element perspective arose. As we have seen, the Five Element model of Chinese medicine was put into written form at the time when Taoism was a predominant philosophy. Taoism is named for the concept of the Tao, the One which is the sum total of all reality: the Great Mystery. Because it is a Mystery, it cannot actually be described. As Lao-Tzu put it:

> *The Tao that can be told*
> *is not the eternal Tao.*
> *The name that can be named*
> *is not the eternal Name.*[12]

Moreover, the nameless Tao is so mysterious that it is both everything and nothing at the same time. Confused? Good. Now you are beginning to get it.

Two

The Tao, the One, exists (or doesn't exist) in a place that is outside the ordinary world of time and space. When the Tao begins to come into manifestation in our world, it does so by dividing into the Two. These two are the opposing but completely complementary forces of a polarity. The Chinese gave these forces the names of yin and yang. These words originally meant shady side of mountain (yin) and sunny side of mountain (yang). Now they refer to all manifestations of shade and sun, light and dark, cold and hot, moist and dry, female and male, low and high, earth and heaven and so on.

There are two important things to know about yin and yang. The first is that they are forever bound together and cannot exist without each other. For example, light only exists in relation to dark, hot to cold and so forth. The second is that they are relative states, not absolute. For example, when I am compared to an 80-year-old woman, I am yang relative to her yin. But when I stand next to a female Olympic athlete, I am relatively yin to her yang.

Three

Yin and yang are the fundamental forces that create our world. But in order for things to happen, for action to take place, there needs to be a moving force between the two poles of yin and yang. This movement derives from something that inhabits and motivates every single particle of our universe. The Chinese called this motivating force Qi (pronounced *chee*). It is a bit hard to translate this in one word. To call it energy is limiting and can be confused with something like electricity. It was considered by the Chinese to be a substance, but not the kind you can box up and sell. It's much more subtle, more resilient, more ubiquitous than anything else you can name. It is the fundamental substance of the universe. Since we don't have any word that can come close to a translation, I will just use the word Qi.

Four

Qi moves but where does it go? It moves out in all directions, to all infinite parts of the compass. But let's say for simplicity that it moves out to the four directions, namely north, south, east and west. To the zenith and nadir, the sunrise and sunset. This is representative of the dynamism of the Tao: that which does not exist comes into existence and moves everywhere throughout creation.

Five

Now we finally get to the five in Five Elements. The Qi moves out in the four directions from a central point. This central point of reference is the fifth Element, the Earth. Meanwhile, the other four Elements are derived from the four compass points. Wood comes from the east, the sunrise; Metal from the west, the sunset; Fire lies at the mid heaven, the highest point of the sun's circuit; and Water lies at the lowest point in deepest night.

If you can imagine looking down on the great pyramid, you would see the apex of the pyramid as a point in the centre with four lines radiating out to the corners. The central point and the connecting arms of the pyramid represent the Earth Element while the four sides represent the other four Elements. The Earth Element acts as a central axis connecting all the other Elements together.

Generation Cycle

As in the above analogy of the pyramid, the Earth insinuates itself into all four points of transition, between Wood and Fire, between Fire and Metal, between Metal and Water, and between Water and Wood. In fact, its energy is palpable at each of these points of change. But if we move the Earth out of the centre and into the place between Fire and Metal, what results is a cycle known as the Sheng or Generation Cycle (see Figure 2.1). It represents a cycle in which each Element gives birth to (generates) the next.

The way this cycle works can be best illustrated by looking at the seasons in nature. (We will look at the seasons more closely in later chapters.) For now, we will see how the five energies feed each other around the circle. We can begin anywhere on a circle, but I'll begin with the Water Element whose seasonal manifestation is winter.

Winter is a time of darkness, coldness, stillness and waiting. Nature is preserving its resources, holding its potential for the appropriate time. This is ideally represented as the seed waiting for the right conditions to germinate. The qualities of Water are quiet, patient waiting, pooling and storing of energy, not rushing to act but waiting for the signal to move. These qualities are what allow the energy of the Wood Element to arise in the spring.

Then, as if a starting gun has gone off, there is sudden, dramatic, dynamic, upward rising in nature and things grow rapidly as temperature and light increase. The strong upward movement in nature allows the seed to quickly manifest its genetic blueprint. The blueprint is the map of where the plant is going, what it will become. These are all qualities of the Wood Element.

Wood moves upwards and creates a strong trunk, which then gives birth to the Fire Element which spreads outwards. This is the energy of summer when everything in nature is bursting outwards to its fullest expansion. Nature is a riot. It is the hottest, brightest, most happening time of year. And the expansion is possible because it has been generated by the Wood.

What goes up must come down. After the zenith of Fire, the energy of the year begins to descend and generates the Earth Element in what we call the late summer season. There is a rounding, drooping, sagging feel to nature, a pleasant heaviness. This is the time of harvest when the fruits of the year are made manifest. The extent to which the Fire has fully flourished will determine the bounty of the harvest and the fullness of the Earth.

As the energy of the year continues to fall, Earth gives birth to Metal and the season of autumn. This is the time of year that nature discards what is no longer of use, and retains what is of greatest value to life. Trees lose their leaves, plants die after dropping their seeds. There is a garnering of what is most precious. This gathering of deepest value is what generates the return to Water.

So far we've seen how each Element gives birth to the next, each generating the next generation. When this system was developed in China, there was a strong Confucian influence which led people to view the world in terms of familial and societal relationships. It was said that each Element is mother to the next Element and in turn is child of the previous Element. This notion gave birth to the Law of Mother and Child. This simple concept has wide ramifications, as we shall see in later chapters. No Element stands on its own, but is a product of its mother and in turn a producer of its child.

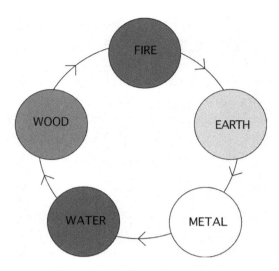

Figure 2.1 Generation Cycle

Control Cycle

If the Generation Cycle was the only one operating, then the energy would spiral out of control; therefore, another cycle operates simultaneously. The Chinese referred to this as the Ke Cycle, or Control Cycle (see Figure 2.2). In this cycle, each Element exerts a restraining or controlling influence on the next but one in a clockwise direction. This provides checks and balances that ensure dynamic equilibrium among all Elements.

By looking once again at nature, we can find analogies for how this works. Water controls Fire the way a bucket of water will douse a fire; Fire controls Metal in the way that heat will soften and shape the hardness of metal; Metal controls Wood in the way a knife will carve or pare wood; Wood controls Earth in the way tree roots will hold earth and soil together; and Earth controls Water in the way banks will shape a river's course or create a dam.

The ancient Chinese also saw the operation of this cycle in terms of familial relationships. It was known as the Law of Grandmother and Grandson. In their society of extended family, the role of the grandparents was to exert a kind but controlling influence on their grandchildren.

When these two cycles are taken together, there is the opportunity for perfect balance and harmony among the Elements. It will also be noted that each Element has a relationship with every other Element. Each Element is mother, child, grandmother and grandson. The Five are entirely interwoven, interdependent and interpenetrating. Again, we will see in later chapters how this principle operates in our lives.

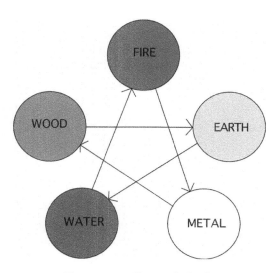

Figure 2.2 Control Cycle

Cycles Within Cycles

There is no absolute manifestation of a single Element. Everything in the universe is a unique combination of Elements.

You have probably seen the kind of picture which shows a person looking at a picture of himself looking at a picture of himself and so on to infinity. The same concept applies to the Five Elements. Water contains within it Wood, Fire, Earth, Metal and Water. In turn, each of these Elements within contains Wood, Fire, Earth, Metal and Water within them. And so on to infinity.

As a specific example of this, imagine being in the garden on a bright, sunny, unusually warm morning in late winter. You are experiencing the Wood (morning) and the Fire (warm day) all within the context of Water (winter). This is a simple example of the infinite possibilities and permutations of the kaleidoscope of Elements in our lives.

This principle of nature also operates within us. Each human being is a unique permutation of the Elements. We are like pixels on the colour wheel used in desktop publishing. There, each pixel is a particular combination of three or four coloured inks in the printer. Similarly, when it comes to human beings, each of us is a unique blend of the Five Elements. No two people are the same.

When we are born, our particular blend has already been created. While our early life experiences certainly shape our personality, direction and preferences, the fundamental cocktail of Elements within us has been mixed. This blend provides us with our uniqueness and shapes the direction, expression and manifestation of our life.

Constitutional Element

The concept of the Constitutional Element is perhaps J.R. Worsley's most significant contribution to the field. Worsley discovered that every person has one Element that has the greatest tendency to go out of balance and that this is also the first Element to go out of balance. Furthermore, he realised that this imbalance causes other Elements to go out of balance in a kind of domino effect. He also concluded that this Element that seems to be present at or soon after birth does not change during the course of a person's life. Worsley called this the 'causative factor', namely the Element that is the original cause of imbalance and disease. Later, Five Element practitioners referred to this as the Constitutional Element, which is the term I use in this book. But the original principle is Worsley's.

This Constitutional Element is not always easy to discover. There are many things that obscure it. Symptoms can be a compelling distraction. So too can behaviours and the stage of life the person is in. To find this Element, the practitioner focuses on four main diagnostic tools: the colour in the face, the sound of the voice, the subtle odour of the body and the predominant emotion in the person's life.[13] Each Element has a particular expression of colour, sound, odour and emotion, and ideally these four all appear in the patient. It is enough to have three of these factors to be sure of the diagnosis, but it is seldom easy and sometimes the Constitutional Element is deduced from fewer than three.[14]

When we do find the Element that is the root of all imbalance, then treatment focuses on that Element to bring it back into health and balance. The result of this is that all the other Elements follow it back to balance. During treatment, the other Elements are not ignored (far from it). But the treatment keeps coming back to this core Element as if it were the hub of a wheel from which all the spokes emanate.

When I refer to treatment, this is usually seen as a patient receiving acupuncture, acupressure or some other Five Element modality. But what I am offering here is a perspective in which all of life can be a source of treatment. As you become practitioner to yourself, every aspect of your life, including what you eat, what you like to do, your preferences, your emotional reactions, your spiritual beliefs – everything – can become a rich source of inquiry into who you are and why you are the way you are.

In this way, we can come to find our own responses and our own relationship to each of the Elements, to see where we are flowing and where we are struggling. And as we discover the Element of greatest challenge, we find our Constitutional Element. While this Element is indeed a challenge, it is at the same time our greatest potential. It is our life's work. It is why we are here. It is the doorway to unearthing our greatest treasure, the truth of who we are.

Chapter 3

The Landscape of the Elements

This chapter introduces you to the important concepts that you will meet in the chapters on the Elements. Here you will get the lay of the land, an overview of the whole kingdom, before you set out on your journey through its five principalities.

The Principle of Resonance

Imagine a great gong being struck. Its powerful, sonorous note passes out into the universe and all things of a similar vibration pick up the note, vibrating in perfect resonance.

Now imagine five great gongs sounding simultaneously, each with its own unique note. Imagine that, according to its nature, every single atom in the universe is resonating to one of these notes. Nothing is left out of this primal harmony.

Similarly, each of the Five Elements acts like the tone of one of the five great gongs, vibrating with its own frequency, a frequency that resonates precisely and profoundly in all expressions of that Element: a season of the year, a colour, a sound, an emotion, an odour, an organ of the body, a sense organ, a set of tissues, a psychological state, a spiritual state. They all pick up the note and resonate with its vibration like a great clan singing the same tone in harmony.

It is as if the Element is like the plucked G string of a guitar in a room full of guitars. The vibration of that string causes the G strings of all the other guitars in the room to vibrate, allowing the particular resonance of G to fill the room.[1] Another resonance that is more familiar to us is the empathic response we feel when someone talks about an experience, an idea or an emotion, and we feel that experience vibrating within us as though it were our own.

If we think of each Element as having a particular vibration, frequency or resonance, then we can understand how all of the associations and correspondences, in fact everything associated with that Element, will have the same vibration.

When we look inside ourselves, we discover that we are not separate from the grand resonant frequencies of the universe, and that, just like everything else, we actually resonate to all five frequencies. When we are balanced, the five frequencies can find their exact vibration within us, and the result is harmony within and between the Elements.

However, if we are out of balance in a particular Element, there is disharmony not only between the Elements, but within all expressions or correspondences of the Element, including the particular organs, emotions and aspects of spirit that are associated with that Element. If there is an off-note in one correspondence, then all the other correspondences of an Element will also be off-note.

The good news is that the corollary is also true. When we address one area of correspondence in our lives, all of the other correspondences will also respond. Thus, we can begin anywhere in our healing and the increasing harmony will flow through to all other areas of the Element. For example, working on the emotion of anger will help to heal the organs of gall bladder and liver, and vice versa. In this example we are bringing the Wood Element into balance, and so all aspects and resonances of Wood will be affected. You can strike the gong at any place and your action will resonate through the whole realm of its Element.

The rest of this section explains the correspondences or resonances of the Five Elements that we will focus on in later chapters. There are many other recognised resonances, but I've chosen nine of them for this book.

Seasons

The seasons of the year are perhaps the most obvious expression of the principle of resonance. Each season has a particular vibration and the way we feel about the season has a lot to do with how its vibration matches our own. Most people have a favourite season and a least favourite season. Some people can't wait for summer to arrive, and feel a sense of loss when it departs, while others hate summer so much they migrate to a cooler climate for those months.

On the other hand, there might be all kinds of reasons why people prefer summer to other seasons. Maybe that is when they go on vacation and get away from a boring job for a few weeks. Or it might be because they love summer sports and can't wait for the warm weather to get out there and play. Or perhaps they adore parties and summer is the time when there are lots of barbecues and get-togethers.

If we look at what is common to all of these activities – relaxing on vacation, playing sports in groups, partying with friends – we see that they all have a similar vibration. They are vibrating in resonance with summer and its associated Element of Fire. The way in which you resonate with activities like these gives an indication of the state of the Fire Element within you.

As you move through the year and pay attention to your responses to the changes in the seasons, you will be getting direct information about the state of health and balance of each Element within you. Often, the vibration of the new season will become palpable even before the change in the weather occurs, so it can be very useful to pay particular attention to how you are feeling at the very start of the season.

The timing of the change of season will vary depending on your location. Each chapter of Part 2 of this book gives some guidelines on when you might expect the new season and Element to emerge. Table 3.1 shows the Five Elements and their corresponding seasons.

Table 3.1 The Five Elements and Their Corresponding Seasons

Element	Season
Water	Winter
Wood	Spring
Fire	Summer
Earth	Late Summer
Metal	Autumn

Colours

Each of the Five Elements has a colour associated with it (see Table 3.2). These colours are another expression of the particular vibration of the Element. And just as we tend to have favourite seasons and least favourite seasons, we have colour preferences too.

Take a look at the colours in your wardrobe. What is the most predominant colour? What is missing altogether? Do you tend to wear different colours in different seasons, or in different weather? Do you choose colours to match your mood for the day, or do you choose a colour to change your mood? These choices indicate the influence on us of the different colours and their differing vibrations.

You can also observe how you respond to the various colours of nature. Do you love the lush green vegetation all around you on a forest walk? Would you rather spend time at the ocean, drinking in its vast blueness? Is your preference for the stark colours of mountains, or the bright red sands of a desert? Perhaps you like many of these colours in nature, but at different times.

As you move through the year, you can pay attention not just to your colour preferences but also to your response to the colours of nature around you as they change from season to season.

The colour resonance is one of the diagnostic tools of the Five Element practitioner. The practitioner looks for the predominant coloration of the client's face, particularly at the sides of the eyes. Finding this colour is one of the keys to discerning the client's Constitutional Element. For example, a yellowish colour around the eyes helps us identify a person's Constitutional Element as Earth. The colour is best seen in good natural light, and is often a subtle hue that is seen with 'soft eyes' when the observer is not really trying.

Table 3.2 The Five Elements and Their Corresponding Colours

Element	Colour
Water	Blue/Black
Wood	Green
Fire	Red
Earth	Yellow
Metal	White

Sounds of Voice

Just as the resonance of an Element creates a certain note, the human voice has a tone that reflects an inner vibration. This makes the quality of the voice very useful as a way of finding a person's Constitutional Element.

The five voices are described as groaning, shouting, laughing, singing and weeping (see Table 3.3). Most voices are a subtle combination of these sounds, but everyone has one that predominates. The Water voice can sound like a deep monotone coming from low down in the body, as if groaning with strain. The Wood voice may be clipped and forceful and have sharp edges. The Fire voice is often light and airy with the hint of a giggle. The Earth voice has the greatest range and sometimes sounds like a song. The Metal voice is falling and often cracked as if hiding tears.

This predominant sound of voice bears a strong correlation to a person's habitual emotional expression. The way a person speaks has a lot to do with how she is feeling emotionally. Everyone has a predominant emotional pattern and this will be revealed in the voice which becomes a vehicle for the emotion. This is usually quite unconscious and influences the sound of voice whatever the subject being spoken about.

Table 3.3 The Five Elements and Their Corresponding Voices

Element	Voice
Water	Groaning
Wood	Shouting
Fire	Laughing
Earth	Singing
Metal	Weeping

Odours

The sense of smell that captures and identifies odours is perhaps our most instinctual sense, the one that is closest to our animal nature. When we smell something, the nerve impulses go straight to the reptilian brain, bypassing the filters of interpretation used by our other senses. We may afterwards interpret what we have smelled, categorising it according to all the smells we know, and associate it with people and places from the past. But the initial 'hit' we get is unadulterated.

There are five broad categories of odour that correspond to the Elements (see Table 3.4). These can best be understood by reference to typical smells of the seasons. The odour of Water is putrid, which refers to the kind of smell you might get from a stagnant pond. The odour of Wood is rancid, the kind of smell you might get from newly cut grass in spring. The odour of Fire is scorched, like that of parched grass on a hot, dry summer day. The odour of Earth is fragrant, the kind of over-ripe smell that comes from fruit dropped under trees and breaking down in the late summer sun. And the odour of Metal is rotten, the smell of decaying, composting vegetation in the autumn.

For the Five Element practitioner, odour is a very important diagnostic tool in determining a person's Constitutional Element. Because smell is our most instinctual sense, the subtle scent of our skin can provide the most direct diagnosis. This is not what we might call 'body odour' from sweating, nor is it the odour of the breath. It is a subtle emanation from the whole body, and can best be sniffed between the shoulder blades, an area that is generally not washed as often as other areas of the body.

The more our health is out of balance, the stronger and more obvious will be our odour. For example, the smell from an unhealthy Wood type will be more like rancid oil than the cut-grass smell of a healthy Wood type.

In addition, the scents of our bodies are created differently from the smells of nature – they derive from the functioning (or malfunctioning) of the organs. Every Element has two associated organs, except for Fire, which has four. When the Constitutional Element goes out of balance, these corresponding organs are the first to be negatively affected, and they in turn affect the odour.

The putrid odour of Water arises because the bladder and kidneys are not processing urine properly. The rancid odour of Wood comes from the liver and gall bladder not breaking down fats as they should. The scorched odour of Fire is a result of the functions of Triple Heater and Heart Protector burning hotter than normal. The fragrant odour of Earth is a sickly sweet smell that is a result of the stomach not digesting food properly. The rotten odour of Metal arises from the large intestine not eliminating waste optimally.

Table 3.4 The Five Elements and Their Corresponding Odours

Element	Odour
Water	Putrid
Wood	Rancid
Fire	Scorched
Earth	Fragrant
Metal	Rotten

Emotions

So far, the resonances we have examined have been at the physical level, but these resonances also appear in more subtle ways, particularly in the emotions. The vibration of each Element corresponds to a specific emotion (see Table 3.5). When we feel a particular emotion, we are like a tuning fork vibrating in resonance with its corresponding Element.

While we all have all of the emotions at one time or another, everyone gravitates to one emotion in particular. It is the emotional groove we tend to fall into much of the time, and we are more familiar with that emotional tone than others. Thus, an assessment of overall emotional temperament provides the fourth and final diagnostic tool used by the Five Element practitioner to determine the client's Constitutional Element. Sometimes these predominant emotions are deeply supressed and are diagnosed by their conspicuous absence rather than by their presence.

Thus, a person whose most common response to life situations is to become fearful or fearless may be expressing a Water constitution. Someone who is habitually angry or who hides and suppresses his anger might be a Wood constitution. A person who is always upbeat and excitedly joyful or alternatively flat and depressed could be showing their Fire constitution. Someone who is overly sympathetic and helpful even at their own expense may be showing an Earth constitution. And a person for whom grief is ever-present or notably absent could be revealing their Metal constitution.

Emotions are seldom absent from our lives. They take up a large space in our consciousness, especially in our relationships. If we want to get to know ourselves and our Constitutional Element better, it is well worth spending some time considering our emotions. We might look at what they are, why we have them, how they serve us and how we can work with them as part of our movement towards greater wholeness.

We will be looking at the emotions in much more detail as we move through the chapters on the Elements.

Table 3.5 The Five Elements and Their Corresponding Emotions

Element	Emotion
Water	Fear
Wood	Anger
Fire	Joy
Earth	Sympathy
Metal	Grief

Tastes

The sense of taste is not one of the diagnostic tools of Five Element practitioners. You may be relieved to hear that they don't taste their clients to determine their Constitutional Element. However, our preferences for particular flavours can give us information about our relationship with the corresponding Elements (see Table 3.6).

Much of Asian cooking includes an attention to balance among flavours, so that a meal includes all of the five flavours of salty, sour, bitter, sweet and pungent. If you find you are craving a particular flavour and can't get enough of it, or if you can't stand a particular flavour and avoid it entirely, these preferences are telling you something about the state of the corresponding Element within you.

We will look at ways we can work with flavours in cooking in the chapter on the Earth Element.

Table 3.6 The Five Elements and Their Corresponding Tastes

Element	Taste
Water	Salty
Wood	Sour
Fire	Bitter
Earth	Sweet
Metal	Pungent

Senses and Sense Organs

In a way, we have already been referring to the senses through the other resonances. We have to use our eyes and vision to see colour, our ears and hearing to detect sound, our noses and smell to identify odour and so on. The senses, and the sense organs that are their instruments, also resonate with each of the Five Elements (see Table 3.7).

The sense of hearing and the ears are resonances of Water. Vision and the eyes vibrate in tune with Wood. Speech (a way we *touch* another's heart) and the tongue are in harmony with Fire. The sense of taste, which we get through the mouth and lips, is in resonance with Earth. Smell and the nose are instruments of Metal.

As we move through the chapters on the Elements, we will explore more fully each of the senses. When we bring a particular focus to one of the senses in its corresponding season, much can be revealed.

A heightened awareness of one sensory channel can illuminate our relationship with that sense. This in turn puts us more directly in contact with the Element of that sense. For example, focusing on vision and the eyes puts us in contact with the Wood Element. We can learn things about the way we see and the way we look at and move through the world. These insights can bring healing that flows through to all the other resonances of Wood. By focusing on one sense, we find that we are also working at subtle levels with the organs, tissues, emotions and even spiritual issues of the corresponding Element of that sense.

Table 3.7 The Five Elements and Their Corresponding Senses and Sense Organs

Element	Sense	Sense Organ
Water	Hearing	Ears
Wood	Vision	Eyes
Fire	Speech	Tongue
Earth	Taste	Mouth and Lips
Metal	Smell	Nose

Organs

Each Element has two organs associated with it (see Table 3.8). Fire has two additional 'functions' which can each be seen as subtle organs. Each pair of organs comprises a yin and a yang organ which function together as a partnership. The yang organs are considered 'hollow' because they are like pipes facilitating the passage of a substance. The yin organs, also called the viscera, are considered to be 'solid' organs that act as reservoirs of Qi.

When all Five Elements are in harmony, the organs function as they should in harmonious symphony. But when an Element goes out of balance and remains out of balance for some time, this disharmony begins to affect the corresponding organs. These disharmonies tend to take time to reveal themselves in the organs, so by the time a serious health issue arises, the Element has usually been out of balance for quite a while.

It follows that when we pay attention to the other resonances of an Element, we can discover imbalances before the organs themselves show signs of disease. As we move through the year, we will look at how we can support all of our organs.

The book *Neijing Suwen* is very clear about the harmful effects of emotion on the yin organs.[2] A habitual emotional state goes deep into the body and is injurious to the deeper organs. Modern psychology now provides us with many ways of working with stuck emotions. We will look at some of these methods in later chapters.

Table 3.8 The Five Elements and Their Corresponding Yin and Yang Organs

Element	Yin Organ	Yang Organ
Water	Kidney	Bladder
Wood	Liver	Gall Bladder
Fire	Heart Heart Protector	Small Intestine Triple Heater
Earth	Spleen	Stomach
Metal	Lung	Large Intestine

Tissues

As well as the organs and sense organs of the body, each Element also has a corresponding tissue with which it resonates (see Table 3.9). If you have a physical condition that afflicts one of these kinds of tissue, then it is pointing to an underlying imbalance in the corresponding Element. Working to improve the balance of any of the resonances will support the healing of the corresponding tissue.

Table 3.9 The Five Elements and Their Corresponding Tissues

Element	Tissues
Water	Bones
Wood	Tendons and Ligaments
Fire	Blood Vessels
Earth	Muscles
Metal	Skin

Gifts of the Elements

So far we have been looking at the resonances of the Elements, the physical and emotional attributes that are affected by the vibration of each Element. In other words, ways in which the Element is expressed in our environment, and in our bodies as sensations or feelings.

What I call the Gifts of the Elements[3] are somewhat different. They represent the essential goodness of the Element, its deepest nature. These qualities are mostly abstract, sometimes difficult to describe. They touch the parts of us that are the higher expressions of our soul. They connect with those places where beauty touches us and where art and music find their landing places within us.

There are many ways of speaking about the Gifts of the Elements, many words to describe the myriad of fine distinctions. Each Element chapter focuses on seven or eight words to convey these concepts and to build up a 'feeling picture' of the essential nature of the Element.

In my groups I show slides that evoke these qualities. We talk about them, discussing the ways they show up in us and affect the ways we feel and act. I call it taking a bath in the Element. The group discussion and the evocative pictures create a field that inspires everyone within it. The essential qualities of the Element begin to soak into us, filling us with the highest expressions of the Element.

In this book I try to convey these qualities in words. You may find it helpful to find your own photographs that evoke the qualities. Doing this practice in a group is very powerful, so it will help to deepen the work if you can find someone with whom to share your exploration.

The Officials

Throughout this book you will see frequent reference to the Officials of an Element. This is a concept that originated in ancient China and was restored to prominence by J.R. Worsley in Classical Five Element Acupuncture. Each meridian (energy channel) and its corresponding organ also has an Official (see Table 3.10). The 12 Officials are personifications of the 12 organs with their functions and responsibilities. The *Neijing* gives them titles and duties as if they were ministers in the imperial court.

When I use the term Official, I am referring not simply to the organ or meridian, but to a whole range of functions and areas of responsibility associated with them. These include mental, emotional and spiritual functions as well as physical.

Table 3.10 The 12 Officials and Their Functions[4]

Official	Duties and Responsibilities
Heart	Lord and Sovereign, radiates the Spirits
Small Intestine	Receiver, assimilator and transformer
Bladder	Storer of the fluids
Kidney	Creator of power, the origin of skill and ability
Heart Protector	Envoy of the heart, bringing elation and joy
Triple Heater	Opener of passages and regulator of fluids
Gall Bladder	Decision-maker, responsible for what is just and exact
Liver	The General, making plans and strategies
Lung	First Minister, policy advisor to the Sovereign
Large Intestine	Responsible for transit of the residue of transformation
Stomach and Spleen	Together, responsible for the storehouses and granaries and for the five tastes

Table 3.11 Summary of the Resonances of the Five Elements

Element	Water	Wood	Fire	Earth	Metal
Season	Winter	Spring	Summer	Late Summer	Autumn
Sense	Hearing	Vision	Speech	Taste	Smell
Sense Organ	Ears	Eyes	Tongue	Mouth	Nose
Colour	Blue	Green	Red	Yellow	White
Sound	Groaning	Shouting	Laughing	Singing	Weeping
Odour	Putrid	Rancid	Scorched	Fragrant	Rotten
Emotion	Fear	Anger	Joy	Sympathy/Worry	Grief
Yin Organ	Kidneys	Liver	Heart Heart Protector	Spleen	Lungs
Yang Organ	Bladder	Gall Bladder	Small Intestine Triple Heater	Stomach	Large Intestine
Tissue	Bones	Tendons and Ligaments	Blood Vessels	Muscles	Skin
Taste	Salty	Sour	Bitter	Sweet	Pungent
Climate	Cold	Wind	Heat	Damp	Dry
Spirit	Zhi	Hun	Shen	Yi	Po

Chapter 4

The Levels of the Soul

Each Element chapter is subdivided into three sections, exploring how the Element is expressed at the levels of body, mind and spirit. These three levels are referred to frequently in our modern age, but what exactly are they? Since we will be spending a lot of time investigating them, I want to spend some time now in considering what they are.

Body, mind and spirit are not separate but arise out of something more fundamental, some core of our being which I call the soul. The soul is the consciousness that is the ground of all experience. It is a medium of awareness. Within this field of awareness there are bubbles of sensations, emotions, thoughts, feelings, images and memories. The soul is our True Nature and it is also the body, thoughts, emotions and patterns. It is the sum total of us, our True Nature and our obscurations.[1]

Body

What Is a Body?

The question 'What is a body?' seems like it would have a simple answer. The human body is a physical structure made up of a head, neck, torso, two arms and two legs. The basic unit of the body is the cell, of which an adult body has about 100 trillion. The body is composed of systems such as the cardiovascular, nervous, digestive, lymphatic, integumentary, musculoskeletal and reproductive systems.

The body is a solid object that moves around, eats, drinks, breathes, talks, plays sports, goes to work and so on. Each person has a body that is separate and distinct from all other bodies. Seven billion separate humans are moving around on planet Earth which is also a separate planetary body distinct from all other astronomical objects.

But discoveries by quantum physicists over the past century have brought this view of solid physical objects into question. One of the most challenging of these is the discovery that more than 99.99% of an atom is empty space. To get a sense of the scale of this, think of a football field and a grain of sand. The football field is the atom while the grain of sand is the matter of the atom. The rest is space. Another way of thinking about it is to consider that if all 7 billion humans on this planet were condensed down to their subatomic particles, the resultant matter would fit in the palm of your hand.

So why is it that when I put my hands together they don't go through one another? How come when a car hits a tree it gets badly dented? That is because while the space is empty of matter, it is filled with electrical fields. When the electrons of one field come within a very small distance of the electrons of another field, they begin to repel each other. This is why things appear to be solid when they are actually not. Theoretical physicist Michio Kaku puts it this way: 'Now you may think that I'm sitting on this chair but actually that's not true. I'm actually hovering 10^{-8} cm over this chair because the electrons of my body are repelling the electrons of this chair.'[2]

If our bodies are almost all space and that space is filled with fields of energy, what is a human body if not a field of energy?

Another discovery of quantum physics is that the observer influences that which is being observed. This is known as the observer effect. Indeed, the observer is a part of the observation and part of what is being observed. Nuclear physicist Jim Al-Khalili explains that an atom only appears in a particular place if you measure it. An atom is spread out all over the place until a conscious observer decides to look at it. So the act of measurement or observation creates the entire universe.[3]

Physicist Amit Goswami asserts that quantum physics shows clearly how consciousness is the ground of our being and that physics enables us to see directly that we can make sense of the world only if we base the world on consciousness.[4] Our consciousness is not separate from physical reality and that includes our own physical body. The way we think, our attitudes, beliefs and emotional reactions all have an influence on the structures of the body.

Already we are beginning to see that the division of the soul into the separate parts of mind, body and spirit is breaking down and that any division is not real, not representative of what is actually happening.

The body is the most dense of these vibrations, therefore changes in body structures take time to develop. Illnesses take time to establish themselves so that by the time they make themselves known through pain and discomfort, or show up in medical tests, they have been developing in the soul for some time. Similarly, it takes time for these conditions to improve once we receive treatment, make lifestyle adjustments, change our attitudes and beliefs or undergo spiritual transformations.

Five Element acupuncturist and medical doctor Leon Hammer stated:

> Characterological signs of disharmony are among the earliest possible indications that the natural function of the [Element] is being disrupted. Generally, they precede by a considerable period of time the signs and symptoms usually associated with disease of these systems and may be thought of as early warning indicators.[5]

The Chinese view of the body can be inferred from the word *shen* used to describe it. It is probably no coincidence that *shen* is also used to describe the Mind of the Heart.[6] Moreover, the word *shen* implies more than just a physical structure since it can also be translated as person, self or life. This implication of holism contrasts with the Western word for body which derives from the Old German word *botah* meaning a container.[7] Our very language embodies the notion that the body is a container in which the mind and spirit dwell.

What Is Qi?

This discussion of electrical fields brings us back to Qi, which has been described, among other things, as bioelectrical energy. The life force that inhabits all living things is an electromagnetic phenomenon.[8] Qi is this life force, that which animates not just life forms but all the forms of the world. 'It is the vibratory nature of phenomena – the flow and tremoring that is happening continuously at molecular, atomic and sub-atomic levels.'[9]

The Chinese ancients believed that Qi is the fundamental substance of the universe that imbues things with existence. In the human body, Qi manifests in different ways for different purposes. There is ancestral Qi which we inherit from our parents. There is postnatal Qi which we derive from food, water and from breathing. (Breath is even one of the translations of the word Qi.) There is defensive Qi which travels at the surface of the body providing a protective sheath. Qi also transforms food into forms that the body can utilise and it transports the nourishment to the body. It also maintains the body's shape through containment.

When the Qi in the body is not flowing freely and smoothly, disorders begin to appear. There can be conditions of excess or stagnation due to emotions, diet, trauma or external pathogens. Conditions of deficiency or emptiness are caused by chronic illness, old age, weak constitution, malnutrition or excessive stress.[10]

Throughout this book we will be developing practices that support this free flow of Qi throughout the body – for illness is nothing more than a manifestation of the impeded movement of Qi.

Mind

What Is Mind?

Mind is the complex of cognitive faculties that enables consciousness, thinking, reasoning, perception and judgement. The big question to have been debated among philosophers, psychologists and spiritual thinkers is the relationship of the mind to the brain and nervous system. Some would argue that the mind is synonymous with the brain and brain activity, while others regard the mind as separate from physical existence. In either case, the mind is what enables us to have awareness, perception, intentionality and responsiveness to the world. It is what allows us to think and feel.

What Is Thought?

What are thoughts and where do they come from? At the moment, neuroscience simply does not know. They are certainly associated with brain activity; some would say they are caused by brain activity. There are conscious thoughts that are part of a cognitive process we call thinking. Thoughts can be idea-like, memory-like, picture-like or song-like.[11]

But there are also many more thoughts that appear unbidden. Anyone who has done any meditation is well aware of the thought stream that flows on and on whether we like it or not. Sometimes we are afflicted by obsessive thinking and cannot stop going over and over an idea. This affects sleep, energy levels and overall functioning. Who or what is doing the thinking?

A study by Benjamin Libet in 1999[12] showed that unconscious processes in the brain precede any conscious thoughts to take action, but that the subject believes the action to be consciously motivated. He found that electrical activity in the brain begins about four-tenths of a second before any awareness of intention to act. This opens the question of how much free will we have in anything that we do. And where are these unconscious thoughts coming from anyway? Who or what is it that is initiating our thoughts to act?

While Western science has no explanation for the origin of thought, the Buddhist and Hindu traditions do provide an explanation. Buddhist philosophy regards the ultimate nature of mind as pure, clear light, but this clarity is obscured by the activity of the false self. The Dalai Lama explains, 'The afflictive emotions and thoughts that arise in the mind are not intrinsic to the mind but rather veil it and inhibit it from expressing its true essence.'[13]

Within the Hindu tradition, it has been pointed out by the Indian sage Gurumaa that all of our experience comes from the five senses and therefore the mind is nothing more than the myriad permutations of these sensory impressions gained in this life and past lives. All thoughts are based on this collection of past impressions. Since the whole world is perceived through this mind, then the world we perceive is created by the mind. So, all of our emotional reactions to the world are likewise creations of the mind. As long as we are bound to these past impressions we will continue to see the world as our own creation.[14]

From the perspective of Chinese medicine, the mind is related to the heart rather than the brain. The concept of *shen*, which is often translated as spirit, can equally be translated as mind.[15] The *shen* resides in the heart. 'The heart is the sovereign of all the organs and represents the consciousness of one's being. It is responsible for intelligence, wisdom and spiritual transformation.'[16] What is more, mind is the most subtle, non-material form of Qi.[17] The functions of the *shen* or mind are consciousness, thinking, memory, insight, cognition, sleep, intelligence, wisdom, ideas, emotions, feelings and senses.[18]

But whatever the origin of thought, what is clear is that mental state influences perception and experience. Therefore, state of mind is a critical factor in determining our experience of joy and happiness and therefore also our good health. Just as our state of mind affects our physical health, so too does our physical state affect our mind. There is a feedback loop in which mind and body are continually affecting each other.

What Is Emotion?

The question of what emotion is has engaged philosophers for centuries, beginning with Aristotle. More recently, psychologists and neuroscientists have joined a debate which continues to this day without a final resolution of the question.

The American philosopher and psychologist William James began the modern debate when he wrote an article *What Is Emotion?* in 1884. His theory is that an emotion is a physiological reaction, a sensory accompaniment to a perceived event; in other words, a bodily feeling. 'My thesis is that the bodily changes follow directly the PERCEPTION of the exciting fact, and that our feeling of the same changes as they occur IS the emotion.'[19]

The idea that emotion is primarily physiological was the dominant opinion for many years until modern psychologists began expressing a view that emotion is 'cognitive', namely that it is an intelligent way of conceiving of a situation. The cognitive view now holds greater sway.

Philosophers have been more interested in the cognitive side of emotion, in particular the connection between an emotion and certain beliefs. Some philosophers have said emotions arise out of particular beliefs, while others have suggested that beliefs are identical to emotions and that emotions cause beliefs.[20]

How much of an emotion is its outward movement (as the word itself suggests) in the form of behaviour? Many psychologists define emotion in terms of how it looks from the outside – for example, as facial expressions, body postures and actions.

We might consider what role culture plays in the analysis. For example, would a person fall in love if she'd never seen or heard about the process before? As another case, Tibetan lamas, on coming to the West, were perplexed by the notion of self-hatred, never having encountered it in their culture.

Contemporary psychologist Martha Nussbaum, putting what she calls a 'neo-Stoic' view, defines emotions as judgements of value and importance. She identifies four characteristics of an emotion: urgency and heat, a tendency to take over the personality, a move to action with overwhelming force and a connection to important attachments. She goes on to argue that all emotions have an object and that the object is intentional and based in the person's perception of it. Emotion embodies a belief about the object, and the object is invested with value for the role it plays in one's life.[21]

The Swiss psychologist Klaus Scherer sought to find an overarching definition of emotion to try to put an end to the 'fruitless debates' generated by James' 'misnomer' of equating emotion with feeling.[22] Scherer's Component Process Model (CPM) regards emotions as the synchronisation of many different cognitive and physiological components. Scherer identified five components of an emotion: cognitive appraisal, bodily symptoms, action tendencies, facial and vocal expression, and subjective feeling. The process begins with appraisal of a situation for relevance, which then triggers bodily reaction, behaviours and feelings.

Modern philosopher and spiritual teacher A.H. Almaas defines emotion very simply as a reaction that is based on a rejection of one's current experience. As such, emotions are of great value on the spiritual path because they reveal the 'holes' where we are disconnected from our True Nature or Essence.

> Essence is something more real and more substantial than emotions. Essence is something as real as your blood. It is not a reaction. But emotions are necessary for us. We need to become aware of our emotions in order to understand and see our Essence. Emotions are a guide and point to where Essence has been lost. Understanding emotions can help untangle the knots of the defences which are attempts to avoid experiencing the holes, and which maintain our separation from Essence.[23]

The emotions not only point to the places where we are disconnected from our True Nature, but are portals to states of Essence because each emotion is a distortion of some Essential aspect. For example, anger is a distortion of True Strength. By fully exploring our anger without rejecting it and without externally expressing it, there can be a transformation of the emotion into the Essential aspect that it is mimicking.

The more you feel Essence, the less you feel emotions. You will still have sensations, and they will be deeper and stronger; but when you feel Essence, your emotions will not be deeper and stronger. An emotion is only a response of the nervous system. Essence is not a response of the nervous system. There is something there filling you. Part of you is present. Some people call the essential aspects 'the real feelings'. But what people usually call feelings or emotions are not Essence. Love, peace, value, strength and will are aspects of Essence. That is the kind of thing you experience. These are Essence. Instead of experiencing anger, you experience strength, calm strength; instead of feeling superior or inferior, you experience value; you experience yourself as a rounded Presence that is full and powerful.[24]

From the above discussion, it becomes clear that emotion is something that spans all three levels of our being: mind, body and spirit. The emotion has a number of cognitive components including appraisal and judgement of relevance and value. There are also responses in the body, namely reactions of the nervous system, changes in physiology, and feelings, or affect (felt sense). And at the level of spirit, emotions point the way to aspects of our True Nature so that understanding them transforms them into 'real' feelings.

Emotions and the Five Elements

The Chinese sage Chuang-Tzu, writing in the fourth century BCE, likened emotions to gales blowing through trees, as if they were some external influence upon the human psyche. 'Joy, anger, sadness, happiness, worry, lament, vacillation, fearfulness, volatility, indulgence, licentiousness, pretentiousness – they are like music issuing from hollows… Day and night they interchange before us, yet no one knows where they sprout.'[25]

A contemporary Chinese philosopher of the neo-Confucian school, Zhu Zi, has a different view. Far from being external influences, he believes emotions to be internal. Simply put, he sees that emotions are the mind in action and the mind is what unites emotions with human nature.[26]

How does all this relate to the Five Elements? Each emotion has a particular vibration and it vibrates at the tone of its corresponding Element. Fear is Water vibrating at the emotional level; anger is Wood vibrating at the emotional level; joy is Fire vibrating at the emotional level; sympathy is Earth vibrating at the emotional level; grief is Metal vibrating at the emotional level. There are many other identifiable emotions which we will explore in the Element chapters, but all correspond to one of these five vibrations.

As we explore the emotional patterns within ourselves, we can come to understand where our experience, perception and expression of a particular emotion are not smooth. This points to an imbalance in the corresponding Element but also shows the realm where we can begin our healing. For example, if anger is the emotion with which we are constantly struggling, then we need to look at how our Wood might be out of balance. We can then work with this Element at all three levels, seeing how the issue of anger is related to body, mind and spirit.

Identifying your primary emotional response to the world may lead you to finding your Constitutional Element. When you work on the issues of your Constitutional Element at all levels of body, mind and spirit, the very core of you is being healed.

In this book I include emotions with the psyche, referring to the psycho-emotional level. While the above discussion demonstrates that emotion is a multi-faceted beast with physical as well as psychological components, I am persuaded that the emotional process begins in the mind.

What Is Ego?

The ancient Taoists were well aware of the false self which clouds and obscures our True Nature. Modern psychologists have mapped the structure of the psyche, and while they don't necessarily see it as a 'false' self, they have come to understand how the individual self is created.

The psychological term *ego* was coined by Sigmund Freud to describe one of the three parts of the human psychic structure. The instinctual part he named the *id*. The *ego* (from the Latin word for 'I') is the part of a person that forms the usual identity or usual self and which seeks to satisfy the id's drives within the confines of societal norms. The third part he called the *superego* which is a controlling, moralistic agency of the mind that acts as a conscience.

The ego is formed during early childhood. At birth, a child is still very much in contact with her origination from the Oneness and no individual self is present. Quickly, though, the child develops a sense of separateness from other individuals, a process that is encouraged by the parents and society at large. By the age of five years the process of individuation is complete and the child's ego has become her identity.

While the ego is useful and necessary for living in the world, it is a structure of the mind and has no inherent reality. When we take ourselves to be a separate person called Bill or Mary and completely identify with that person as who we are, we are seeing the world as one of separate objects. This is the usual view and is absolutely part of human development. But what we need to come to understand and realise is that this view is inherently not real and merely a mental construct.

The ego is very busy. It is constantly in motion, thinking, imagining, planning, comparing, remembering, hoping, desiring, wanting things to change. It actually needs to keep active in order to support the myth of its existence.

> The activity of ego is taken to be the activity of a person – an entity – who has desires and hopes. So here ego is seen as taking oneself to be a person, separate from the rest of the universe, who was born to a set of parents, who was a child, who grew up, in time, to his present status of an adult who has his hopes, desires and goals. The belief that this separate individuality is one's identity, one's self, is seen by some teachings as the main barrier to the ultimate reality which is an impersonal and universal Being, or alternately, the Void.[27]

Spirit

What Is Spirit?

The answer to the question of what spirit is will vary widely depending on the respondent's religious, spiritual and philosophical views. Most definitions would agree that it is a part of us that is non-corporeal (i.e. something that is not part of the body). Some see that the spirit is the part of us that survives after death, though whether this includes consciousness or personality is a matter of difference. Some definitions regard the spirit as equivalent to the soul, while others see an overlap between soul and spirit.

The English word 'spirit' comes from the Latin *spiritus* which means breath or breathing as well as spirit, soul or ghost. This notion that breath and spirit are connected is an ancient one. One of the best-known verses in the Old Testament is 'And the Lord God formed man of the dust of the ground, and breathed into his nostrils the breath of life; and man became a living soul.'[28]

While the ancient Chinese were not theists, they had a similar notion that the breath is what animates life. They believed that Qi is the animating life force and one of the translations of this word is breath.

The Five Spirits

The Taoists had a notion of spirit that is somewhat more complex. They believed that a human being does not have one spirit but five, each relating to one of the Five Elements and each having a different role to play in life and in death.[29] Moreover, these ancient philosophers did not believe that the spirit animates the body, but that 'spirit and body are nothing but two different states of condensation and aggregation of Qi'.[30] This is truly a holistic perspective.

We have already seen that *shen* can be translated as mind or spirit and that it resides in the heart. *Shen* is also the spiritual aspect of the heart which is the yin organ of the Fire Element. The other four spirits are also associated with the yin organs. *Hun* (Ethereal Soul) is the spirit of Wood and resides in the liver. *Yi* (Intellect) is the spirit of Earth and resides in the spleen. *Po* (Corporeal Soul) is the spirit of Metal and resides in the lungs. *Zhi* (Will) is the spirit of Water and resides in the kidneys. We will examine these spirits in detail in later chapters.

It is worth noting here that the *hun*, spirit of Wood, and the *po*, spirit of Metal, are considered to be two aspects of a polarity that is the soul of the human being. At death it was believed the *hun* ascends to the stars while the *po* disintegrates and becomes part of the earth. This is just one illustration of the concept that humans are between heaven and earth.

The Virtues

I am indebted to Lonny Jarrett, Five Element acupuncturist and classical scholar, for his book *Nourishing Destiny*,[31] which illuminates the importance of virtue in leading a life that is in alignment with the Will of Heaven. In a way, the virtues are like the Gifts of the Elements (see Chapter 3) but with a more profound significance for our lives.

The ancient Chinese philosophers used the term *ming* to convey the concept of destiny, which implies a Heavenly mandate. *Ming* is conferred when heaven approves our cultivation of virtue. The character *te* is the term for virtue, personal character, inner strength or integrity. The Chinese character has three components, suggesting action that is perfectly right, unswerving and transparent.[32]

The concept of virtue crosses both Taoist and Confucian thought. The Taoist classic the *Tao Te Ching* can be translated as the *Book of the Way of Virtue*. But it is the Confucian and neo-Confucian philosophy which sees virtue as a defining quality of a person's life. Jarrett states:

> Heaven mandates a unique mission for each of us to fulfil in this life. Recognising and accepting this mandate is only the first step in fulfilling the contract. Only through continually bringing our original nature into the world may we cultivate virtue and preserve our *ming*. *Ming* is the source of each individual's power and authority.[33]

The Confucian scholar Mencius (c. 371–289 BCE) observed that *ming* is the conduit for the Will of Heaven as it operates through humankind. By aligning his own will with the Will of Heaven, a person becomes a conduit for the divine Qi and thus is true to his True Self.[34]

In 79 BCE there appeared a scholarly work, the *Bai Hu Dong*, interpreting the writings of Confucius. In this, the Confucian virtues were first paired with the Five Elements. These Elements were wisdom (Water), benevolence (Wood), propriety (Fire), integrity (Earth) and righteousness (Metal).

The value for us here is to contemplate for ourselves the presence or absence of these virtues in our lives. Of particular value is an inquiry into our relationship with the virtue of our Constitutional Element. The virtues 'emerge when the destiny of a specific constitutional type is being fulfilled. As a given virtue erodes, an habitually occurring behaviour arises depending on the presence of an excessive or diminished emotion (e.g. fear, joy, anger, longing, sympathy).'[35]

Put another way, the virtues of our Constitutional Element most exalt us if we cultivate them, and make us most ill if we do not.[36]

Spiritual Issues

When a soul is born into a human life, she emerges from the sea of Oneness and coalesces into this world of form. At the moment of conception a shift begins to take place from formless to form. What some call the Fall has begun. By taking form in a human life, we begin to lose contact with the Oneness from which we emerged and in so doing we begin to forget our True Nature. As the ego develops, the connections to source begin to fade. By about the age of five years, the child has completely forgotten where she came from. For most people, this state of affairs continues unless, at some point in adulthood, the spiritual instinct awakens a desire to know our true origins once more. This is the beginning of awakening, the beginning of the Return. For most people it is a long journey of gradually dissolving the patterns that bind us to ego, for while any part of us is operating from ego, we are disconnected from our True Nature.

The five spiritual issues are a differentiation of the Fall in the same way that the Elements are differentiations of the Tao. As with the Elements, everyone has all five spiritual issues as part of their journey (see Table 4.1), but there is one in particular that is deeply challenging. This is the spiritual issue of the Constitutional Element. It is the issue that is the greatest challenge, but at the same time it is the way back to the Source. It is the primary pathway of the Return.

Table 4.1 The Five Elements and Their Spiritual Issues

Element	Spiritual Issue
Water	Returning to original nature
Wood	Finding true path
Fire	Knowing true self
Earth	Cultivating true purpose
Metal	Recognising the preciousness of now

The Diamond Approach

Each of the sections on the Spiritual level of the Elements includes the perspective of the Diamond Approach. This teaching is a complex mapping of the terrain of the soul and her spiritual journey. For the most part I will be looking at the essential aspects and how they intersect with the Five Elements. The essential aspects are qualities of True Nature that manifest in us and can be directly perceived at a subtle level. Examples are will, strength, love, compassion and value. These aspects could be regarded as the Gifts of the Elements at their deepest essential nature. The teaching also shows that the emotional reactions of the ego mind are actually doorways to directly perceiving these qualities of Essence.

'Not only is Essence the pure and authentic presence of our Being, the ontological beingness of our soul, but this presence manifests itself in and as various experiential qualities that are clearly discernible.'[37]

Almaas uses the terms Essence and Presence largely interchangeably. Presence (not to be confused with being present) is the ontological reality of consciousness and is felt as a medium that is homogenous, unified, whole and undivided, like a body of water. This medium is consciousness that is aware of itself not by reflecting on itself but by being itself.[38] From this perspective, Essence or Presence is the fundamental nature of the universe, the ground of Being.

> Golden Elixir is another name for one's fundamental nature. There is no other Golden Elixir outside one's fundamental nature. All human beings have this Golden Elixir complete in themselves. It is entirely realised in everybody. It is neither more in a sage, nor less in an ordinary person. It is the seed of the Immortals and the Buddhas, the root of the worthies and the sages.
>
> LIU YIMING (1734–1821)

Chapter 5

Activities and Practices

This book is designed as a guide to using the model of the Five Elements in daily life. While it's a wonderful theoretical model for how energy moves in the world, it can also be very practical. There are lots of activities and practices throughout the book where you can put the theory into action. I encourage you to try each of them. They are all things that I have tried in my own life and trialled with groups.

There are six kinds of practices that are indicated by their respective icons. Here I talk in general about how they are used in the Element chapters.

Journaling

I spent a whole year journaling my personal relationship to the Elements before beginning the actual writing of the book. When the idea of a book sprang into mind, the first thing I did was to go to an office supply store and buy five A4-size journals in the colours of the Elements. The colour of each book I was writing in matched the season and Element, helping to keep these in my consciousness. I found that at the beginning of each season, the ideas of the Element began pouring forth. As the season waned, so did the ideas. When the energy of the next season arose, I switched to writing about the new Element in a different coloured book and once more the ideas flowed.

Towards the end of the spring of that year I found the ideas for the Wood chapter were beginning to dry up and journal entries were becoming sparse. One morning I realised that the Wood energy was no longer around and that the Fire energy of summer had become palpable. So I closed the green journal and reached for the red one. Immediately, the insights began to flow and writing recommenced at its former pace. Also I noticed that the very words I was using were the language of Fire. I wrote about my enthusiasm and about digesting and assimilating which are functions of the small intestine, one of the organs of Fire. I even noticed that my handwriting became bigger and more expansive, as if the spirit of Fire had taken over my pen.

What had happened was that by taking off my green glasses and putting on my red ones, I began to see and experience the world through the lens of the Fire Element. I began to access those aspects of myself that resonate with Fire. This was a huge discovery and convinced me more than ever that the more we become immersed in an Element, the more it reveals its perspective, lessons and gifts.

Journaling is one of the main practices of this system and provides a central location for your reflections as you engage with the material. It is a place where you can answer the questions posed as well as write about whatever is arising in your experience. I recommend having separate journals for each season. If you can't find the right colours, make some covers with coloured paper. It will contribute to your immersion. While it is not necessary to write every single day, I suggest making regular entries, even if you feel there is nothing to say or if you feel out of touch with that Element. In fact, exploring resistance and stuckness can open the inquiry process in a way that often leads to insights.

Entries don't only have to be written. Draw or paint your entries if that is your preferred medium. Cut out images and stick them in. You might even collect materials from nature that reflect the season: leaves, flowers, pollens, twigs, rocks, feathers, insects…the list is yours to complete.

Why is it important to have it all down? Why not just think about it all? Journaling is not just about the act of writing but represents a whole process of self-reflection. It forces you to crystallise your thoughts and thereby deepens the thought process. Journaling promotes clarity. Sometimes you think you are clear about something, but when you come to write it down, you realise that it wasn't so clear after all. The process promotes honesty. Since the journal is for you and your process, you are not writing with a gloss for an audience. This allows you to get closer to what is true about yourself and truth has a way of revealing more truth.

Another important aspect of journaling is that you get a chance to explore different parts of yourself and give these parts an opportunity to speak up. For example, you might have a part that wants and desires something that another part thinks is bad and wrong. The journal allows both parts to have their say. The parts might even get to have a conversation on the page.

Dream journaling is another important part of this work. By going through the self-reflective process, it is likely that your dreams will become more vivid and memorable because you are opening yourself to learning more about the parts that are as yet unconscious. Recording these dreams then gives the unconscious parts the green light to reveal more of themselves to you.

These days most of us write using a computer. Indeed, that is what I am doing right now. Why then am I suggesting that you write using pen and paper? I believe the act of writing by hand is more intimate and has the capacity to be more real and immediate. There is no cutting and pasting, no retrospectively deleting parts which don't fit with a self-image or the dictates of the inner critic. If you want to delete something, you have to scribble it out and that too is part of the realness.

Handwriting is a reflection of the writer's internal state at the time of writing. The size and shape of the letters, whether the lines are straight or angled, points of emphasis such as circling, underlining, scribbling in the margin – all of these aspects add to the picture of where you are at the time.

Since you will be spending a year with your journals, take all the time you need in choosing them. Take time also to choose a pen or pencils that feel really comfortable for you. They are going to be the instruments of the expression of your soul for the next year.

Inquiry

We have already introduced the concept of inquiry by discussing the self-reflective inquiry of the journaling process. This can be extended to inquiry in the company of others. This can be done with one or two other people. It is a process of thinking aloud in the presence of people who are supportive of you finding out more about yourself.

Inquiry is open-ended and has no goal other than to discover more and more of the truth of who we really are beyond ego structures. It is a process that is never-ending because the discovery of truth leads to more questions which lead to deeper levels of truth.

My own experience is that while individual inquiry is very useful, inquiry done with others can be profound. Having others as supportive witnesses to our process provides a field that encourages deep exploration. It also keeps us focused and on track. And at the end of our inquiry, our inquiry partner(s) can offer feedback that might allow us to see things or make connections that we could not do on our own.

Group inquiry helps us to follow the thread of our unfolding experience, identify and describe ego structures which operate upon our thinking and behaviour, recognise the inner critic when it arises and be able to disengage from it, recognise what is in the way of our being our deepest, truest self, and in the process make contact with essential states of Being. In addition, by working with others we learn to listen attentively and non-judgementally, to follow the thread of someone else's experience and to give feedback that helps to further the other's inquiry. These skills then become helpful in being attentive and wise to our own inquiry process.

This method can be used in answering the questions posed in various places in the text. It can also be used to inquire into a particular issue or situation in your life. Or it can be done to simply inquire into where you are right now at this moment. Over time, inquiry becomes an ongoing practice in which we are constantly attuned to and interested in all that we experience internally.

Inquiry is a practice that takes time to learn. At first it might feel awkward or artificial. As with any other skill, it takes time to master. In a way we are always beginners because no matter how far we have come in our self-understanding, we are still at the beginning of what we do not yet know about ourselves. Since we live in an infinite universe, all things are infinite, including our unfolding.

The Inquiry Process

Inquire in groups of two or three. Choose a time period you want to inquire for (e.g. 10 or 15 minutes). Each person has the same amount of time. Set a timer for this period. Decide who is going to inquire first. Each person takes turns to talk aloud about her internal process while the listener(s) listen attentively without comment or interruption. At the end of the inquiry period, the listeners can then offer feedback that helps the inquirer to further her process of understanding. Five minutes is a good time period for this.

Some things to pay attention to as the inquirer are:

- Notice your body and how you feel in different parts of it.

- If there is a sensation or pain that catches your attention, stay with it and notice what happens as you simply sit with the sensate experience; follow the changes.

- Notice your emotions. What are you feeling emotionally? Is it in a particular part of your body? How do you feel about having this feeling? Notice what happens to the feelings as you pay attention to them.

- Notice your thoughts as you inquire. Are there thoughts that tend to take you away from the focus of your inquiry? Do you become foggy, forgetful or sleepy? How do you feel about having these reactions?

- Notice if your inner critic comes in and tells you that you are a bad person, or this inquiry is stupid or that what is happening is not the right thing. Whatever is happening is perfectly fine since there is no goal and no rules about what should be achieved. Whatever is happening is simply what is happening.

- Notice your reactions to what is happening. Are you rejecting what is occurring in your experience? Are you trying to hold on to a particular state or experience?

- Try to allow all of what is arising, including the rejection. If you are rejecting, then don't reject the rejection. Allow it all.

Some things to pay attention to as the listener are:

- Half of your attention is on the inquirer and her process, tracking what she is saying.

- The other half is on yourself, noticing your internal responses and reactions to what is being shared.

- Notice the same kinds of things you were paying attention to when inquiring, only this time you are listening instead of talking.

- By following these guidelines you remain self-aware while someone else is speaking.

- Things you notice while listening may become food for your own later inquiry.

Diet and Lifestyle

Scattered throughout the chapters are pieces of information and advice on how to best support the Elements through diet and lifestyle. Some of this information comes from Chinese medicine, some comes from Western medicine and naturopathy, and some comes from psychological and spiritual traditions. These are not prescriptions for everyone but rather guidelines and suggestions. Ultimately, you are your best doctor in knowing what you need to eat and how you need to live to best support a healthy body, mind and spirit.

In the Garden

I am a keen gardener and one of the great joys of my life is to work with the Five Elements in my garden. By getting my hands in the dirt, contacting the living earth, the plants, the trees, the produce, the worms and the compost, I stay deeply in touch with the seasons. Over time the gardener learns the rhythms of nature in a profound way, not just externally as the seasons manifesting in nature, but through an internal resonance with this natural rhythm.

I have included a section in each chapter about garden activities as they relate to the seasons and the Elements. If you are already a gardener, you probably already know these things. Even so, it can be instructive to look at your gardening year from the perspective of the Five Element cycle.

If you don't have a garden, I encourage you to begin one so you can gain the support of the seasonal rhythms in a direct way. Even if you live in an apartment, there is always the opportunity to grow plants in window boxes or plant pots. If you are renting, this is a great way to ensure that you can take your garden with you.

For the ambitious there is the option of building raised-bed gardens, which do not even need bare soil. You can start one on a slab of concrete, build a box and fill it with soil and organic material. Here, too, the garden is transportable if you move.

Nowadays there is a lot of interest in community gardens, some privately organised, others sponsored by local governments. Even if you do not have the space or the permission to dig a garden at your house or apartment, you may find the opportunity to have your own plot in a big garden shared with others. Or maybe one of your neighbours has a big patch of ground doing nothing. Why not ask if you can develop the ground in his yard in exchange for a share of the produce?

Each season in the garden brings its own tasks, delights, challenges and lessons.

These will be reflected in the garden sections of the Element chapters. I hope that these sections will encourage you to be like those ancient Chinese naturalists whose intimate contact with the seasons inspired the very development of the Five Element model.

Acupressure

Each of the organs has an energetic pathway (meridian) through the body. This pathway has two parts. There is a superficial pathway that passes just under the surface of the body, through the muscles and other tissues. Also there is a deep pathway that links the superficial pathway with its related organ and tissues. At places where the superficial pathway rises closer to the surface, the energy can be accessed and treated by needles, pressure, heat or other methods of stimulation.

These locations are the traditional acupuncture points lying along the meridians, whose pathways are on both sides of the body. Apart from the Triple Heater and Heart Protector, each meridian is simply named for its primary organ (e.g. the meridian passing through the lung is called the Lung meridian).

When an Element is out of balance, the imbalance will tend to show itself as congestion in the Qi along the pathways that correspond to the organs of the Element. While it takes years of study to become skilled at finding and treating these energy blocks, knowledge of the locations of these basic pathways is very helpful in making connections among the various resonances. For example, if you have an ongoing pain in the big toe which is on the path of the Liver meridian, and you also suffer from blurred vision and feelings of irritable anger, together these things probably indicate that the Wood Element is out of balance.

In each of the Element chapters you will be introduced to the pathways of the associated meridians. In addition, you will learn a few acupressure points that are supportive of the physical organs and tissues, the emotions and the spirit.

In the sections on the physical level, it is the source points that are most useful. Not only does the source point directly treat the related organ, but it is completely safe to use. Whether the meridian is in excess or deficient, the point brings the energy back to balance.

In the sections on the psycho-emotional level, I have chosen the points on the front of the body called the *mu* points or alarm points. These are helpful in releasing stuck emotions that are related to the Element. In the sections on the spiritual level I have chosen points on the back known as the outer *shu* points. These are very effective in balancing the meridian at the level of spirit.

There are many other points I could have introduced, but I wanted to make it simple.[1] If you have an interest in learning more, there are many acupressure and acupuncture books and websites you can consult.[2] Another thing to note is that all of these points have an effect on the whole of us. As discussed above, there is really no separation between the levels of our Being. While the source points are great for easing the organs, the effect flows on to mind, emotions and spirit. Likewise, the *mu* points and outer *shu* points have effects on all levels.

In locating points on the body, the measurement known as cun is used. This is sometimes referred to as a body inch. It is a proportional measurement based on a fraction of a body part. For example, there are 16 cun between the knee and the ankle. For our purposes, a simple method is this: one cun is the distance across the knuckle of the thumb; 1.5 cun is the distance across the knuckles of the index and middle fingers; 3 cun is the distance across the knuckles of all four fingers. Always use as a measure the hand of the person receiving the treatment.

Meditation

One of the most supportive practices for inner exploration is to have an ongoing meditation practice. You may already have an established practice, yet you may still find something useful in the sections in the Element chapters which offer ways to focus the attention that are in accord with the nature of the Element. Each of the Five Element meditation practices is a different way of focusing our awareness that evokes the spirit and flavour of that Element.

If you are looking for a basic, ongoing meditation practice, here are some suggestions for a simple practice and tips to support its continuation.

What is the point of meditation?

There are many motivations for taking up meditation. For some people it is a way to relax and reduce stress; for others it is a kind of self-hypnosis that supports lifestyle changes. Some people use it to focus on achieving a particular outcome, such as healing someone or achieving world peace.

When we meditate as a support for deep inner work, we are not doing any of these things. We may experience positive outcomes like relaxation, less stress, ease in life, inner and outer peace, and so forth, but these are not the aim. In fact, the aim, if you can call it an aim, is to do as little as possible, and ultimately to do nothing at all.

The point of meditation is to unhook from the regular thought stream of our ordinary world. It is like uncoupling the baggage cars from the engine so that we are not hooked into and run by our endlessly active mind, often called the 'monkey mind'. It is this ceaseless chatter of our ego structure that is in the way of coming back to who we truly are.

A daily meditation practice reminds us that who we really are is not our body, our thoughts or our emotions. This daily reminder helps us to take this perspective into our life in the ordinary world.

Establishing Support for Practice

If you have decided to start meditating, it is important to set up conditions that will support your ongoing practice. It is not easy to maintain a long-term practice and so we need to do whatever we can do to support ourselves on this journey.

First of all, find a place in or around your home that is dedicated to meditation and not used for another purpose. This does not have to be a whole room but can be a corner of a room. It needs to be a place that will be relatively quiet and away from others, unless they are meditating too. Have a chair or a cushion placed there that is only used for your meditation. This is a sacred space and it might help to decorate it as such. You might have spiritual icons, statues, art, flowers, fruit or crystals. These can serve as reminders that this is a dedicated space and it reflects your own dedication to your practice.

Once you have set up your space, it is time to establish a routine. While meditation can be practised anywhere at any time (in fact, ultimately you will be meditating everywhere, all the time, whatever you are doing), it is good at the beginning to set up a regular time. Figure out where it can be fitted into your day in such a way that the rest of your life will not pull you away from meditation. Early mornings are a good time because the mind is not yet fully hooked into the Ten Thousand Things (Taoist terminology for the world of manifestation) that will engage its attention during the day. But if you find that you do better with another time of day, that is fine. Just try to make it the same time every day.

Now that you have the place and the time set aside, how long will you meditate? At first, I suggest you start small. Try five minutes to begin with and work up from there. While this might seem very short, believe me, when you begin meditating, your ego will find a million ways of distracting you so that five minutes can feel like an eternity. Another possibility is that you might find it easy at first, but later it becomes more difficult. It is a good idea to start with the bar low so that you have a good chance of success. Failure to keep up a regular practice makes it even more difficult to pick it up again. Meditating every day for five minutes is much better than 35 minutes once a week.

If after a week at five minutes you are doing well, then move to ten minutes for another week or two. Gradually increase the time until you are meditating for 20 or 30 minutes a day. If you find you reach these levels but have trouble keeping your commitment for some reason, then go down a step or two until you feel you have re-established your practice.

It is best to use a timer for the period of meditation. I have recently started using a phone app that rings a Tibetan bell at the start and finish and find that it peacefully supports my practice. Try to find a timer that is not too loud because this can be startling at the end of the period. The reason for the timer is that you need to have a fixed time for your meditation, neither more nor less, the same every day. You do not want to be opening your eyes to check the clock as this will be yet another distraction. There will be plenty of those already!

Support of Others

While meditation is your own internal practice, it is important that you have the support of others in that practice. First of all, it is important that others in your household respect what you are doing. They may not be joining you, they may not even understand why you are doing this, but it is important that they respect your practice. Let them know when you are meditating and perhaps put a sign or symbol on the door so you won't be disturbed.

It is also invaluable to be a part of a group that is meditating. Even if the group only meets once a week or once a month, when you are a part of a group, then a field of support is generated that carries over beyond the meetings. There are many kinds of meditation groups you can join, some of which have a particular spiritual path, some of which don't. You can also establish your own meditation group among your friends where you get together weekly or monthly to meditate together and support one another in your practice. This also creates a field of support.

From my own experience, I know how very hard it is to maintain the focus and discipline of a daily practice over a long period. Do not underestimate the power of belonging to a group.

A Basic Practice

Now let me suggest a basic meditation practice. There are many ways of meditating, many paths up the mountain. This is just one way.

First, sit on your chair or meditation cushion. If you are using a chair, have your feet flat on the floor and rest your hands on your thighs or in your lap. If you are cross-legged on a cushion, let your hands rest gently in your lap, palms up. Make sure your back is upright but not rigid. Close your eyes, or, if you prefer, have them very slightly open and looking down.

Now that you are settled, bring your attention to your lower abdomen. There is a place about two fingers' width below the navel and the same distance below the skin. This is an important energy centre. It has many names: hara, dan tien, k'ath, second chakra, belly centre. It is an organ of perception, the place where our gut tells us what is true. It is low down in the body and is a good place to focus if only to bring us down out of the head. But it is far more than this. With regular attention to this centre, it is activated and becomes a subtle centre of perception that is beyond the usual five senses.

As you breathe, feel your breath going down into this place and feel your abdomen rise and fall. In actual fact, the breath doesn't go any further than the lungs, but your attention brings the Qi of the breath to this area. This is called belly breathing as distinct from chest breathing where only the chest rises and falls.

This is the essence of the practice. You spend the whole meditation just breathing in and out with your focus on the belly centre. Sound simple? Well, pretty soon the monkey mind comes in and gives a hundred reasons why this is stupid, a thousand other ways we should be spending our time, and bringing us a million memories of the past and plans for the future. This is normal. It is what the ego mind does. We just need to try to let it do its thing without being taken over by it. When you notice that your thoughts have taken you away, come back to the breath in the belly. Try not to judge yourself for going away, or berate yourself for it. It is simply what happens. Imagine your mind is like an energetic and enthusiastic two-year-old who is all over the place and needs gently to be guided. Bring that gentleness to yourself.

There are a couple of things that can help you to focus. The first is to place one palm over the belly centre and the other palm over it. You can even put your thumb on the spot, pressing lightly. This uses bodily sensations to focus the mind. If you find yourself wandering too much, use this technique until you are refocused and then let your hands go back to their resting place.

A second focusing technique is to count your breaths. This gives the mind something to do that overrides other thoughts and can be really useful in the beginning stages of establishing a meditation practice. As you breathe into the belly, count 'one'; as you breathe out, count 'one' again. Breathe in again for two, out for two. Continue counting like this up to ten. If you make it all the way to ten, congratulations! Then you start again from one. If you find that you have become distracted by a thought, or if you lose count, you begin from one again. This will almost certainly happen, so don't be discouraged when it does. Just remember the two-year-old you are guiding and training.

When the timer rings, your meditation is done. It is nice to finish with a ritual gesture such as a bow or hands together at the heart centre. As you get up out of your seat, try to take this more centred place with you into the day. Even if it only makes it to the door, that is fine. Over time you will bring your meditative state into the rest of your life, and your awareness of yourself and your surroundings will gradually widen and deepen. Life becomes a meditation. Meditation becomes your practice of life.

Seasons of Life

After all this examination of Five Element theory, resonances, gifts, levels of the soul and the different kinds of practices, you are now ready for the journey through the cycle of the Five Elements over the next year. The more you engage with the Elements, the more they will repay you with their wisdom.

What season are you in right now? If it is winter, start with the Water chapter on the next page. If it is spring where you are, go straight to the Wood chapter. Are you in the warmth of summer? Fly right through to the Fire chapter. Is it the late summer or harvest time in your neighbourhood? Swing along to the Earth. And if it is autumn or fall you are experiencing, drop into the Metal chapter.

Put on your appropriately coloured glasses and begin to pay attention to all you see, hear, smell, taste and feel that resonates with the Element you are exploring. Write, draw, sing, dance, walk, run, dig, play, work, eat, drink, do and be according to the Element of the season. By so doing you will be exploring the depths of this vibration within yourself. It will teach you where you are healthy and whole, and where you are in need of healing and growth.

But most of all, play with it and have fun in the process. The journey is your reward.

Part 2 ——————————————————

THE JOURNEY

Chapter 6

Water

The Nature of Water

The movement of Water is inwards. As the most yin of the Elements, Water will always find the lowest point and come to rest there.

In a sense, Water is the most fundamental of the Elements. It is the most abundant compound on the earth's surface, covering about 70% of the planet, and its continued presence on earth led to the development of life. It continues to be significant in the sustaining of life: water comprises about 60% of the human body. The percentage is greater in newborn babies and less in ageing bodies. The decline of water in the body parallels the decline in vitality and health as the body ages.

Water stores heat efficiently and it bonds to itself and to other substances. It is known as the universal solvent because many other substances can dissolve in it and be held in suspension. All of these properties are necessary for the biochemical processes of the body and make water crucial to life. Without water, the body cannot survive more than a few days.

The various ways that water behaves offer insights into the qualities of the Water Element. It is the only natural substance that is found in all three physical states – liquid, solid and gas – at the temperatures normally found on Earth. Thus, we all have direct experience of the changing nature of water to ice and steam and can observe its indestructibility.

In all its forms water reveals its power, from the capacity of ice to gouge gorges and sink ships, to water's power to erode land and turn turbines, to steam's capacity to drive engines and cause explosions.

In its liquid state, water takes many forms that are very different from one another. Think of the parts of a river, from its beginnings as a spring in the hillside, as a gently babbling brook, as rapids and waterfalls in the mountains, to the broad, powerful, meandering river of the plains and finally to the vast-moving depth of the ocean. Think, too, of puddles, ponds, lakes and wells which show other characteristics of stillness and depth.

In short, water appears in the form of its container, whether it be as a river, lake or ocean; a cup of tea, a bath or a swimming pool; or displaced by a hand, a body or an ocean liner. Water is nothing if not adaptable.

The Chinese character for Water is *shui* (see Figure 6.1). The central stroke represents the main flow of a river while the other four strokes are the whirls, eddies and back currents of the river.[1]

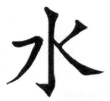

Figure 6.1 The Chinese character for Water

The Resonances of Water

The Season: Winter

The Water Element is most easily observed in nature as the season of winter. It is the time of year when there is little or no growth, a time of waiting, resting and hibernating. Nature has retreated to its lowest ebb, shrunk to its most minimal, conserving its resources through the long cold night of the year. Temperatures are much lower and in some locations drop below freezing, producing ice and snow.

Winter is the coldest time of the year because at this time the sun's rays hit the Earth at a shallow angle. These rays are more spread out, which minimises the amount of energy that hits any given spot. Also, the long nights and short days prevent the Earth from warming up. Cold and dark are yin qualities and therefore intrinsic to Water.

When does winter begin? This depends on your location on Earth and your prevailing climate. In temperate zones, you can expect to feel the beginnings of winter in early November or early May depending on your hemisphere. This is a month earlier than what is traditionally regarded as the beginning of winter, but the first hints of a season tend to have a greater impact upon us. Many people struggle with this transition from autumn to winter which is indicative of an imbalance in the Water Element.

This point of transition from autumn to winter was celebrated in Gaelic tradition on 1 November as Samhain, marking the end of the harvest season and the beginning of winter. Christian tradition later marked it as All Hallows' or All Saints' Day and its modern celebration appears as Halloween on 31 October.

This point lies roughly between the autumn equinox and the midwinter solstice and marks the beginning of the darker half of the year.

If you live closer to the equator, winter will come later, while if you live closer to the poles, your winter will be earlier. You can look for the signs of winter within yourself: a desire to spend more time indoors where it is warm and cosy, more reluctance to get out of bed when it is dark and cold, reaching into the closet for scarves, gloves, hats and extra layers.

The Sense: Hearing

The sense of hearing is closely related to the Kidneys, which are organs of the Water Element. It is said that if the Kidneys are healthy, the ears can hear the five sounds.[2] Its tendency to decline with age is a result of the lifelong decline in the Kidney Qi.

Hearing is a sense of rapid response. While it might take a full second to notice something with your eye, turn towards it, recognise and respond to it, the same reaction to sound happens at least ten times as fast.[3] This is because hearing has evolved as our alarm system, operating below consciousness, and even during sleep. When we are startled by a sound, a chain of neurons from the ears to the spine takes the noise and converts it into a defensive response in a tenth of a second. We'll see later how this alarm response relates to Water's emotion of fear.

Listening is different from hearing. Hearing is simply the act of perceiving sound by the ear. If you are not hearing-impaired, this just happens. Listening, however, is something you consciously choose to do. Listening requires attention and concentration in order to derive meaning from hearing. While hearing is a sense, listening is a skill. You could say that people tend to be hard of listening rather than hard of hearing. There are none so deaf as those who are determined not to listen.

The Colour: Blue (Black)

Some authorities say blue is the colour of the Water Element, others say it is black, while still others call it blue-black, or even a dark, purplish colour.[4] All agree it is a dark shade.

Water in large quantities, such as rivers, lakes and oceans, is blue because the water reflects the blue of the light spectrum, and also reflects the sky which is often blue. No light penetrates into deep water so there the water appears black.

Blue is often regarded as a peaceful colour, one that brings down frantic energy and calms the spirit. This corresponds with the descending nature of the

Water energy. Blue – or 'having the blues' – is also a euphemism for sadness and depression, states where there is too much sinking energy.

Blue was a relative latecomer to art and decoration because of the difficulty of making blue dyes and pigments from natural materials. These were derived from the plants woad and indigo and the minerals lapis, azurite and later cobalt.

In modern fashion, dark blue is considered conservative, especially in the form of the business suit. Navy blue refers to the dark colour of blue worn by seamen, beginning with the British Navy in the eighteenth century. Another watery connection.

What is your relationship with the colour blue? How do you feel when you wear it? Do you wear it at particular times; does it alter your mood? How much do you have in your wardrobe? How much blue is in your home? Too much blue can be depressing for some but it is good to have some of this colour. According to feng shui principles, it is beneficial to have something blue on the Water wall of a room, the one in which the entry door is located.

In Five Element diagnosis, blue or black at the sides of the eyes or under the eyes can be indicative of a Water imbalance and may derive from Kidney deficiency. People can get this look when they are very tired, run down or depleted, or if there is some pathology of the kidneys. For example, those on kidney dialysis have this appearance. People of a Water constitution will display this colour even when they are well. Sometimes it looks as if the person is wearing a Zorro mask, the dark colour completely surrounding the eyes. It is often dark blue to black, but can appear as a lighter, sky or powder blue.[5]

The Sound: Groaning

The sound of voice that represents the Water Element is the groaning voice. This is a sound that is sinking or falling in tone and which can be indicative of stress or strain. It is a deep note, and one which has little modulation. Of all the sounds of voice, it shows the least variation. It is as if all the normal tones of a voice have been flattened out. It can sometimes sound like water running over gravel. Sometimes it is as if the voice has been stretched out into a longer sound like an old cassette tape that has stretched.[6]

The sound of the groaning voice carries the emotion of fear, which we will look at in detail later. Imagine how it is to dread something happening. The groan is the feeling of dread being expressed as a tone: oh no, not that. This groaning sound was comically expressed by Neil in the 1980s television sitcom *The Young Ones* whose catchphrase was 'Oh no!'

The sound can also reflect an imbalance in the Kidneys, which store the *jing* or Essence of life. When there is insufficient energy to power the life, a groan of effort is the result. Imagine the sound you might make when getting out of bed after insufficient sleep or anticipating the arrival of a person who is difficult to deal with.

The sound of someone's voice is diagnostic of their Constitutional Element. People who are of a Water constitution will demonstrate this long, low groaning sound in their everyday speaking voice. Thea Elijah calls this the dial tone or the voice of doom.[7] Like water, it is a sound that finds the lowest level. The flatness of the Water voice can sometimes be confused with the type of Fire voice which is characterised by a lack of laugh.

The Odour: Putrid

The resonance of odour is the third of the diagnostic tools in determining a person's Constitutional Element. Those of a Water constitution have an odour emanating from their skin that can be described as putrid. When the person is in good health, this odour is slight and resembles the smell of fresh water. When there is an imbalance in health, the odour is stronger and can be like a stagnant pond or even the smell of urine or ammonia.

The odour arises from the organs of the Constitutional Element not doing their job adequately. In this case, the bladder and kidneys, the 'waterworks', are not functioning well enough to manage the fluids of the body and the emanating putrid odour is the result.

The Emotion: Fear

The movement of Water is inwards, so it is natural that its emotion is one that sinks and contracts.

Fear is deep, visceral and is experienced low down in the body, affecting the low back, pelvis and legs. In cases of extreme fear, the force of descending energy is irresistible and a person can lose control of bladder and bowels.

Many of the idiomatic expressions for fear are suggestive of its cold, watery nature: a chill down the spine, bowels turning to water, breaking into a cold sweat, blood turned cold, frozen with fear, shaking like a leaf.

All humans experience fear in some way at some time. It is a normal and natural response to danger or threat. It is an instinctual emotion that has helped us survive as a species. However, when fear becomes extreme, goes beyond a reaction appropriate to the circumstances, becomes paralysing or traumatising, or interferes with normal functioning, this indicates an imbalance in the Water Element.

Another kind of imbalance occurs at the other extreme. When there is a conspicuous absence of fear in circumstances where it would be normal, or when the person repeatedly engages in risky activities without regard for common safety, this is also an imbalance in the Element. The legendary daredevil Evil Knievel who holds the record for the most broken bones in a lifetime (over 433) was a classic example of this type of behaviour.

Emotion is the fourth diagnostic tool in Five Element work. A person of Water constitution will exhibit a relationship to fear that is unusually significant. Fear becomes the predominant emotion of the person's life. The fear will be either very evident or strikingly absent. Overall there is something that strikes the observer as not quite right or 'off-note' around the emotion of fear.

It must be noted that people who have experienced severe shock or trauma can seem to be Water types. Unresolved traumatic experiences that are held in the bodymind[8] can profoundly affect the Water Element. The emotion of fear can appear to override the emotion of the Constitutional Element. In such cases the other diagnostic tools must be relied upon. (We look much more closely at all of these issues in the section 'The Emotional Landscape of Water'.)

The Gifts of Water

When we are in harmony with an Element and the Element is in balance within us, then we have access to the positive qualities of that Element in our lives. There are many such qualities and this list is by no mean a complete one. These are some of the more fundamental of these qualities. As you read about these qualities, consider how easy it is for you to access them in your own life. Your answers will tell you much about the relative strength or deficiency of the Water Element within you.

Not Knowing

We live in a world of unknowns. Nothing is certain. Life is an unfolding mystery. Yet most people try to create a sense of certainty in their lives in order to feel safe. The unknown can be a scary place, so we try to know as much as we can in order to avoid any nasty surprises. However, no matter how much we know, this sense of certainty is an illusion. We can never be sure what the next moment will bring no matter how much we try to protect ourselves.

Another way to be that is more real is to become more comfortable with not knowing and to hang out for a while in the unknown. One of the concepts of Zen Buddhism is *beginner's mind*. This is an attitude of openness, eagerness and lack of preconceptions when studying a subject, even at an advanced level. It's like coming to something as if for the first time. Such a place of not knowing arouses curiosity and interest in the world, making it appear new, bright and fresh in every moment.

We can learn to bring this practice of open curiosity to all of our life. The longer we can remain in the unknown of a situation, the more the limitless potential of Being is available to us. The Water Element is comfortable with the unknown, with the hidden depths.

The Water Element, as the Greater Yin, is the Element closest to the deepest places within us. It is a gateway to our unconscious, to the Tao and our place within it. As humans, we are all waves in the great ocean of the Tao, arising as forms out of the ocean, and falling back into the formless. We are both formless and form, constantly manifesting and dissolving.

As we comprehend this universal truth and begin to have our own experiential glimpses of this reality, we come to realise that nothing can be known, and that being in the unknown is the deepest wisdom. We see that the more certain we are of what we know, the more we are cut off from all we don't know. As the Zen master Shunryu Suzuki succinctly said, 'In the beginner's mind there are many possibilities, but in the expert's there are few.'[9]

When we begin to live in not knowing, we find that we are not *taking* action but that action arises anyway. The more we are in contact with the fundamental ground of the Tao, the more we are able to watch our actions arising like waves out of the ocean. We become spectators, marvelling at the unfolding of our own lives.

Staying in the deep Water of not knowing, without the impulse to move to action, allows the fullest transformation from potential to manifestation.

> *Not knowing is true knowledge.*
> *Presuming to know is a disease.*
> *First realize that you are sick;*
> *then you can move towards health.*
> *The Master is her own physician.*
> *She has healed herself of all knowing.*
> *Thus she is truly whole.*[10]

What gets in the way of being in a state of not knowing? Remember a time when you experienced beginner's mind.

Knowing

Water finds its way to the deepest places. It is at home in the depths. From the depth arises innate knowing. Lao Tze in the *Tao Te Ching* taught that all of manifestation arises out of the nothingness of the void. Likewise, knowing arises from the mysterious depths of Water. All knowing is grounded in not knowing.

In our bodies, this place of knowing is the belly centre, known in various traditions as the hara, lower dan tien or k'ath. This centre is an organ of perception, a place of true knowing. It is where we get our 'gut feelings' of what to do, when to act and what best serves the unfolding of our life. Cultivating this centre through meditation and hara breathing strengthens the capacity to know directly.

True knowing or direct knowing is not an activity of the mind. It is not about factual information, reasoning, deducing or forming conclusions. It is not an intellectual capacity at all. Rather, it is direct understanding. This is close to what Aristotle and other ancient Greek philosophers were referring to when they used the word *nous* which referred to intuitive understanding as distinct from sense perception.

True knowing is not something that can be written down and studied by future generations. Nor is it something that is unchanging, that can be held on to and pointed to as fact. True knowing arises moment by moment as is appropriate to that particular moment. Like the wave which arises out of the ocean and falls back, only to be replaced by another wave, this kind of knowing arises in a way that is relevant to what is here in this very moment.

True knowledge exists in knowing that you know nothing.

SOCRATES

Spend some time contacting your belly centre using the hara breathing technique. (See the basic meditation practice in Chapter 5.) From this place, ask yourself the question, 'What do I know in this moment?' Continue to ask the question for as long as you are curious.

Potential

Nothing illustrates the concept of potential more completely than a seed. Whether it is a lettuce seed, an apple seed, an acorn or something else, this tiny package contains the blueprint for a plant, a flower, a bush or a tree. The seed is not the plant or the tree, but it has the potential to become that. What is required are the right conditions of soil, moisture, temperature and sunshine for the seed to germinate and begin its path of growth.

Potential is possibility and latency. It carries a sense of waiting with patience for the right time for things to birth and sprout into life. It suggests a promise of things to come. And as with the seed, there is a sense of fullness, of a huge amount of energy packed inside, just waiting for the chance to burst forth. This notion is contained in the expressions 'filled with potential' and 'pregnant with possibility'.

For humans, life begins with the meeting of the egg and sperm of our parents. They carry the DNA, the ancestral imprints that will determine the potential of our particular life. A baby's birth is often greeted with great joy of seeing such potential in a new life, a recognition of infinite possibilities.

Potential is not confined to youth. As adults, we have this potential in our life no matter what age we are. Each day, indeed each moment, is filled with potential and the possibility of becoming.

 What potential do you recognise in yourself? As you explore this question, what is the feeling in your bodymind?

Power

We have all experienced the incredible power of water. It is visible in the immensity of the ocean, its waves, tides and currents. Who has not felt its power while swimming, felt the force of a breaking wave, the pull of a tidal current? Water power is observable in a river as it drops over a waterfall or pounds its way through rapids. Surges in river levels cause flooding which can unleash great destructive power.

The power of water derives from the fact that water finds its way to the lowest possible level, pulled by gravity towards the deepest point it can find, ultimately the ocean. Much power can be harnessed from these gravitational movements of water, through hydroelectric power generation.

The same water power resides within the human body in the form of stored energy. From the perspective of Chinese medicine, this energy is stored in the Kidneys and has the potential to power our personal engine for 80 years or more.

This power resides not in the actions that we take in life, but in the stored energy that is available to carry out those actions. Power is action waiting to happen. It is the petrol in the tank that fuels all activity. And it is the strength of the Water Element that provides this capacity.

Recall a time when you felt powerful. Notice the sensations in your body and where they are located. What emotions are there?

Stillness

Water is so adaptable that it can be an ocean or a waterfall in constant motion, yet can also be a deep and quiet lake or an underground pool that is perfectly still and dark. Darkness, depth and stillness are emblematic of Water's deep yin nature.

Many of us live in a culture that values activity and production but rarely encourages stillness. It is beneficial for us to contact this quality of stillness in our own life in order to counteract these endless demands to be active. Even within ourselves, there is the ceaseless drive of the ego to be doing something at every moment. Ego's inherent nature is of endless, spinning activity. Even without the pressures from outside to be active, there is an inner activity that strongly resists any move towards stillness.

We appropriately take vacations from work in order to rest and restore. It is also healthful to take time off from the inner activity of thinking, planning, remembering, obsessing and worrying. Winter provides ample opportunity to dwell in stillness, offering us long dark nights to sit or lie in quiet reflection. Watching the fire, listening to relaxing music or sitting in candlelight are all ways to support stillness. Perhaps most beneficial is a regular meditation practice which provides the space to unhook from the thought stream of mental chatter and to become like the underground pool of quiet stillness.

Make a list of all the ways you could be more still. What gets in the way of your inner stillness?

Trust

Trust is the confidence or faith that someone or something is reliable and will not be a danger to us. In relationships, the degree to which one person trusts another is a measure of a person's belief in the honesty, fairness or benevolence of the other person. Trust is the antithesis of fear.

The emotion of fear is critical for our survival. Without it, we wouldn't run away from danger or turn to defend ourselves from attack. Adrenaline, which powers these survival responses, is a crucial part of our hormonal system. However, when fear overwhelms us to the extent that trust is lost, the Water Element becomes unbalanced.

It is said that trust needs to be earned. We trust someone if they demonstrate that they will not harm us. We trust a situation that we've learned is not dangerous. These are examples of conditional or relative trust. At the deepest level is something known as Basic Trust, a trust that no matter what happens, we will ultimately be all right. Even if we are hurt, even if we die, there is still a trust that everything will turn out for the best. This is a trust in the basic goodness and benevolence of the universe. When we are deeply in contact with our own depth, this kind of trust becomes available to us.

Think of some of the people and situations that you trust deeply. How does that feel?

How much are you in contact with Basic Trust?

Wisdom

The classics tell us that the Kidneys are the Essence of the Water Element, and wisdom proceeds unceasingly from them without any doubt or uncertainty.[11]

Scholars of the Five Elements say that true healing and balance in the Water Element come from transforming fear into wisdom as represented by the archetype of the Sage.[12] Mahatma Gandhi is a good example of this archetype. The Sage has learned a lot from his long life as well as from the accumulated wisdom of the ancestors. He understands that fear is transformed by accepting and embracing the unknown. He has come to accept and even welcome fear. By not resisting fear, the Sage is able to be steady and courageous in the face of the unknown, even when facing the greatest unknown: his death.

Wisdom is the virtue that empowers us to stand firm when things are unknown, and to chart a steady course through uncertain waters.[13] We do this through the clever utilisation of our inner resources which are inherent in our Kidney Qi. This includes knowing our limits, when it is time to conserve and when it is time to utilise resources for the greatest benefit. This is the path of wisdom engendered by a healthy Water Element.

Who do you know who embodies this gift of wisdom? Recall a time when you were in contact with this kind of wisdom.

Will

The Chinese classic *Nei Jing* teaches, 'When Intent becomes permanent, we speak of Will.'[14] The spirit of Water is *zhi*, often translated as Will. The will we are speaking of is not the driven willpower of the ego, which exerts effort to achieve its ends, but rather a real force that underpins all life. At its core, it is the will to live, an immensely powerful force. Remember, Water is the most yin Element, so here Will is also yin. Lori Dechar describes it as 'the yin fire, the pilot light that ignites the flame of all organic processes'.[15]

Inherent in the gift of Will are the qualities of steadiness, solidity, dependability and determination. When we are in touch with the quality of Will, it can feel like being a big mountain with deep roots, solid and immovable. It is felt as a substantial presence in the lower body.

Will is the power that lies behind continuous action. It engenders perseverance and persistence, the ability to just keep moving forward. Like Old Man River, it just keeps rolling along.

But whose will is it? When we see ourselves as a discrete entity that is separate from everything, then the will is merely the effort of the ego to maintain its separate identity. True Will derives from the mandate of Heaven. As we begin to align our personal will with the Will of Heaven, the less effort is needed to move through the world. There is conservation of Kidney Qi and there is balance and health in the Water Element.

Think of a time when you experienced this kind of True Will. How did it show up in your life? How does it feel now to recall it?

And More...

The gifts we've explored here are just some of the many qualities that the Water Element offers. Below are some others to ponder. Think or write about the extent to which these qualities appear in your life and how much access you have to them.

Capacity	Genius	Persistence
Concentration	Inquiring	Reassurance
Confidence	Listening	Resolve
Courage	Memory	Resourcefulness
Determination	Mystery	Resting
Endurance	Patience	Silence
Flow	Perseverance	Steadfastness

Journal Entry: 24 June 2012

Like the ancient river, winter thoughts meander slowly across the open plain of mind.

Of all the Elements, Water is the greatest yin. It expresses most strongly the characteristics of yin: deep, dark, cold, moist, slow. We've been living with these qualities in nature for some time. The winter gives the opportunity (invites me) to be with, to explore these qualities in, myself.

I write this by the window in the pale light of a late afternoon in mid-winter. The wood stove makes a slight hiss and an occasional pop. There is overall a quiet stillness.

These expressions of deep yin invite me to sit here, to stay with myself, to contemplate, or, rather, to just *be*. The time for doing will come soon enough. For now, I sink down into being, drawn down to my depths on this sinking current of Water, dropping down to that measureless cavern that is me and which is all.

The Physical Level of Water

Now that we have an understanding of the resonances and qualities of the Water Element, let us look at the ways they manifest themselves in the physical body. The extent to which we are out of alignment with the Water Element will determine the ways in which imbalances will be expressed in our organs and tissues.

Organs and Tissues
The Bladder
WESTERN MEDICAL PERSPECTIVE

The urinary bladder is a hollow, muscular organ located in the pelvic cavity behind the pubic bones. Its function is to store the steady drip of urine that flows from the kidneys, through the tubes known as the ureters and into the urinary bladder. As a storage pouch, it is designed to swell in order to accommodate the urine, going from spherical to pear-shaped as it becomes more distended and rising up into the abdomen. At the lower end of the bladder is an opening to another tube called the urethra through which the urine is passed to the outside when the bladder is emptied. This flow is controlled by sphincter muscles.[16]

The average capacity of the bladder is about 750 ml, as much as a bottle of wine, though well before this capacity is reached, sensory nerves alert the brain of the need to urinate. This is known as the micturition reflex. While this can be voluntarily overridden, at some point the involuntary reflex wins out.

Ageing affects the bladder as its tissue becomes less elastic and can no longer hold as much urine. In addition, the sphincter muscles become weaker with age. The urethra can become blocked in men as a result of an enlarged prostate gland, and in women due to prolapse of the bladder or vagina.

CHINESE MEDICINE PERSPECTIVE
The Bladder has a wider sphere of activity in Chinese medicine. While it stores and excretes urine, it is also involved in the transformation of fluids that is necessary for the production of urine, and it does this in conjunction with several other organs.[17]

The Small Intestine, which separates the pure from the impure, passes the clear fluids to the Bladder which then transforms them into urine using Qi and heat. The energy for this heat is produced by the Kidneys. The Heart also is involved in the process as Heart Qi needs to descend to assist in the excretion of urine.

The Triple Heater also plays a role by ensuring that the lower burner is open and free for the transformation and excretion of fluids. The Liver also assists because the Liver channel flows around the end of the urethra, and a free flow of Qi in this channel ensures smooth urination. Finally, Lung Qi descends to assist the transformation; its failure to do so causes urine retention, a problem that is common in the aged.

The Kidneys
WESTERN MEDICAL PERSPECTIVE
The kidneys are two reddish-coloured organs that resemble kidney beans in shape and which lie towards the back of the body above the level of the waist and partly protected by the lower ribs. They are 10–12 cm (4–5 in) in length, 5–7.5 cm (2–3 in) wide and 2.5 cm (1 in) thick.[18]

While we can manage with one kidney, if both fail, then the body is no longer able to eliminate the toxic wastes of metabolism. While kidney dialysis can do some of this work, without intervention, kidney failure results in death.

The primary function of the kidneys is to maintain body homeostasis by controlling the volume and composition of blood. This work is carried out by nephrons which act as a filtration network. They selectively retain or expel water and minerals, and remove toxic wastes such as ammonia and urea as well as essential materials that are surplus to requirements. All of this forms as urine to be passed on to the bladder. Other functions of the kidneys are to control blood pH, regulate blood pressure by secreting renin and participate in the activation of vitamin D.

The adrenals are small glands that are located on top of each kidney. While they are a part of the endocrine system, they have an important relationship to the kidneys. One of the hormones secreted by the adrenals is aldosterone, which acts upon the kidneys to increase their reabsorption of sodium and to increase the excretion of potassium. This process controls electrolyte homeostasis in the body.[19]

CHINESE MEDICINE PERSPECTIVE

From the Western perspective, the kidneys are certainly important organs with complex functions; however, in Chinese medicine their significance is profound, for they store Essence and as such are the root of life itself.

Dr Leon Hammer puts it this way: 'Kidney energies are the inherited energies that unite past, present and future and bind all three, in the individual person, to cosmic forces, to the secrets and mysteries of the universe.'[20]

Essence or *jing* is the fuel for life. This precious substance derives partly from the parents (prenatal Essence) and partly from the Qi extracted from food and air (postnatal Essence). This powerful energy is stored in the Kidneys and the health of these organs is linked to the strength of Essence.

Prenatal Essence, that which is inherited at conception, supports the development of the foetus, controls growth after birth, sexual maturation and fertility. It also determines our basic constitution, strength and vitality. Later in life it provides the material for the formation of sperm, ova and menstrual blood. All of these functions are directly related to the Essence inherited from the parents.[21]

Postnatal Essence is the Qi which we ourselves derive from the food we eat and the air we breathe during our life. This is added to our inherent store of Essence in the Kidneys. The more healthy is our diet and breathing, the more Qi we extract to add to the fuel tank.

Essence is also used to produce Marrow (as opposed to bone marrow) which fills the spinal cord and the brain, and therefore influences intelligence, memory, concentration and thinking. When the Kidneys are healthy and Essence is strong, these capacities of the brain will also be strong.

The Kidneys also have a direct influence on urination and are seen as the 'gate' which controls this function. Moreover, they control all fluids in the body including the fluids required by other organs such as the intestines, spleen and lungs.

It is clear that the basis of good health is to maintain the health of the Kidneys and Essence. We will look at ways we can do this later in the section on diet and lifestyle.

Ears

The Kidneys are said to open into the ears and that when the Kidneys are healthy, the hearing will also be healthy.[22] Conversely, when the Kidneys are weak, hearing may be impaired and tinnitus may develop. Repeated ear infections can also be indicative of Kidney weakness.

It has been observed that the ear is similar in shape to the kidneys, which may provide a connective link from the organ to its sense organ. It can also be seen that the ear is shaped like a foetus. Indeed, it is this parallel that underlies the principle of ear reflexology. The head of the foetus corresponds with the ear lobe, while its bottom corresponds with the tip of the ear. Needling of points in the ear can help to heal corresponding areas of the body.

Bones

The Water Element is the deepest yin, so it makes sense that the tissue of Water is the deepest tissue of the body, namely the bones. A balanced and healthy Water Element will allow for strong bones. Problems with bone growth in childhood are indicative of Kidney weakness. Likewise, osteoporosis in later life is evidence of a decline in Essence and Kidney health.

The teeth are also considered to be the tissue of Water, bones which have risen to the surface. The strength of the Water will determine the strength and health of the teeth. It is worth noting here that individual teeth relate to specific meridians so that defects in a particular tooth can suggest areas of weakness in the energetic system. These meridian tooth charts are readily available on the Internet.

Hair

The hair of the head is considered to be the external manifestation of the Water Element. It relies on the Kidney Essence for its nourishment and growth. Thus, if the Essence is strong, the hair will be full, luxurious and glossy. Conversely, if Essence is weak, the hair may become prematurely grey, brittle, thin, dull in colour and may fall out.

Diet and Lifestyle

Foods That Support Water

Blue is the colour that corresponds to the Water Element. Black is also considered to be a correspondence by some traditions. Therefore, foods that are blue or black in colour are supportive of this Element.

Fruits of this colour include blackberries, blueberries, black grapes, blackcurrants, plums, figs, prunes and raisins. Vegetables include eggplant, black beans, purple potatoes, blue corn and black rice. Other foods are dark miso, soy sauce and tamari, all of which not only have the colour but also the salty flavour of Water.

It has been discovered that eating blue foods such as these can reduce the risk of heart disease and diabetes, as well as lowering blood pressure and waist size. Also the anthocyanins that are typically found in these foods can help prevent urinary tract infections such as cystitis by stopping bacteria from sticking to the urinary tract wall.

Good intakes of anthocyanins have also been linked to improved balance, coordination and short-term memory in old age.[23] It is interesting to see how many of these benefits relate directly to the organs and functions of the Water Element.

Some suggestions to get more blue/black food in your diet:

- Add a handful of blueberries, blackberries or raisins to your morning oatmeal or cereal.

- Blend fruit smoothies with blackberries and blueberries.

- Bake an eggplant, halved, scored and covered with crushed garlic and salt.

- Enjoy stewed black plums with yoghurt.

- Choose black grapes over green for snacks.

- Try a sandwich filling of soft cheese and blueberries.

- Cook up a pot of delicious ratatouille with lots of eggplant.

- Go for black beans over red beans when eating Mexican food.

- Make a hearty winter stew of black beans and root vegetables.

The flavour of Water is salty; therefore, foods that are salty are also supportive of the Element. As with any flavour, its use must be moderate. In this case, too much salt can create problems with the heart by increasing blood pressure. The ancient Chinese were aware that overconsumption of the flavour of one Element can result in imbalances in the Element that is its grandson.[24] In this case, too much salt affects the Heart, which is the primary organ of the Fire Element.

Foods that are salty include sea salt, miso, soy sauce, tamari and seaweed. There are far fewer salty foods than any other flavour and no vegetables or fruits are naturally salty with the exception of sea vegetables such as arame, dulse, kombu and nori. However, salt is added to most prepared food so it is important to limit consumption of highly salted processed foods such as pizza, potato chips, soups, cured meats, canned fish, sauces and pickles. Salt is often used as a preservative which is then masked by adding lots of sugar, resulting in a double whammy for the body.

Blood closely resembles seawater in its composition of elements, minerals and trace minerals.[25] The body's cells are permanently bathed in the ocean from which we came. We should therefore use sea salt in our diet, not table salt which is simply sodium chloride and which has been denuded of the other minerals. Himalayan salt is best because it was formed from seawater millions of years ago and is therefore unpolluted. If you are concerned about reducing salt in your diet, take note that only 5% of people react to salt with higher blood pressure.

Water, water everywhere, nor any drop to drink.

SAMUEL TAYLOR COLERIDGE

The body contains more water than anything else, and we cannot live for long without it. Good health relies on being well hydrated with clean, fresh water. How much should we drink? In recent years there has been a rule of thumb that we need eight glasses a day, or about 2 litres. However, there are so many variables to consider that this figure is not right for everyone. People with bigger bodies need more. Those living at altitude need more. Living in a hot climate or exercising vigorously requires more. If you are taking medications that are diuretic, or drinking a lot of coffee or tea, then you will need more water to replace the loss. Conversely, those who are less active or who live in cold climates may need less than the conventional eight glasses.

Drinking more water does not necessarily mean you are being hydrated. It is common for people to go long periods without drinking water, then when the thirst response is triggered, they drink a lot all at once. Much of this water is not absorbed into the cells and just gives the bladder a workout. Much better is to drink small amounts frequently.

There is a fascinating story that illustrates the healing power of hydration. Fereydoon Batmanghelidj, an Iranian doctor, was imprisoned in Tehran during the 1979 Iranian revolution. With no medications at his disposal, he treated his sick fellow prisoners with regular intake of water and discovered that many degenerative diseases were cured by this regimen. He later wrote that a dry mouth is not a reliable indicator of dehydration. The body signals its water shortage by producing pain. Dehydration actually produces pain and many degenerative diseases, including asthma, arthritis, hypertension, angina, adult-onset diabetes, lupus and multiple sclerosis. Dr Batmanghelidj's message to the world is, 'You are not sick, you are thirsty. Don't treat thirst with medication.'[26]

The quality of drinking water is just as important as the quantity. These days many water sources are polluted with toxic chemicals. Most town water supplies are treated with chlorine to kill bacteria, but the chlorine can create its own health risks. The prevalence of agricultural pesticides and herbicides in the environment results in these harmful chemicals finding their way into the water supply. It is therefore beneficial to filter water in a way that removes these chemicals. It is also good to put filters in your shower and bath in order to reduce chlorine intake through the lungs and skin when you wash.

Bladder Health

There are two main problems that can affect the bladder, and both influence urination: the first is infection, the second is weak muscles.

Lower urinary tract infection, also known as cystitis, is an inflammation of the bladder and urethra. It is characterised by a painful, burning sensation when urinating and often frequent or urgent urination. Urine is often cloudy, smelly and even bloody. Other symptoms that can be experienced are low back pain and low-grade fever. Women are much more susceptible to infection than men because of the proximity of the urethra to the anus.

When infection is severe, antibiotics are often used to treat cystitis, but there are other remedies available. Diluted cranberry juice (pure, not sweetened) has been found to be helpful. Colloidal silver and garlic combat infection, while probiotics restore friendly bacteria.[27] Drink a lot more water, especially barley water, to flush out the bugs. And avoid all sugar, which supports bacterial growth. Herbs that soothe the bladder include buchu, crataeva and uva ursi as teas or in capsules.

Urinary incontinence is a common condition in which there is a loss of voluntary control of the bladder. It is usually related to weak musculature of the pelvic floor. Causes of this include ageing, being overweight and childbirth. Strengthening these muscles is quite simple and effective for many people. They are often referred to as Kagel exercises after the gynaecologist Arnold Kagel who first recommended them in 1948.

Sit, stand or lie with legs slightly apart. Tighten the muscles around the front and back passages, as if trying not to go to the toilet. Imagine you are drawing the muscles up inside. Hold each squeeze as tightly as you can for 5–10 seconds. Do this up to ten times, resting for 5–10 seconds between squeezes. Then do up to ten fast squeezes. Do this whole routine about five times a day. Don't hold your breath or tighten your stomach muscles. Start slowly with fewer repetitions and shorter contractions, then increase as your muscles get stronger.

Kidney Health

Winter is an important time to support the kidneys as these organs are more susceptible to problems during cold weather. Keeping the low back warm is important. Keep your shirt tucked in, wear a singlet or even get a kidney warmer. Important, too, is to stay hydrated by drinking sufficient water to aid the kidneys in filtering the blood and flushing out toxins. There are many herbs that support kidney function including green tea, nettle, dandelion and uva ursi as well as many Chinese herbs including ho shou wu and ginseng.

Pathological conditions that affect the kidneys are various kinds of kidney disease and kidney stones.

Upper urinary tract infection or pyelonephritis affects the kidneys and ureters, the tubes which take urine from the kidneys to the bladder. This condition can be quite serious and therefore requires medical help. Symptoms include high fever, shaking chills, pain in the side or low back, nausea and vomiting.

Other kidney diseases are: glomerulonephritis, an inflammation of the filtering units of the kidneys; Bright's disease, which is characterised by blood protein in the urine and oedema; and uraemia, which is the presence of toxic waste in the bloodstream. All of these are serious conditions that need medical attention.

Kidney stones occur when accumulations of mineral salts formed in the kidneys become lodged in the urinary tract. This is extremely painful (possibly the only way a man can understand the pain of childbirth!). The pain is often accompanied by vomiting and consequent dehydration which requires medical attention. Most kidney stones are composed of crystallised oxalic acid, so those who are prone to kidney stones, or whose parents were, would be advised to reduce consumption of foods which are high in oxalates, foods such as spinach, beet greens and chocolate. Dehydration is another cause of kidney stone formation, so adequate hydration, especially in hot weather, is an important preventative measure.

A Healthy Back

Back pain is one of the leading causes of pain, disability and absence from work. The Bladder meridian runs like a double set of railway tracks down the back, parallel to the spine, a total of 36 acupoints on each side of the body. So a healthy back reflects a balanced Bladder meridian. What is more, many of these points (shu points) relate to and can be used to treat other meridians and organs. Pain, tightness and other symptoms at specific places in the back can be diagnostic of imbalance in other meridians. Here are some ways to maintain a strong and healthy back:

- Hara breathing (see basic meditation practice in Chapter 5) builds Kidney Qi and also strengthens the lower abdomen and lumbar spine.

- Build core strength with abdominal strengthening, pelvic tilts and lifts.

- Pilates-style exercises that focus on engaging the abdominal muscles, pulling them down and in. Imagine you were about to be punched in the belly and how you would contract your muscles.

- When lifting, engage the abdominal muscles, bend the knees, push down into the floor, use your leg strength to assist the lifting and do not make the back do all the work. Maintain a straight back. Take a long breath in before lifting and breathe out as you lift and straighten.

- Spinal twists rotate the spine as well as the spinal nerves and ligaments. These exercises are excellent for maintaining the health of the discs that separate the vertebrae and help to avert disc shrinkage that causes height loss as we age.

- The spine, also known as the vertebral column or backbone, is an integral system composed of 24 articulating vertebrae as well as the sacrum and coccyx or tailbone. The movement of each vertebra affects all the others because the spine operates as a functional unit. For example, when you turn your head to the left, the cervical vertebrae of the neck turn left, but at the same time the lumbar vertebrae and sacrum turn to the right. This is why spinal twists have a beneficial effect on the health of the spine.

- Make sure your bed is supportive and comfortable. Like humans, ageing beds begin to sag and are not good news for backs.

Winter in the Garden

If you are beginning your cycle through the seasons in winter, it may be too early to start your garden outdoors, but there are other ways you can begin right now. You can start with seed trays that can be kept indoors on a window ledge on the sunny side of the house. If your climate is not too severe, you can build a greenhouse. This doesn't have to be a large glass shed but can be a frame covered with polythene plastic, or even a large glass bottle with the bottom cut off. (See below for a neat way of creating these mini greenhouses.)

I have recently discovered that kale seeds can germinate as low as 4ºC (39ºF), and once they're up they don't mind a frost. I've just put a tray of seeds in the bathroom window, which is a lovely suntrap on the north side of the house, and they sprouted in four days.

While waiting patiently for spring to arrive, winter is a good time to mulch the ground to prevent weeds from taking over, for cleaning and oiling garden tools, sorting through the seed collection and discarding out-of-date seeds. Since the seed is a particular totem of the Water Element, paying attention to seeds and contemplating their potential in the coming year is a great Watery activity.

Winter solstice is not a day; it is a precise moment in time. In 2015 in Adelaide it was 2.08 a.m. on 22 June. This marks the shortest day, but, more precisely, it marks the lowest angle of the sun, its greatest distance from the Equator. This is a time to deeply contemplate the depth of winter and the Water Element, feeling the deepest yin of your particular location. It is a great day to walk in nature. This year I marked the occasion by circumambulating a local hilltop regarded by local aborigines as a sacred site. While I've done this walk many times before, the fact of doing it at the time of the solstice made it special and I found myself being more present and aware of everything around me.

How to Make a Mini Greenhouse

Take a large glass bottle. A 2-litre wine or olive oil bottle works well. Tie a piece of thick string around the bottle, positioning it as close to the bottom as possible. Carefully soak the string with methylated spirits. Light the string with a match, turning the bottle so the flame catches all round. Hold up the bottle like a torch until the flame has burned out. Immediately plunge the bottle into a bucket of cold water. If you are lucky, you will hear a satisfying crack as the bottom of the bottle breaks off. You may have to repeat the process until this happens.

Now you have a little greenhouse that can go over a seedling in the garden, allowing you to plant out several weeks earlier, protecting the plant from low temperatures and frost at night and magnifying sunlight during the day.

Activity: Fire Gazing

About 300,000 years ago our human ancestors learned to control fire, a discovery which changed their lives dramatically.[28] They had a source of heat to keep them warm, to keep them safe from animals and to cook food which allowed for a higher calorie intake. All of these things were especially beneficial in wintertime when the nights were long, cold and dangerous. In addition, the fire became a focal point for family and community. I wonder if our love of watching fires puts us in touch with deep ancestral memory that evokes a sense of safety and belonging.

Fire can be a source of deep relaxation, meditation and contemplation, activities which are very supportive of the Kidney Qi and the adrenals. Watching a fire can take us out of our busy minds, away from thinking, planning, worrying and judging, putting us more in touch with the unconscious mind and the realm of the Water Element.

If you have access to a fire, whether indoors or outdoors, try this exercise. If you don't have a fire, you can try lighting some candles and gazing into their flames.

It is best to do this at night when you can turn off all other sources of light. This way the fire can become the complete focus of your gaze. Also turn off any music or other sound disturbance. It's best to do this alone, or, if you are with others, in silence. This reduces distractions. Simply watch the flames, whether they are leaping and dancing or soft and licking, or watch the glowing embers pulsing with heat. Allow your thoughts to wander; let your imagination loose. Soft gaze, soft eyes, soft thoughts, soft mind. Let yourself drop deeper and deeper into this space that is below conscious thought. Maybe you see images in the flames, maybe your thoughts wander off by themselves, or maybe you just zone out and there are no thoughts at all. Whatever happens is fine. Don't try to make anything happen. Don't try to make anything not happen. In this way fire gazing becomes a form of meditation.

After a period of fire gazing, most people become much more relaxed and sleepy, less troubled. Chances are you'll be ready for an early night and a long and restful sleep.

Meridian Pathways

The Bladder and Kidney meridians are the energy pathways of the Water Element. The Bladder meridian is unique in several ways. It is the longest of the meridians and has more points (67) than any other. And it has a dual pathway running parallel to the spine along which lie the shu or transporting points. Each shu point relates to one of the 12 meridians and is directly connected to its corresponding organ. The inner line of points affects the organs themselves while the outer line affects their psycho-emotional and spiritual aspects. The implication of this is that any work on the back, whether it is acupuncture, acupressure, massage, chiropractic or another modality, will affect all the organs and systems of the body. It also explains why back problems are so common, because any kind of imbalance can appear as an energy congestion in the back.

The Bladder meridian begins in the inner corner of the eye, above the tear duct. It travels up and over the top of the head, down through the back of the neck and onto the back. Here it divides into two streams, rather like a river that flows around an island. The inside stream lies 1.5 cun (body inches) from the spine, while the outer stream is 3 cun from the spine. The streams join up again at the back of the knee, from where the meridian continues through the calf, swings under the outer ankle bone and along the outside of the foot to end at the little toe. Figure 6.2 shows the Bladder meridian's pathway.

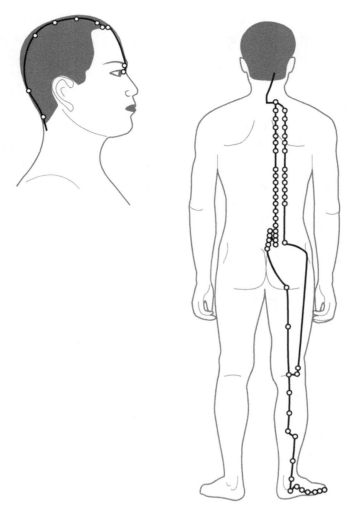

Figure 6.2 The pathway of the Bladder meridian

The Bladder meridian's partner, the Kidney meridian, begins on the sole of the foot in the deep hollow below the base of the toes. It travels around the arch of the foot, does a circle around the inside ankle bone and proceeds up the inside of the leg and onto the abdomen. There it runs very close to the midline and when it reaches the ribcage, goes wider to run alongside the sternum to finish under the clavicle. Figure 6.3 shows the Kidney meridian's pathway.

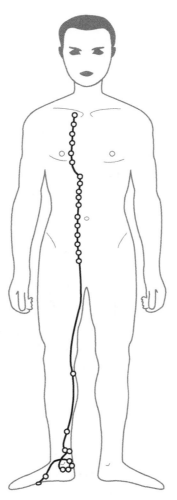

Figure 6.3 The pathway of the Kidney meridian

If you feel pain, discomfort, congestion or other symptoms along these pathways, or if you have issues that relate to these organs, you can help free the energy by doing a visualisation practice. Imagine a ball of blue energy or light passing along the length of the meridians, freeing up any blocks in the energy flow. You can use your breath to support the practice by breathing out as you pass down the Bladder meridian and breathing in as you bring the energy up the Kidney meridian. You may also use your hands to stroke along the pathways, though it can be difficult to reach the points of the Bladder meridian along the back. Do this several times. If you find a place where it is difficult to move the energy through, stay there and focus your mind, hand and breath to help free the block.

Organ Awareness

After doing the meridian visualisation practice, you can then bring your attention specifically to the organs themselves. Beginning with the bladder, place one hand over the pubic area, then place the other hand over it. Tune in to this organ which has been a lifelong servant in service of your urinary system. Bring to mind the colour blue, maybe the colour of the ocean or a blue sky. Allow this colour to infuse your bladder. Men might also see the colour infusing the prostate gland which lies right below the bladder. Acknowledge your bladder for its steadfast work of holding and controlling urine. Send love and gratitude to your bladder. Notice how it responds to your attention and recognition. Notice how you feel as you do this.

When you are ready, move your attention to your kidneys. Sit in a way that you can comfortably place the palms of your hands at the base of the ribcage in your back where your kidneys are. Again bring the blue colour to mind and allow it to sink deeply into all the cells of these organs. Send the colour also to the adrenal glands that lie perched above each kidney. Acknowledge these organs for their ceaseless work in filtering blood and regulating fluids and mineral composition. Send love and gratitude to your kidneys. Notice how they respond to your appreciation. Notice how you feel as you make this connection.

Acupressure for Physical Health

After the meridian visualisation and organ awareness practices, you can focus specifically on the source points for each meridian. The source point heals the organ directly as well as balancing the meridian. They are powerful points while at the same time being very safe. The source point has the effect of tonifying the meridian if it is deficient, or sedating it if it in excess. It is a very smart point. Hold each point with steady pressure for 2–3 minutes, first on the left side, then the right.

KI 3 *Taixi* Supreme Stream
The Kidney source point lies behind the inner ankle bone in a hollow between the bone and the Achilles tendon (see Figure 6.4).

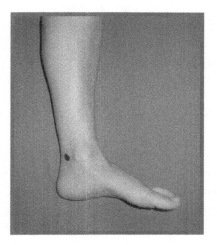

Figure 6.4 The Kidney source point (KI 3 *Taixi* Supreme Stream)

BL 64 *Jinggu* Capital Bone
The Bladder source point lies on the outside of the foot just below the head of the fifth metatarsal bone, the large bump about halfway along the foot (see Figure 6.5).

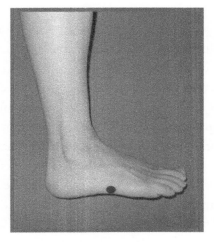

Figure 6.5 The Bladder source point (BL 64 *Jinggu* Capital Bone)

The Psycho-emotional Level of Water

Having explored the ways in which Water shapes us at the physical level, let's now look at the ways it shows up in our mental and emotional life. Thoughts and feelings are of a finer vibration than the body and so their energies are swifter and can change rapidly. But in another way, our emotional patterns, beliefs and attitudes can become fixed and entrenched. Here we will look at the ways in which the Water Element can appear in us.

The Emotional Landscape of Water

Fear

Of all the emotions, fear is the most primal since it is intimately connected to survival. When our sense of survival is threatened, fear is the normal response. This response comes from the animal, instinctual nature. Life clings powerfully to itself, so when we perceive that our life is under threat in some way, instinctual fear arises. A serious illness, a physical attack, a near miss on the freeway – these are some of the things that can provoke this instinctual fear.

Fear is often labelled as a negative emotion, probably because it can feel so unpleasant. But it is actually a very necessary part of the emotional matrix. Its purpose is to prompt us to take action. The steadfastness, determination and power of Water provide the means to take appropriate action to avoid danger. Without an instinctual fear response, we would be much more at risk of moving into dangerous situations that could be life-threatening. Fear is one of the things that has kept our species alive and flourishing.

However, we can also become afraid for much more minor reasons, in situations that are not life-threatening – for example, seeing our superannuation sink along with the stock market, worrying that our partner might leave us, or committing a social faux pas that raises fears of social ostracism. Countless things from large to small can create fear. In such situations our life is not directly threatened, but some part of us believes it is. This is the response of our ego structure, that collection of ideas, memories and beliefs that crystallises into who we take ourselves to be (see Chapter 4). Whenever this structure feels under threat, fear arises because the structure feels that its very existence is being undermined. This fear seems all the more real because we experience the effects in our body.

Since the ego identifies completely with the body, these physiological manifestations seem very real indeed. The rising heart rate, the quaking, the feeling that our insides are dropping down, the diminished control over the bladder and colon, the feeling of being frozen or paralysed, the irrepressible desire to run as fast and as far as possible – these unconscious physical reactions all stem from the core belief that we are destructible.

This ego – this 'I' – is based on the fundamental belief that we are separate individuals, that we are separate from other individuals, separate from nature, separate from the Tao. From the Taoist perspective, this is a distorted view of reality, for there is no separateness and we are all manifestations of the same fabric of the Tao. In short, fear arises as a result of our disconnection from the ground of True Nature, from Tao. Underpinning all fear is a fear of death and the belief that death means destruction.

The Taoist sage Chuang Tzu saw the emotions as powerful winds, the breath of the universe, and human beings as trees. The winds blow through the trees and move their branches, blowing through all the cavities and hollows, and making music, the music of the Earth. The sage recognises this and sees that when the winds have passed, he can settle again, unmarked by these emotions.

Fear is not a problem unless it becomes lodged in the body. If we can feel the fear and allow it to run its course – in other words, observe it as we would observe the wind in the trees – then its effects are short-lived and do not remain. However, when the wind of fear blows through us and we do not settle, the fear sinks like cold water and pools in the Kidneys. This diminishes our Qi, causes fatigue and depletion and reduces access to the Water qualities such as resolve, resilience, determination and will.

When there is an underlying imbalance in the Water Element, there will be an inherent instability around the emotion of fear. Fear becomes the lens through which life events and experiences are interpreted. When Water is the Constitutional Element, this becomes the core imbalance. From birth onwards, or even in utero, there will be repeated emotional responses to fear which becomes the dominant response to life. The character structure then crystallises around these emotional responses to the world and the emotion of fear becomes the guiding principle in life.

Even if you are not of a Water constitution, you may still find that fear is a strong determinant in your life. Therefore, consider to what extent you find yourself described in the following sections.

THE LOSS OF GROUND
When Water is the core imbalance, the world is a scary place. There is a fundamental loss of connection with the universe as a ground of holding Presence, a profound loss of Basic Trust. (We will look more closely at these concepts in the section 'The Spiritual Level of Water'.) This loss of connection with the ground, both

inner and outer, means that there is nothing safe to stand on. Any ground that appears is experienced as fleeting, shifting, unstable and not to be relied on.

A child who is fearful naturally seeks reassurance from her parents, looking to them to provide the ground that has been lost. Yet no matter how much the parents reassure, there really is nothing that can be provided that will substitute for the loss of the inherent ground of Being. Parents who do their best to provide reassurance will certainly help the child be less afraid than those parents who are insensitive to their child's fears. But when this is a core imbalance, it will structure beliefs, perceptions and behaviour for a lifetime.

When some kind of danger is actually present, fear is a normal and necessary response, prompting us into survival behaviour. If we are being chased by a dog or attacked in the street, then the adrenaline rush that arises helps us to survive the danger by running away or turning to fight. In our modern world there are many more subtle dangers that provoke fear, like losing a job, a house or a retirement income. All of these fears tell us that our survival is threatened and that we need to take action. But when the Water Element is deeply imbalanced, fear is the response not just to these but to most situations in life.

The personality patterns that arise from a fearful response to life will tend toward either of two polarities. One polarity is more yin, where the energy moves downward and inward; the other more yang, moving upward and outward. Both are responses to the same emotion, and you may find both polarities in the same person at various times.

THE YIN RESPONSE: FEARFUL, CAUTIOUS, PARALYSED

The fearful person is constantly vigilant, scanning the environment, alert for danger. This often manifests as a perpetual planning ahead for all eventualities, covering all the bases just in case something goes wrong. There is a belief that nothing is safe unless we make it so. Lots of energy is channelled into this preparation for disaster. Paradoxically, this extreme caution can be paralysing, placing severe limits on the ability to take action. There is a lack of drive and will to act.

The compulsive attention to all the things that might go wrong, and having alternate plans from plan B to plan Z, is an exhausting and impossible task. There is always going to be something that you didn't anticipate and account for. And there are many factors that are beyond our control, even if we do account for them. When one of these unanticipated events occurs and something does go wrong, this reinforces the belief that the world cannot be trusted.

The lack of trust in the world and the self may prompt the fearful person to cling to an authority figure such as a guru, a teacher, a teaching or a health practitioner. This person or belief system is idealised and trusted completely. This pattern arises out of a desperation to find a ground, to find something stable and solid to rely on to replace the ground that is missing. However, the idealised authority figure usually does not and cannot live up to this unrealistic, misplaced trust. As a result, the world becomes even less trustworthy than before, and the core structures are further strengthened. This can prompt a repeated, ongoing and never-ending search for the 'right' authority.

This personality pattern, when it develops to its extreme, becomes focused on phobias and paranoias. Phobias arise out of an intense fear of specific objects or situations which the person goes to great lengths to avoid and which, when encountered, cause extreme anxiety and distress. One well-known condition is agoraphobia, literally fear of the marketplace, where a person is afraid to go out of doors and leave the safety of the home environment.

Paranoia is an even more extreme case of fear response. Here, the person believes he is being persecuted by others or sees conspiracies behind perceived threats to his safety. Authorities may become hated and/or feared. There may be the belief that 'everyone is out to get me' or that accidents and coincidences are intentional. All of these responses are evidence of a severe imbalance in the Water Element.

THE YANG RESPONSE: FEARLESS, DRIVEN, GRANDIOSE

For some people with a Water imbalance, the feelings of fear are so unbearable or unacceptable that a defence is needed. As a result, a layer of fearlessness becomes superimposed over the fear. This defence forms the outermost shell of the personality, making unconscious the fear within. The yin response to the fear has changed to the yang response as a way of coping with the difficulty of the emotion. This is sometimes referred to as the counter-phobic personality, which instead of fleeing the source of fear, actively seeks it out in an attempt to overcome the original anxiety.

This kind of person appears unusually fearless and tends to enjoy risky activities. He is the daredevil who, over and over again, proves to himself and others that he is not afraid. He may take up extreme sports, enter dangerous occupations, choose the riskier path over the safer one and glory in that rush of adrenaline. But this need to prove again and again that he is unafraid is actually a reaction to the underlying, unconscious fear.

Another expression of the yang response is drivenness. Here the need to achieve, accumulate, succeed and win are driven by the unconscious fear of not surviving in a dangerous world. The belief is that we must 'kill or be killed'. Such people can become very successful in business and accumulate great wealth and power in their quest to make themselves safe.

This need to get ahead and stay ahead of others can lead to extremes of social behaviour that are intimidating and bullying. This can be seen in the schoolyard bully demanding money or toys, the office boss who uses his position of authority to intimidate and threaten employees or the dictator who ruthlessly kills his perceived enemies. All of these behaviours are created out of an intense reaction to fear.

Grandiosity is another trait that can appear in the yang response. It arises as a defence against the low self-esteem that often accompanies the painful lack of an inner ground of self. Grandiosity is an unrealistically positive view of one's abilities, a certain imitation of God. It is the ego self that assumes, without thinking, that it is the centre of the universe. There is a profound loss of connection with the Oneness of the Tao.

RETURNING TO BALANCE

A lifetime of living in reaction to fear places great stress on the organs and systems of the Water Element. The kidneys, the bladder, the adrenal glands, the ears and hearing, the bones and the lumbar spine are all subjected to stresses that weaken their functions. Overall, there is an ongoing depletion of Kidney Qi, the well of the life force. Conditions that may then arise include kidney stones, kidney disease, adrenal fatigue, hormone imbalance, exhaustion, urinary tract infections, urinary dysfunction, infertility, impotence, ear and hearing problems, tinnitus, loss of bone density, low back pain and lumbar disc protrusion.

If you have a number of health conditions in this list, while it is important to address these physical conditions medically, it is also important to look for underlying causes. Consider the possibility that anxiety or fear may be at the root of these problems. Understanding and acknowledging the connections between emotions and their physical manifestations is a very good start to healing both levels.

Likewise, if you recognise some parts of yourself in the above descriptions of the various personality forms that a fear imbalance can take, then you have already taken the first step to healing them. Winter is a great time to work with these imbalances, since the Water Element is most available and most supportive at this time of year.

Depending on whether you tend to respond to fear with caution and paralysis or fearlessness and drivenness, there are different strategies you can employ.

If you are the kind of person who responds to fear with paralysis:

- When you feel fear, take some deep breaths into the belly centre (hara), drawing in the Qi from the breath and building your store of *jing*.

  As with all of these exercises, do not try to dismiss the fear or push it away. Such resistance will tend to make it stronger. Try to be with the fear and observe it as much as you can. Imagine you are watching a movie of yourself. Take a step back from yourself. Reverse zoom the camera, taking you out of the centre of the fear.

- Make fists and rub your lower back with your knuckles.

  Massage your lumbar spinal muscles with vigorous strokes up and down. This brings warmth and life to the kidneys and helps to melt the freeze response in the body.

- Put your attention on your big toes.

  This may sound silly, but the big toes are the parts of the body that are furthest from the head where much of the anxiety response is going on. This exercise brings your attention away from the thinking mind and into the feet.

- While standing, put your attention on the middle of the soles of the feet.

  There is an important Kidney point on the sole (K1 Bubbling Spring). Imagine you are drawing the supportive energy of the Earth into your body through these points. When you feel some activation in the points, perhaps warmth or a tingling or pulsing, then draw the energy up the insides of the legs, up the abdomen and into the chest. You can use your inhalation to assist the process.

- Soak your feet in a basin of warm water with Epsom salts for 15 minutes.

  This can be very helpful before bedtime to help induce relaxed sleep.

- The Emotional Freedom Technique or tapping has been proven to be very effective in calming anxiety.

  This practice involves tapping lightly on specific acupressure points while making positive statements. There is a wealth of resources on the Internet for this method.

- Imbalances in the Water Element can be effectively addressed by working with a Five Element acupuncturist or acupressure therapist.

  Treatments for the Water Element are particularly effective in winter when the ambient energy of the season supports the work of balancing the Element.

- Psychotherapy can be very helpful in working with anxiety and phobias by exploring the origins of these patterns.

  Jungian analysis, Gestalt therapy, psychodynamic work and Internal Family Systems therapy (among others) can bring mental and emotional understanding that supports the energetic balancing of the Five Element treatments.

- Personal work, such as journaling, work with dreams, meditation, yoga, body awareness practices and Qi cultivation practices such as qigong, will also contribute to the lasting healing that results when we start examining and understanding our lives.

- The thing that is needed most of all in our journey is kindness towards ourselves.

  Understanding is not enough – our wounded parts cannot heal without compassion. True healing only occurs when we can combine the wisdom of our understanding with the loving kindness of the heart.

If you are the kind of person who responds with fearlessness and drivenness:

- Are you in contact with your belly centre?

  Take time to do some hara breathing, taking Qi into the belly via the breath and building a store of *jing*. This practice may get you in touch with feelings in this centre that you were not aware of.

- Are you the most fearless person in your family or group of friends? Are you mystified by the way others are afraid in situations that hold no fear for you? Perhaps you can begin to look at why this is. Are you overriding normal and natural survival responses?

  Instead of dismissing the fears of your friends, ask them why they are afraid. Maybe they have a good reason to be fearful.

- Make a list of all the daredevil things you have done in your life.

  Consider your reasons for behaving in these ways. Why did you choose to act in dangerous ways?

- Remember that fear is a normal and natural emotion that has helped the human race survive. It continues to be a normal, instinctual response.

  If you do not feel fear at all, what is it that is covering up your normal fear response? Take time to journal about this, talk to others, perhaps talk to a counsellor or therapist.

- Keep in mind that for some people the fearlessness is directed towards those in authority.

  There is a challenging of authority figures, from parents and teachers to police and government. Unfortunately, the prisons are full of people like this who have lost fear of the consequences of challenging authority. This is not to say that the status quo should not be challenged, but if this challenge is made out of a fearlessness which is out of touch with the natural fear response, then the consequences can be serious. If you are reading about yourself in this paragraph, spend some time considering what is in the way of your normal survival responses.

- If you are the kind of person who lives a life continually on the go, always doing, never resting, this can be a way of keeping fear at bay.

  Consider why you are so driven, single-minded, ambitious and compelled to succeed. Ask yourself why you are unable to come to rest, and what would happen if you did.

- Soak your feet in a basin of warm water with Epsom salts for 15 minutes.

  This can be very helpful before bedtime to help induce relaxed sleep.

BEING CONSCIOUS OF FEAR

All fear arises from a sense of danger to our health, happiness or our very existence. Sometimes the fear is blown out of all proportion to the circumstances. It can be useful to examine our relationship to fear as in the following exercise.

Below is a list of words that reflect many of the points along the fear spectrum. They are not in any particular order.

Shaky	Fearful	Anxious
Foreboding	Horror	Dread
Trepidation	Nervous	Scared
Angst	Afraid	Panicked
Uneasy	Apprehensive	Afraid
Edgy	Alarmed	Frightened
Jumpy	Agitated	Terrified

Now take the following steps:

1. In your Water journal, arrange these words in order from lowest intensity to highest intensity.

   There is no right way to do this. It will be different for everyone depending on their personal history and their associations with the words. If some words don't make sense to you, leave them out of your list. Add in any other words you can think of.

2. Take the words one by one and write a sentence about when you might get this feeling. If your first word is shaky, you might write: I feel shaky when I'm running late for work in the morning.

   Do this for all of the words on your list. Leave a line between each statement. Take your time. I'm encouraging you to feel the feeling as fully as possible. This exercise might take you all day or even all winter!

3. Continue each sentence with 'because I imagine that…' So your sentence may now read: I get shaky when I'm running late for work in the morning because I imagine that if I'm late, I won't get the promotion I'm hoping for.

4. When you've written all your sentences about all of these feelings, take some time to write about how the process was for you.

   Was it easy, challenging, enjoyable, painful or insightful? Do you feel differently now in relation to your fear? Remember, what we're trying to do here is to bring more conscious awareness to our fear so that it can be expressed and managed in healthy ways. Knowing that you are afraid and why allows the emotion to flow through and not get stuck in the bodymind.

Journal Entry: 25 May 2011

Fear

A cold, rippling, trickling, like water in the gutters on a drizzling day, grey and chill.

Deep, deep down in the lowest part of my psyche is an underground pool with a dark, dribbling overflow that attracts my attention.

Low in my body, the dark pooling around my perineum, anus and genitals; chilling, shrivelling, limiting, castrating, disembowelling, organs turning to slush, draining away uselessly.

The dark, black, velvet ground opening up, retreating out of view.

The outer wall of the space-lock opening, pulling me out to the cold vast space of annihilation. Fear of nothingness. Fear of not existing. Fear of non-me.

These are the fears of bodymind that freeze me into inaction. Like the children's game of statues. Water frozen, incapable of rising to feed Wood. Frozen soil cannot feed the tree.

HATRED ARISING FROM FEAR

Fear is certainly the primary emotion of the Water Element, but there are other emotions, attitudes and behaviours that are derived from fear. Indeed, some authorities regard fear as the key emotion that underlies all other emotions. Philosopher and spiritual teacher A.H. Almaas says, 'Fear is the underlying motive of all the defensive manoeuvres of the ego.'[29]

A particularly strong emotion that arises out of fear is hatred. Hatred is distinguished from anger in that hatred is cold and anger is hot. Anger is an instantaneous, explosive and uncontrolled reaction that wants to stop something. Hatred is controlled, methodical, slow, emotionally cold and wants to cause pain. Hatred intends to destroy.

Consistent with the nature of Water, hatred is cold, hidden and secretive, the stab in the back, the assassin's knife. It is cold-hearted and mean, entirely cut off from loving kindness.

Hatred is one of the more difficult emotions for us to acknowledge. Because its intent is to destroy, we are often loath to admit that we have a part of ourselves that wants to harm or even kill another human being. So feelings of hatred are most often kept well concealed, even from ourselves. Ironically, we tend to hate more those whom we love; hence, the term 'love-hate relationship'.

Difficult as it is to acknowledge our hatred, the more we can do so, the more we can feel the intense feelings of wanting to hurt and maim, to kill or destroy, the less likely we are to act them out in the world. It is when these feelings are unconscious and go underground that they are more likely to come out sideways, taking us by surprise. This unaware hatred can manifest in cutting remarks that are designed to wound another, actions that are calculated to destroy another's pride, reputation, relationship, business or in some way diminish them.

Revenge is a kind of hatred and one which is a culturally sanctioned feeling. The wide popularity of revenge movies is testament to this. These movies allow the viewer to contact his own feelings of hatred in a way that is safe and will not be considered abnormal. Retributive justice, the belief in an eye for an eye, is likewise a form of revenge. Revenge expresses hatred without acknowledging it.

Envy and jealousy are also emanations of hatred. Envy is the act of coveting what someone else possesses (e.g. their looks, their wealth, their job). This emotion derives from the fear that what I have is not enough for me to survive on, that I need what the other has in order to be safe. Jealousy is arguably the stronger emotion of being apprehensive or vengeful out of fear of being replaced in the affection of someone you love or desire. Who has not felt this pain of jealousy and the desire to hurt the one who is threatening, or even to hurt the loved one?

 Below are some other emotions, attitudes and behaviours that arise from fear. Consider the degree to which you observe them in yourself.

Ambition	Grandiosity	Separation
Animal survival	Hard-hearted	Sexual domination
Atheism	Insistent	Suspicion
Bullying	Isolated	Traumatised
Collapse	Intimidating	Urgency
Delusions of grandeur	Lack of will	Wilfulness
Driven	Megalomania	Trauma
Emptiness	Mistrust	
Exhausted	Overwhelm	

Trauma

Trauma is caused by physical accident or injury, exposure to stressful events or ongoing situations, and by physical or emotional abuse. However it is caused, trauma profoundly impacts upon the Water Element, the Kidneys and the *jing*. While the initial shock of an event impacts the Heart and the Fire Element, it is the ongoing impact of unresolved trauma upon the adrenals that places long-term stress on the Kidneys and the Water.

WHAT IS TRAUMA?

Definitions of trauma have changed markedly over the years. The word itself derives from the Greek and means wound. The medical definition of trauma is a physical wound or injury from an external source.[30] This excludes the majority of traumas which are not physical in origin. Meanwhile, the psychiatric definition is limited, including only extreme events that most people would not encounter in their lives, things like war, violent assault, serious injury or overwhelming shock.[31]

The main limitation of these definitions is that the focus is on the event as opposed to the response to the event. Modern definitions are now focusing on the psychological and physiological impacts on the individual of a much broader range of events.

In looking at the impacts of post-traumatic stress disorder, acupressure therapist Iona Teeguarden explored how the nervous system is hyperaroused in response to an event.[32] If the brain and nervous system are unable to calm down from the original shock, the brain becomes rewired and the arousal from the shock is unresolved. Such a perspective recognises trauma as the lasting results of an event, as opposed to the event itself.

Neurologist Robert Scaer's 2005 work *The Trauma Spectrum*[33] challenges the old view of trauma as an occurrence outside normal human experience. He widens the definition of trauma to include any negative life experience that affects the body and brain. This is challenging to the medical and psychiatric models in several ways. First, his thesis is that trauma is a spectrum, meaning that it is a condition that lies on a continuum of severity. Second, events that many people would not find traumatic can be very traumatising for some individuals; the event itself is not the issue but rather the impact it has on the individual. Finally, his most challenging idea is that trauma, particularly childhood trauma, contributes to much of our illness in adult life. In particular he attributes it to autoimmune disorders such as fibromyalgia, chronic fatigue syndrome, irritable bowel syndrome, gastrointestinal reflux and multiple chemical sensitivities, as well as to migraines, myofascial pain, tics, premenstrual syndrome, chronic pelvic pain, cystitis, thyroid, adrenal and other endocrine disorders, sleep disorders, attention deficit disorder and the list continues.[34] In short, the conditions that prompt most visits to the doctor can be seen in Scaer's list.

A modern pioneer in working with trauma is Peter Levine, whose work over 30 years has perhaps contributed more to a modern understanding of trauma than any other. His books *Waking the Tiger*[35] and *Healing Trauma*[36] outline his ideas that offer hope for healing. 'Somatic Experiencing' is the name he has given to the process of unwinding trauma in the body. The name itself reveals the fundamental principle of his work, namely experiencing the sensations in the body. He states: 'The healing of trauma is primarily a biological process, a bodily process and not a psychological one.'[37]

Levine's work was profoundly influenced by watching how animals shake after undergoing a frightening experience – for example, a deer that has escaped a predator or a polar bear that has been captured for tagging and then released. It is as if they are shaking out the fear that has accumulated during the experience. The basic premise of Levine's work is that trauma results when the hyperarousal produced by a triggering event remains undischarged and uncompleted. The fight-or-flight response, which is natural in all animals as a survival mechanism, in humans often becomes frozen into the body and needs to be released. This undischarged energy is available for discharge at any time, and this is done through awareness of bodily sensations.

Since we know from Chinese medicine that stored fear injures the Kidneys and hence the *jing*, it is therefore clear that any kind of unresolved trauma will negatively impact the Kidneys and the Water Element. And if we accept Scaer's definition of trauma as any negative life experience that affects the body and brain, then almost everyone can find themselves somewhere on the trauma spectrum. Consider these experiences as examples of trauma:

- Hospital birthing practices like separating the child from the mother.

- Routine medical procedures like skin cancer removal, colonoscopy and even routine pelvic examinations that are done insensitively.

- Life-threatening illnesses like being told you have cancer.

- Child-rearing practices that include routine smacking, food deprivation or separation.

- Harassment; this could be by neighbours, at work, from stalking and so forth.

- Witnessing violence, abuse or death. It doesn't have to be you experiencing the violence. Witnesses can also be traumatised. In families where one member is being abused, the whole family has the potential to be traumatised because the underlying fear is *am I next?*

- Daily involvement with others' trauma. Emergency services workers are at great risk of being traumatically impacted by daily witnessing.

- Childhood developmental trauma that can include lack of love and holding, separation from parents, loss of a parent, instability at home, rejection and criticism.

SEXUAL ABUSE TRAUMA

Recent investigations into sexual abuse in church and institutional settings have begun to reveal how widespread this is in the community. It is estimated that one in three girls and one in six boys are victims of sexual abuse before the age of 18 years.[38] The impact upon the psyche of such an experience is often deep and lifelong. The younger the victim, the closer the relationship with the perpetrator and the more frequent the abuse, the more devastating are the consequences.

The effects of such betrayal are felt strongly by the Heart and Heart Protector (see Chapter 8). The impact on the Kidneys is to undermine the sense of trust both in individuals and in the world at large. Such trauma erodes basic trust that the world is a safe place. Most common is a freeze response that becomes locked in the tissues and has a profound effect the person's relationships, especially those of an intimate nature. Often, memories of abuse are sealed away, especially when the victim is very young. In this case the behaviours that arise in response to the abuse remain but are not understood. Recovering such memories later in life is usually deeply distressing and challenging, and takes a long time to come to terms with.

POST-TRAUMATIC STRESS DISORDER

Post-traumatic stress disorder (PTSD) is the condition that occurs when the response to a traumatic event persists for more than a month after the event and causes flashbacks, extreme anxiety, avoidance or numbness.[39] This can result from an actual or perceived threat to one's own life but can also occur from witnessing death or injury to others. Many of the symptoms of PTSD mirror an imbalance in the Water Element. Examples of this are being easily panicked, panic attacks, anxiety, numbness, hypervigilance, being easily startled, having ongoing fear or terror, phobias and paranoia.

This condition is common among war veterans, refugees and victims of violence, yet it can also be seen in those who have suffered ongoing punishments at home or school, been bullied in the playground or workplace, been emotionally abused by a parent or spouse – indeed, any situation where there is ongoing attack of some kind. While a single occurrence of such events may be considered minor, when the events are repeated often, trauma can result. A graphic illustration of this is the experience of a woman who spent four years in a repressive convent school named, ironically, Holy Wounds, where corporal punishment, often random, was a daily occurrence. As an adult, she developed the habit of checking for danger whenever she entered a room. One day when checking out the back room of a bookstore, she encountered a Vietnam veteran who asked her, 'What war were you in?'[40]

WORKING WITH TRAUMA
Working with trauma involves revisiting the experience from a place where there is holding for it, the kind of holding that was not available at the time. In fact, if there is adequate holding at the time of the event, then trauma does not result. So working with the trauma means going back and working with it in a way that provides holding retroactively. You engage your present capacities and those of your therapist, recovering the memories and feeling the feelings while being held in a safe environment. This process takes time, patience and kindness, and it needs the help of others.

Some form of therapy is almost always necessary in coming to understand the origins of the trauma, its impact on the present life and healing from it. Specific therapies that work well with trauma are Somatic Experiencing, Hakomi and other forms of somatic therapy. Also the Internal Family Systems method has been found to be particularly effective in working with the parts of the psyche that split off at the time of the traumatic event as a form of protection. A method called Eye Movement Desensitisation and Reprocessing (EMDR) has a proven record in reducing the effects of traumatic memories. Bodywork that provides safe, gentle, therapeutic touch also can be enormously supportive of the healing process.

All of these methods work on reversing the changes to the brain that were caused by the original event. The structure in the brain called the amygdala is the one that is most drastically altered by trauma. Studies have shown that it actually enlarges in those with PTSD. It is the part of the brain most associated with emotion, and especially with fear. It makes associations between sensory stimuli and triggers the responses to those stimuli. When there is an unresolved trauma, the amygdala responds to anything associated with the original traumatic event by triggering a fear response. It becomes sensitised to pain, fear, panic and terror. But just as the amygdala became sensitised to negative experiences, it can be retrained to become sensitised to positive experiences.

One essential requirement for doing such work is finding a therapist with whom you feel safe. Since the primary damage is to a sense of trust, then a feeling of safety is crucial to re-establishing trust in the world. A second requirement is that the work proceed slowly and carefully, working with the experiences a little at a time in a way that is manageable. It is most important to not become overwhelmed by the memories because this can lead to re-traumatisation, which counteracts the healing. Levine uses the term 'resource' to describe a positive memory or experience that can act as an oasis of safety from which to work and to which to return as needed. Resourcing helps to avoid the pitfall of re-traumatisation, which severely limits healing from trauma.

The third, perhaps most important, requirement for the work is kindness towards yourself. It is common for people who have been abused as children to take responsibility for their abuse, as if they were to blame in some way. Shame and guilt are common responses, especially around sexual abuse. The child is never to blame, never responsible for the abuse. Having kindness towards these very hurt and damaged parts of ourselves is key to success in working with trauma.

Even when you are working with a therapist, most of the time you are on your own. Here are some suggestions on how to maintain self-support in the process.[41]

- Identify situations where you become re-traumatised and disengage from those situations. This may mean removing yourself from particular locations or relationships. This shows the wounded parts that they are being taken care of.

- Taking action to support and protect yourself engages strength and will in a way that was not possible at the time of the traumatic event.

- Always go slowly in the work. Err on the side of caution. If you are in doubt about doing something, then don't.

- Do not continue to work with a therapist if you feel they are triggering re-traumatisation.

- Do not share your trauma with anyone unless you are sure they are compassionate and sympathetic towards your experience.

- An ongoing meditation practice is very beneficial as it strengthens the sense of the larger holding ground of True Nature, which is the ultimate support.

Some people hold the view that it is better to leave the past in the past, just get on with life and not wallow in the suffering of what is past. To them I would respond that the past is not the past when it is still present in your body. Actually, the body doesn't know anything about time, and as far as it is concerned, unresolved traumas are still happening now. You cannot make these things go away by pushing them down or just by wishing them away. Unprocessed hurt and unresolved suffering will still show up in unconscious behaviour that will affect the life of the individual and those around her or him.

Meeting the Challenges of Water Out of Balance

Table 6.1 shows the challenges of Water being out of balance and how those challenges can be addressed.

Table 6.1 How the Challenges of Water Being Out of Balance Can Be Addressed

Challenge	How to Meet the Challenge
Overwhelmed	Temporarily withdraw, simplify, conserve, rest and restore. Contact your *zhi* (Will). Remember a time when you called upon your reserves for a successful outcome.
Driven	Cultivate periods of stillness frequently during the day. Meditate each morning. Set a time-out timer.
Isolation	When the need for withdrawal becomes extreme, consider the fears that are underneath.
Facing the Unknown	Contact the wisdom that lies in the belly centre, grounding in the feet and legs. Become comfortable with not knowing.
Chronic Fear and Mistrust	Seek reassurance from those you trust; reality check whether fears are justified. Talk about your fears, what is at the bottom of the fear (e.g. fear of survival, abandonment, loss of love). Remember a time when you were afraid and nothing bad happened. Mindfulness practice: recognising the fears and noticing what else is present, holding the fears in a compassionate space. Hold outer Kidney shu points (see page 130).
Trauma	Trauma is fear that has been frozen in the bodymind. Recognise, name and come to accept the trauma rather than push through it. See it as a normal experience. Get help from a therapist and/or a somatic bodyworker. Take baby steps in the work so as to build success. Allow the freeze to melt, feel the shaking.
Separation from True Nature	Cultivate faith in the truth that the universe is fundamentally loving. Connect with the ground of Being, the unity of reality. Remember past spiritual experiences.

Acupressure for Psycho-emotional Health

The points I have chosen to support psycho-emotional health are known as the front mu points or alarm points of the Water meridians.

GB 25 *Jingmen* Capital Gate

The Kidney alarm point actually lies on the Gall Bladder meridian. GB 25 *Jingmen* Capital Gate is a powerful point for supporting and mobilising the Kidney Qi and regulating the Water pathways. As the alarm point of the Kidney lying on a Wood meridian, Capital Gate will bring forth the Kidney Qi and make it available for action. Thus, it is capable of restoring the Will and counteracting fear and timidity. Its effect can be magnified by holding it in conjunction with the source point K 3 learned earlier. GB 25 is located at the free end of the twelfth rib (see Figure 6.6). On the back, find the lowest rib and palpate laterally until you find the tender point at the end of the rib, almost to the side of the body.

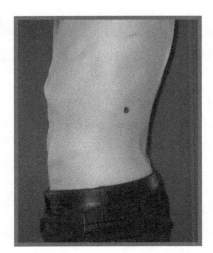

Figure 6.6 The Kidney alarm point (GB 25 *Jingmen* Capital Gate)

CV 3 *Zhongji* Middle Pole

CV 3 *Zhongji* Middle Pole is the alarm point of the Bladder meridian and lies in the lower abdomen. The central pole referred to in the point name is that of the Pole Star of the northern hemisphere around which all other stars revolve, implying the point is of central significance. It is a good point for grounding in the belly and lower body, especially when there is fear and a feeling of being on shaky ground. It calls upon deep reserves of Qi, tapping into a powerful energy source that strengthens the whole body, mind and spirit. This point can be further strengthened by holding it together with the source point BL 64 learned earlier. The two alarm points can also be held in combination to good effect, balancing both yin and yang of the Water Element.

CV 3 is located on the midline 1 cun above the pubic bone, or one-fifth of the distance between the pubic bone and the navel (see Figure 6.7).

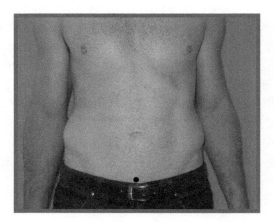

Figure 6.7 The Bladder meridian alarm point (CV 3 *Zhongji* Middle Pole)

The Spiritual Level of Water

Our spiritual nature is that which is not the body, thoughts, emotions or personality. If there is anything that remains of us when we die, it is this. Here we examine how the Water Element influences spiritual life.

The Spirit of Water: Zhi

The character *zhi* has two parts. The upper part depicts a growing plant, suggesting development, while the lower part depicts the heart. This illustrates the profound relationship between *zhi* and *shen*, Kidneys and Heart, Water and Fire. This is the significant axis of the Greater Yin and the Greater Yang, each mutually supporting the other.

The most usual meaning of *zhi* is will, though it has also been translated as ambition, purpose, determination, knowledge, mind and memory.[42] The will that is referenced here is not that of willpower and effort where there is an unnatural pushing and drivenness to achieve goals. Rather, it works independently of a person's volition, operating virtually below the level of consciousness, a force which moves a person towards his destiny without much conscious thought.[43]

Kaptchuck describes it as 'the will that can't be willed', meaning that it is the kind of will that allows the person to move forward without pushing the river.[44] A person with strong Kidneys has a strong Kidney spirit, a drive to be alive; one with less Kidney strength may have a lack of drive but overcompensate by pushing themselves.

Underpinning the *zhi* is the innate power of life itself, life that wants to live, strives to stay alive and survive. It manifests in the human drive to reproduce and thrive, something we've been remarkably successful at as a species.

The classics say that the Kidneys house the *zhi*;[45] therefore, anything that injures the Kidneys will also injure the *zhi*. Fear that does not flow freely and release from the body will dwell in the Kidneys. Chronic fearfulness, trauma, ongoing stress, penetrating cold, addictions, overwork and insufficient sleep will all contribute to draining the Kidney Qi and therefore the *zhi*. The saying 'burning the candle at both ends' is an apt expression of such depletion.

If the *zhi* is imbalanced, the result is a move to one of two extremes. At one extreme there is a collapse of will, resulting in a lack of drive and determination, listlessness and passivity, weakness, withdrawal and even despair (deficient kidney yang). At the other extreme there is a restless, unrelenting activity that derives from strong ambition and hyperdetermination (deficient kidney yin). Put simply, there is either lack of drive or overdrive. Both are symptoms of *zhi* out of balance.

Other possible outcomes of *zhi* imbalance are forgetfulness and memory lapses, the overuse of stimulants to provide false fuel for activity, addictive patterns, insomnia and nervous breakdown.

What does *zhi* look like when it is in perfect balance? Such a person moves forward without seeming to move, as if propelled by some invisible force. This kind of will is unobtrusive and tends to go unnoticed because it is so natural. It is well expressed in the Chinese concept of *wu wei*, or the action of non-action. *Wu wei* refers to the cultivation of a state of being in which our actions are quite effortlessly in alignment with the ebb and flow of the elemental cycles of the natural world. It is a kind of 'going with the flow' that is characterised by great ease and awakeness, in which, without even trying, we're able to respond perfectly to whatever situations arise.[46]

Ultimately, the highest form of Will arises when the personal will is in alignment with the Will of Heaven, which is stored in our Essence (*jing*) and exists within as a blueprint for our highest development. We must align our personal will with this blueprint if we are to manifest our greater destiny. The situations that life presents us with provide the opportunities for understanding the need for this alignment to occur. The more balanced is our *zhi*, the more there will be the inner knowing of how this alignment can arise.

The Virtue of Water: Wisdom

The classics teach that wisdom is the virtue of Water.[47] Wisdom is therefore the quality which reflects and expresses the harmony of the Tao through the facet of the Water Element.

We normally think of wisdom as the accumulation of knowledge through life experience. The virtue of wisdom is not knowledge or experience per se, but rather a contact with deep, inner knowing that lies below conscious thought. It is a knowing that is comfortable with being in the unknown and trusting that ultimately truth will be revealed. Kaptchuck suggests that the word *faith* is the closest meaning of wisdom. Not a religious faith, but a trust that can embrace the unknown.[48] This is the yin aspect of wisdom, the province of the Kidney Official. Its yang counterpart, expressed through the Bladder Official, is the clever utilisation of resources stored in the Kidneys in a way that will most optimally support progress through life. When these two officials are in balance and harmony with each other, the deep, innate knowing is resourcefully translated into wise living in the world.

The ancients understood that as a human loses contact with his True Nature, then the purity of the virtue of an Element is also lost. When this happens, the virtue begins to degrade into the emotion of that Element. Thus when wisdom is eroded, it turns to fear. This is expressed either as excessive fear or as repressed fear.

All fear is a reaction to the unknown. The greater the unknown, the greater is the propensity to react with fear. (Death is the greatest unknown and that which tends to inspire the most fear.) When our Water Element is out of balance, we either under-utilise or over-utilise our resources in order to avoid contact with the unknown.[49] Both of these approaches lead to depletion of inner resources.

The only way to return to wisdom is by going through the fear. Since the virtue of wisdom has degraded into the emotion of fear, it is necessary to go back through the fear to find wisdom. Fear therefore becomes the doorway through which we must step in order to recover the lost virtue. The sage, the wise man or woman, has spent a lifetime developing wisdom by facing the fears that arise from life situations. By meeting fear head on many times in his life, he has returned to the inner knowing that nothing is separate from the Tao. From this place, he faces all fear, including his own impending death, with calm equanimity.

The journey through fear to wisdom is a challenging one for all on a spiritual path. For people of a Water constitution, this passage is most confronting, for it requires a plumbing of the depths of the very emotion that is most difficult to face. In a sense, this is the life work of the Water type.

The early Taoists regarded wisdom not simply as an abstract concept, but as a psychic substance that forms a bridge between instinctual will and conscious awareness. Wisdom was seen as an inner light that resolved the paradox of spirit and matter, transforming the false self into self as Tao.[50] Surely as succinct a definition of enlightenment as you could find.

The Spiritual Issue of Water: Returning to Original Nature

The *Tao Te Ching* elegantly teaches that the Tao cannot be named, is unknowable, eternal and a Great Mystery. It is the void out of which all of manifestation – the Ten Thousand Things – springs, and yet it is both void and manifestation. The Tao is everything and nothing at the same time. Great Mystery indeed!

As soon as we incarnate in the material world of the Ten Thousand Things, we begin our separation from this eternal unknowable. Newborn babies are closest to the Tao, in contact with it yet unconscious of it. As the child grows, he develops an ego, a sense of himself as a separate entity, and with that, the separation from his original nature is complete.

All spiritual traditions have their teaching stories that describe the separation of man from his True Nature. The fall from grace, the eviction from the Garden of Eden, the loss of the precious pearl, and this Sufi parable which likens the loss of original nature to amnesia induced by drinking the waters:

> Once upon a time Khidr, the teacher of Moses, called upon mankind with a warning. At a certain date, he said, all the water in the world which had not been specially hoarded would disappear. It would then be renewed, with different water, which would drive men mad.
>
> Only one man listened to the meaning of this advice. He collected water and went to a secure place where he stored it, and waited for the water to change its character.
>
> On the appointed date the streams stopped running, the wells went dry, and the man who had listened, seeing this happening, went to his retreat and drank his preserved water.
>
> When he saw, from his security, the waterfalls again beginning to flow, this man descended among the other sons of men. He found that they were thinking and talking in an entirely different way from before; yet they had no memory of what had happened, nor of having been warned. When he tried to talk to them, he realized that they thought he was mad, and they showed hostility or compassion, not understanding.

At first, he drank none of the new water, but went back to his concealment, to draw on his supplies, every day. Finally, however, he took the decision to drink the new water because he could not bear the loneliness of living, behaving and thinking in a different way from everyone else. He drank the new water, and became like the rest. Then he forgot all about his own store of special water, and his fellows began to look upon him as a madman who had miraculously been restored to sanity.[51]

Why is this issue of separation from original nature of particular relevance to the Water Element? In many ways, Water is the fundamental Element, the point on the cycle which is both beginning and ending, a point of turning. It may even be considered as the space between ending and beginning. It is 'the worldly manifestation of the first stage in the movement of Tao'.[52] The substance of water is the primordial medium from which all life on earth arose. Likewise, the Water Element is the phase in which the Tao begins its movement towards manifestation in the world.

As we've already seen, the Kidneys store Essence (*jing*) and are also the source of all yin and yang in the body. Therefore, the Kidneys are often referred to as the Root of Life.[53] That which has emerged out of the Tao and into this particular example of the Ten Thousand Things, namely our own life, is carried as an imprint in our *jing* which is stored in the Kidneys. In this way the Water carries the nature of Tao, expressed within the flow of our life, even as it carries us away from our original nature.

Water is the primordial Element; therefore, its spiritual issue is the core of all spiritual issues. Winter is a special time to explore the ways in which we are separate from original nature as well as the ways we are in contact with the Oneness. The energy of deep winter 'provides a natural access to the core of our spiritual self'[54] and is deeply supportive of this inquiry.

Just as Water is the beginning of the movement away from our True Nature, so too it can be the portal through which we begin our return to that nature and to the direct knowing that we are one with all creation. This means not simply that we are connected to everything, but we *are* everything. This deep understanding may seem a long way off for many of us, but as we hold it as a possibility and begin the deep exploration of inner space, exploring the watery world of human existence, we make ourselves open to directly experiencing and knowing this truth. It may come about as a result of deep meditation, contemplating a koan (a paradoxical riddle without a solution), reciting a mantra, inquiring into current experience, communing with nature, or as a flash of insight while doing something as simple as going through a doorway.

It is the recognition that while we appear to be separate entities and seem to have a separate and independent existence, in reality our body, mind and spirit are arising moment by moment out of something infinitely bigger, the Tao, and that every other separate entity is similarly arising. Our nature is the Tao itself.

In what ways are you disconnected from your True Nature? How do you experience the Oneness of all creation?

The Diamond Approach
True Will

From the perspective of the Diamond Approach, the quality of will is one of the five primary essential aspects of our nature, perfections of the human soul. It provides steadfastness, determination and staying power which are necessary capacities for spiritual practice. Without staying power, no practice will work. The reason that practice works is that by staying with it we actualise our will. At the same time, practice is the expression of our will.

Without will we don't have the support for any process. Will is what allows us to continue and sustain our attention in the face of difficulties. When there is will, there is no indecisiveness. In fact, there is no need for decision, for things simply happen, supported by this will.

What most people regard as will is a kind of effort that is actually the will of the ego. This is false will, which can be confused with real will. False will is a distant approximation of real will, the ego's attempt to mimic the essential aspect of True Will. It is characterised by determined effort and trying to control either oneself or the environment.[55] It derives from a contraction in the body, a tense, hard place that is used as a platform for action.[56]

While determination is a quality of True Will, it doesn't derive from ego effort. Rather, it is sense of Presence infusing an inherent confidence in one's capacity that something will be done. Without trying to make it so, there is commitment, steadfastness, certainty and discipline. It is like being a mountain that is solid, unswayable and deeply supportive of living in the truth of who and what we are. True Will gives a sense of capacity, not just that I *can*, but I *will*.

What is in the way of finding this True Will? First, there is the delusion that the small self has the capacity to do it all by itself. This delusion is actually a defence against feeling our lack of will. The false will is a major defence against not having True Will. When we delve into this absence of will, we might feel a sense of collapse, as if our bones have gone soft or we are turning to jelly. There might be a feeling of emptiness in the belly or an absence of feeling in the lower body. Feeling this lack of will is the doorway to contacting True Will.

As we do this work, fear naturally arises.

> We see that will and fear are connected. The loss of basic confidence makes us block our will, which then creates a fear that without the false will we'll have no support. We feel we will be vulnerable and defenceless, unsupported, groundless, with nothing under our feet. We feel our needs will just collapse under us if we let go of the false will. This might actually happen momentarily, until the True Will is felt. With the True Will, you do not feel as if you are being supported, you simply feel the absence of the fear and of the need for support.[57]

True Will moves us towards what is real. It acts as support and as a rudder, supporting the direction towards truth. It is complete openness to what is happening right now and an implicit grounding that serves as a confidence that things will flow.[58]

> Ultimately, True Will manifests as an understanding. It's not as if something is there that will do something for you. It's an understanding that the organism, the life force, knows what needs to be done in the best, most efficient way. It's a confidence in yourself. If the True Will is operating you experience it as confidence and trust.[59]

One practical way we can evoke True Will is by keeping determined commitments. Commitment is a steadfastness of engagement. This applies to commitment to spiritual practice as well as keeping agreements with others. Failure to keep commitments erodes our will. Often the keeping of commitments is challenging and reveals what is still in the way of contacting True Will.

 Consider the strength of your commitments to work, hobbies, family, friends and yourself.

What gets in the way of making commitments? What gets in the way of keeping commitments?

Living Daylight

All fear arises out of a misunderstanding that we are destructible. If we take ourselves to be separate entities, which is the perspective of normal consciousness, then it is natural to assume that we are destructible, for we are vulnerable to injury, hurt, pain and eventually death. This view misunderstands the reality that we are not separate but rather a wave in an infinite ocean of consciousness.

To be truly ourselves, there needs to be a basic trust in reality; otherwise, we will be too scared to be ourselves. How can we be so trusting when the world seems so unpredictable and at times unsafe? If you want security from external situations, then you'll be waiting forever. We need to understand that it is the universe itself which holds us, not the external environment. The universe is actually a benevolent, loving presence which Almaas calls Living Daylight.

The extent to which we can contact this loving presence depends a lot on our early experiences of holding. If during childhood there was loving, supportive holding by our parents and carers, then it is easier to relax and believe that the world is to be trusted. But if our early experience was one of lack of security and holding, then it is more difficult to develop an inner trust that things will be all right.

> Living Daylight, this tender and loving presence, is experienced as the origin of all states of consciousness, as well as the origin of everything. If this loving presence is seen as the True Nature of everything that exists, the universe is seen as benevolent since it is made up of benevolence, and is therefore something you can trust. The soul feels held by the universe, taken care of in a loving, appropriate way, provided for, supported and loved.[60]

When we have an experience of the Living Daylight, this loving presence of the universe, it allows us to relax in a very deep way. It is the ultimate antidote to fear. Moreover, once we have had an experience of it, our fears relax and we are actually able to perceive the loving presence even more deeply, which further relaxes us.

We understand that Living Daylight emerges from the environment as a whole. It is a gentle, smooth, soft sense of lovingness and lightness which suffuses the world. The more trust there is, the more we see the Living Daylight, which in turn allows more trust. Then we can relax whatever the situation.

Journal Entry: 18 July 2011

Reflections on Time

The sense that time is linear, that the past is gone, the future yet to come, that we are travelling along a road, is an illusion.

When did time begin? There is no place you can say time began. Similarly there is no place where time will end. It is beginningless and endless, as big a mystery as the universe itself.

I heard an astronomer recently who said that looking into space is like looking backwards in time, and that there is a limit to what we can see in any direction. There is a horizon beyond which it is impossible to see.

Hameed's *Death and Dying* talks[61] suggest that life, living and death are not a continuum, but that each is its own thing. It is what is happening in the moment. Birth is birth. Dying is dying. Death is death. They are each their own thing.

Such is every moment.

Acupressure for Spiritual Health

Here we look at the outer shu point of the Kidney meridian, located on the back of the body along the outer line of the Bladder meridian. This point is particularly effective in healing at the level of mind and spirit. The effectiveness can be increased by using the point in combination with the source points and the mu points learned earlier.

BL 52 *Zhishi* Residence of the Will

BL 52 *Zhishi* Residence of the Will is located at about the level of the navel and four fingers width out from the spine (see Figure 6.8). It is level with the space between the second and third lumbar vertebrae.

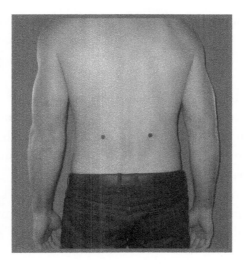

Figure 6.8 The outer shu point of the Kidney meridian
(BL 52 *Zhishi* Residence of the Will)

This point influences the spirit of Water, *zhi*, translated as Will. This is not the willpower of the ego or small self, but rather the Will of Heaven, mandated to us by the Tao. When we are in balance, we understand that we are not separate individuals, but drops of Tao manifesting the Universal Will.

When we lose contact with this truth, we start to believe that we have to do it all by ourselves, that it is all up to us, and that nothing will happen without us doing it. There is a loss of contact with the ground of the Tao.

There are two main responses to this loss. One is to be overwhelmed by the need to do it all ourselves, and to collapse into paralysis. The other is to take on an expansive, driven grandiosity. These reflect the yin and yang responses as discussed in the psycho-emotional level above.

One of the translations of the point name *Zhi Shi* is Ambition Room, which brings to mind the words of Macbeth. Macbeth is one of literature's monsters and a sobering illustration of grandiosity at its extreme.

> *I have no spur*
> *To prick the sides of my intent, but only*
> *Vaulting ambition, which o'erleaps itself,*
> *And falls on the other.*[62]

Macbeth's ambition to be king drove him blindly and heartlessly to regicide. His lust for power destroyed his compassion and filled him with hatred.

At the opposite extreme, a collapse of the Will leads to an absence of ambition, fearful holding back, a collapsing downwards and depression with no will to recover. Getting cold feet, both literally and figuratively, is emblematic of this second response. Residence of the Will helps both of these extremes return to balance, calming an insistent, relentless urgency or strengthening a fearful, paralysed impotence.

There is another important balancing function of the *zhi* which can be seen in its Chinese character. The lower part of the left-hand character represents the heart. The relationship between the *Zhi* of the Kidney and the *Shen* of the Heart is paramount in maintaining the Water/Fire balance which in turn is central to a person's yin/yang balance.

This balanced connection allows the Will of the Tao to be mediated by and expressed through the human heart. Harmonious action naturally arises as a willing surrender to the dynamic force of the Tao.

Meditation: The Belly

This meditation focuses on building the Qi in the belly centre and circulating that Qi around the Central Channel. It both cultivates and circulates Qi. The practice can be done alone or in a group. When done as a group meditation, the group field can powerfully strengthen the holding ground of Presence.

Find a comfortable sitting position. Bring your awareness to the hara, that place two fingers' width below the navel and the same distance inside the body. Just notice the sensations in that area. Sensations of temperature or movement. Maybe there's no sensation at all. Just notice what is there. Now as you breathe in, imagine you are drawing in the universal Qi, the Heavenly Qi, with your breath and bringing it down to that place in the belly. As you breathe out, imagine you are holding the energy that has been captured from the breath. Breathe in, draw the Qi; breathe out, hold the Qi. Do this for a few minutes.

Now that the energy that has been gathered in the hara, allow it to fall like a slow waterfall downwards to the perineum, the soft place in the very floor of the pelvis. Then as you breathe in, imagine that the energy is being drawn up the spine and over the top of the head. As you breathe out, watch the energy move down the front of the body like a slow waterfall down to the perineum. Breathe in up the back and out down the front. You may see it as a ball of light, a ball of energy; maybe you feel it as a movement of energy, or maybe just watch and imagine in your mind that it is moving along that circuit. Do this for a few minutes.

As you finish the next cycle, bring your attention back to the hara and notice the sensations that are there now. Notice any changes in your body and mind.

When you are ready, open your eyes and come back into the room.

Transition from Water to Wood

As winter draws to a close, there is a transitional period of a few weeks in which the ambient energy of nature is stirring awake, like a hibernating bear stretching his paws, yawning and thinking of food. There is a sense of buoyancy, as of something rising to the surface of the water.

Even though the temperatures are low, it still gets quite cold at night and the sun still gets up late, something has changed. The days are warmer and some days the warmth is so inviting that you want to find a nice sheltered place and soak up the warmth. Nature is starting to bud and shoot as it responds to this warmth. Overall there is a sense of things quickening and slowly picking up speed.

But what really characterises this transition is its erratic nature. For a few weeks it feels as if nature cannot quite make her mind up whether it is winter or spring: stop – start – hot – cold – yes – no – maybe. The movement is jerky, like an old train starting its journey where the carriages are jerked a few times before there is a smooth forward movement. In many climates this period is accompanied by gusty winds and driving rain. Some people find this weather exciting and exhilarating, while others find it disturbing. If you have an extreme reaction towards this transition to spring, your Wood is probably calling for attention. (The next chapter will probably be an important one for you.)

So, when you begin to feel these changes, when you feel the uprising energy within your body as well as observe it in nature, it's time to begin the work of the Wood chapter. Are you ready? On your mark. Get set. Wait for it, wait for it…

Go!

Journal Entry: 27 July 2012

We're in the final phase of winter. Another week of cold, wet days should see it out. Already we're getting hints of spring waiting in the wings. I think of Henry V's speech to his troops at the siege of Harfleur, stirring his men to action:

> *I see you stand like greyhounds in the slips,*
> *Straining upon the start.*[63]

But what is this doing in Water, by Harry?

On, on to Wood, to Green and to Spring!

(Exeunt, Alarum and chambers go off)

Chapter 7

Wood

The Nature of Wood

The movement of Wood is upwards. The nature of Wood includes all forms in the plant kingdom, but the quintessential icon of Wood is the tree which sprouts from its seed and rockets upwards in search of light. Its branches splay outwards to fill the space, but the fundamental direction is up.

The many forms that plants and trees take can give us insight into the nature and qualities of Wood. The tiny plant that forces its way up through a crack in the pavement demonstrates Wood's ability to find ways around obstacles to growth. In its early stages, a plant grows rapidly and vigorously, yet also in a jerky series of growth spurts which is another feature of Wood. The weeds that proliferate in the garden show the sheer unstoppable nature of Wood. Bamboo, which bends easily in the wind, is a great illustration of the flexibility of Wood.

Trees can also show us what Wood is like when it is not healthy. Old trees become stiff, brittle and break in the wind. Plants suffering from drought become stunted and gnarled, unable to manifest their full potential. And trees that have died leave their grey bones in a pile, fuel for the next fire.

The Chinese character for Wood is *mu* (see Figure 7.1). The central vertical line represents the trunk of a tree, the horizontal line its branches, the slanting lines its roots. The fact that much of the tree is below the ground is a reminder that a healthy tree and a healthy Wood Element are deeply rooted.

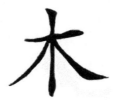

Figure 7.1 The Chinese character for Wood

The Resonances of Wood

The Season: Spring

The Wood Element is most easily observed in nature as the season of spring. Indeed, the very word spring conjures up images of things jumping up suddenly and rapidly, bounding, leaping forth as if from nowhere. Following the quietness, darkness and dormancy of winter, it is as if nature is waking up after a long rest, stretching her arms, feeling her muscles and tendons as she prepares for movement.

We know when the season of spring has arrived because its evidence is everywhere in nature. The grass suddenly takes off and we have to dust off the mower in the shed. The deciduous trees begin to bud and their leaves sprout. The veggie garden starts to take off, not just the veggies but all the weeds too. We notice the birds beginning to court and nest, magpies become aggressively territorial and dive-bomb us on our hikes. And we ourselves begin to feel something rising within in response to this uprising surge in nature, akin to the sap rising in the trees. We start to feel more energy, more interest in getting outdoors, tackling projects and making plans. If we are in tune with the rhythms of nature, this call to movement and action is irresistible.

When does spring begin? This will depend on your latitude and climate zone. Traditionally, in northern China spring began on 1 February, corresponding to 1 August in the southern hemisphere. Interestingly, this is almost the same as the cross-quarter day of Candlemas in the European tradition, and Groundhog Day in modern American culture. It is the point roughly midway between the winter solstice and the vernal equinox, a time when the lengthening of the days begins to accelerate. This rapid increase in the daylight hours begins to quicken movement in nature and in us.

The higher the latitude in which you live, the later the spring will arrive. But you can begin to look for its signs sometime in February in the northern hemisphere or August in the southern. Most importantly, look for the signs within yourself. Pay attention to your predominant focus as it turns from the inward-looking yin qualities of the winter to the outward-looking yang qualities of spring. This shift will be accompanied by an inner sense of something rising upwards in your body. You may feel the bubbling sensation of something coming up the inside of your legs and up the front of your body, filling and expanding your chest with an energy that demands expression.

When you pay close attention to yourself, you will know when spring has sprung. You won't need to look at the calendar or the thermometer, you'll know it from within.

The Sense: Seeing

As winter turns to spring, the spotlight begins to move from the sense of hearing to that of seeing. If we have heeded the suggestions of nature and have spent more time looking inwardly during winter, our eyes have been less active. Now, with the longer days, stronger light and much more going on around us, our eyes are called upon to be much more focused.

Just as hearing does not automatically imply listening, so looking does not necessarily mean seeing. Our eyes give us the ability to receive visual input. But in order to really see, we must engage in a conscious way with that visual input. This is the difference between dull eyes and bright eyes.

When we become jaded or bored by life, or we are just going through the motions in a routine way, our looking becomes dulled and we do not really see. The arrival of spring and its Element of Wood gives us the support to see our world with fresh eyes. Try this: walk out of your front door, look around you, imagining that you are seeing everything for the very first time. Look at things closely as if you've never seen them before. Imagine you are a toddler coming across this scene for the first time in her life. What wonder you might experience then.

Often, when we look at something that we've looked at many times before, we don't really see it. We are actually seeing a memory of it. We see a memory of the table where we have eaten breakfast a thousand times; we see a memory of our car that we drive to work; and we see a memory of our colleagues with whom we interact at work. Imagine how different everything would seem if we were able to bring fresh eyes to everything we see. Why, we might even fall in love with our partner every single day!

The Colour: Green

Since the Element of Wood is best represented by the trees and the plant kingdom, it makes sense that green should be its colour. Green is the predominant colour of vegetation. The spectrum of green includes the bright green of new leaves, the emerald green of the fields of Ireland, the dark greens of the northern European forests. It includes the blue-green of the ocean, the bright green of a tree frog, apple green, lime green, pea green, the green gemstones: emerald, jade and tourmaline.

Green means go! Green is environmentally conscious. Green signifies nature, life, youth and hope.

How much green do you have in your wardrobe? Apparently, green is our second favourite colour, so chances are, quite a bit. If all your clothes are green or you have no green at all, it may be that you need some balance in this.

An extreme attitude to the colour green, either an aversion to or an abnormally strong liking, may indicate some imbalance in your Wood.

What about in your home? Do you have green plants in the house? Some green in the home is important for balance. According to feng shui principles, it serves to have some green on the Wood wall of a room (i.e. the wall to your left as you come into the room).

In Five Element Acupuncture diagnosis, the colour green at the sides of the eyes indicates a Wood Constitution. Sometimes this green can look a little yellow, making it difficult to distinguish between Earth and Wood Constitutions. In this case, other diagnostic indicators become more important to make the distinction.

The Sound: Shouting

The energy of Wood is a strong uprising force that demands expression. Of all the sounds that a voice can make, the shout is the most forceful. It gets attention.

When our desires in life are not met in the ways that we would like, we may become frustrated. When we find obstacles in our path that frustrate our forward movement, we may become angry.

The shout is a way that we can discharge some of this frustration. It also lets other people know about our angry feelings. We may even use it to get what we want from others. Sometimes we just need to shout to be heard above the hubbub of everyone else. The shout says, 'Hey, what about me?'

The shouting voice carries the emotion of anger. We all have times when we shout, but when the predominant sound in a person's ordinary speaking voice is a shout, it indicates that they have a Wood Constitution. The shouting voice is not necessarily loud, though it may be. The significant factor is its force and emphasis. It may sound jerky or clipped with an emphasis on final consonants.

Many Wood people actually have a voice that is very quiet, and we may have to strain to hear their words. This is called a lack of shout. It comes about when the uprising and forceful energy of Wood is so suppressed that it disappears from view and from hearing.

The Odour: Rancid

The resonance of odour is the third of the diagnostic tools of the Five Element practitioner. This is the subtle odour that emanates from a person's skin. People of a Wood constitution have what is called a rancid odour. When the person is in good health, the odour is not very evident and has a light smell like freshly cut grass. But when the person is out of balance, the rancid odour becomes more evident and can smell like old oil or fat.

The odour derives from the fact that the organs of Wood, the gall bladder and liver, are not functioning optimally in their job of processing oils and fats in the body.

The Emotion: Anger

Of all the emotions, anger is probably considered by society to be the most negative. This is probably because anger that goes out of control can be so destructive. People can get hurt or even killed. Property can get smashed. Others can become terrified and traumatised.

Because of these potential negative consequences of the acting out of anger, the emotion of anger is seen as negative. Yet the emotion itself is no more negative than any other feelings that we may have. In fact, it is the energy of anger that fuels so much activity in the world.

Wood energy is a dynamic, unstoppable force for action. When that force meets an obstacle, the energy builds up and the consequent force finds a way around the obstacle to achieve its goals and desires. Without this force, no action would ever be accomplished. We would just collapse at the first hurdle in our path.

So if we relabel anger as an unstoppable force for action, it doesn't seem so negative. We can feel all the frustration and anger we like as long as we don't turn it into a weapon that harms others. In fact, the more we can stay with the feeling itself, the more it becomes a powerful strength to be ourselves in the world. (We examine this in much more detail in the section 'The Emotional Landscape of Wood'.)

Emotion is the last of the four primary diagnostic tools of the Five Element practitioner. When a person's predominant emotional perspective is from the realm of anger, that indicates they are of a Wood constitution. For the Wood type, anger is the most difficult emotion with which to come to terms. For this person, anger responses to life are extreme. At one end of the scale, there may be a response of fury and rage at the least provocation. At the other end of the scale, the person is unable to be angry even when it is appropriate – for example, when they are being unjustly treated. It is difficult for the Wood type to be in a place of balance around anger.

The Gifts of Wood

When we are in harmony with an Element and the Element is in balance within us, then we have access to the positive qualities of that Element in our lives.

There are many such qualities and this list is by no means a complete one. These are some of the more fundamental of these qualities. As you read about these qualities, consider how easy it is for you to access them in your own life. Your answers will tell you much about the relative strength or deficiency of the Wood Element within you.

Vision

The ability to see the world in all its colours and shapes is indeed one of the greatest gifts of a human life. Of all the senses it is the one that most people say they would find hardest to lose.

But Wood's gift of vision goes far beyond the ability to take in visual information through the eyes. It is also about the capacity to *envisage*, to see a future possibility with the mind's eye.

People who have this gift most strongly are called visionaries. Their imagination and foresight help them to make creative leaps that see future possibilities projecting out from current circumstances.

In the modern era, Steve Jobs was repeatedly described as a visionary for his ability to see technological possibilities and pursue their production. Martin Luther King's 'I Have a Dream' speech is particularly illustrative of this quality of Wood. He had a vision of a world of racial equality which is slowly being realised.

How is your vision for your own future? How clearly do you see the path before you in your own life?

Planning

Once we have a vision for our future, we need to find a way to get there. We need a map, a plan, a flowchart, a series of connected steps that will allow us to follow a path. This quality of Wood is the province of the Liver Official who is sometimes personified as the General.

Imagine this General's headquarters where the room is strewn with maps, plans, lists of troop units, transport, all the information that is needed to form the big picture. From this place, removed from the battles themselves, the General can formulate an overarching strategy, a grand plan.

In our individual lives, planning is incredibly important. Each day we need to plan what we are doing that day and the order in which we are going to do things. We need to prioritise, organise and strategise. Without these steps of pre-planning, our day can become chaotic, we might waste time and energy backtracking, and the day just doesn't run smoothly.

We need to plan each day, but we also need to have a sense of where we are going in a longer time frame. What are our plans for the next month, the next year, the next stage of our life? At various points in our lives we pause and take stock, reassess our direction, make a new plan, draw a new map.

When the Wood is not strongly available to us, we might have difficulty making plans. We might have difficulty even knowing what it is that we want, so we can't even begin to plan. Some of us get lost in details and have problems seeing the big picture. We can't see the wood for the trees!

 How do you feel about the direction your life is taking? What are your plans for the next year, five years, ten years? How flexible are you in changing plans when circumstances change?

Decision-making

Once we have our plan and a map of where we are going, we set out on our journey. The journey begins with a first step and proceeds through a series of steps until we reach our destination. While the planning itself is the province of the Liver Official, the actual implementation of the plan on the ground is the function of the Gall Bladder Official, sometimes personified as the General's Chief of Staff.

While the General holds the overall plan, the Chief of Staff makes the step-by-step decisions about how that plan is put into operation. The capacity to decide is a fundamental one for Wood. When the Wood is healthy, decisions are made easily and quickly because things are clear. The plan is clearly understood and the best way to carry out the plan is obvious. All the information is taken in and organised, and the way of action naturally arises.

Some of us are good planners but not so good at carrying out the plans. Others are good at managing details but not so good at seeing the big picture. When our Wood is in balance, we have access to both of these aspects.

 How bold are you at taking the first step? What stops you from making a decision?

Good Judgement

It is one thing to make bold decisions, it is quite another to make wise ones. Some people move so quickly into action they find that their decision has not been a considered one. The consequences of rash action can be very counterproductive. The ability to be a good judge of a situation, whether concerning a person or a course of action, is one of the qualities of a healthy Wood.

Like a judge in a court, we need to be able to consider all the evidence with impartiality, weigh this evidence for truth and validity, and come to a judgement that gives consideration to all factors. When we've looked closely at all sides of a situation, the best course of action becomes clear and we can take action.

Difficulties arise when the judging phase takes too long and we go back and forth between options, vacillating in an agony of indecision. Healthy Wood is able to judge soberly and decisively.

How well are you able to judge a person when you meet them? Do you tend to make judgements quickly or slowly?

Clarity

When we can see clearly, our field of view is wide, we take in all the components of a situation and everything becomes transparent and obvious. The greater the degree of clarity we have, the more truth we recognise. Clarity brings objectivity.

When we are clear, we not only see clearly with our eyes, but we think clearly and we are able to express ourselves clearly. The way forward in the world becomes clear to us and we are able to act without prevarication.

When we are in this place of clarity, it is as if the fog has lifted, revealing a bright sunny day. Our thoughts are sharp, clear, quick and clean, without anything weighing them down. The upward movement of our Wood is unimpeded.

How clearly do you see? Do you notice everything around you? Is your vision wide or narrow?

Imagination

In 1971 John Lennon invited us to 'Imagine' a world of peaceful brotherhood. This iconic song has certainly captured the imagination of succeeding generations. Imagination is an amazing thing. We see something in our mind's eye that is not present to the senses, but in our inner world it becomes vividly real.

The imagination actually has powerful effects on the body. Studies have shown that people who imagine they are at the gym going through their exercise routine are having beneficial effects that are almost equal to the actual exercise.[1] We imagine ourselves in the arms of a lover and we experience the same rush of endorphins as if he or she were really there with us. And if we imagine that we are in danger, our adrenals produce adrenaline to help us react to the imagined danger as if it were real.

Imagination is a kind of waking dream. It is a fundamental faculty through which people make sense of the world and it plays a key role in the learning process. Storytelling, so much loved by children, is a basic training for the imagination. And child's play is often an expression of the imaginative process.

Do you have a vivid imagination? Do you tend to imagine optimistically or pessimistically?

Creativity

If imagination is all in the mind, creativity is imagination in action. It is the way in which original ideas find concrete application in the world. In short, it is the process of invention.

The whole of human history is the charting of invention. In prehistory, it meant the discovery of fire and its applications to cooking, safety and toolmaking. It meant the fashioning of increasingly complex tools and weapons, the discovery of the principle of the wheel, the development of language.

Each succeeding generation learned from and built upon all past discoveries, adding to the expanding pool of human creativity. And now in our modern time this process is growing exponentially as human creativity rapidly develops human potential in all areas of physical, mental, emotional and spiritual life.

Does your imagination flow easily into creative activity?

And More…

The gifts we've looked at here are just a few of the many qualities that the Wood Element has to offer. Here are some more to consider. Think or write about how much these qualities show up in your life and how much they are available to you.

Action	Design	Flexibility
Growth	Individuation	Inventiveness
Negotiation	Perspective	Visualisation
Cleverness	Direction	Goals
Hopes and Dreams	Ingenuity	Lucidity
Organisation	Strategy	Will to Become

The Physical Level of Wood

Let us now look at the ways in which the resonances and qualities of the Wood Element reveal themselves in the physical body. The body is the densest form in which our nature manifests. Our shape and size, our posture, our organs and tissues, and the way we move are all expressions of ourselves at the body level. The particular ways that Wood is expressed in us will have a great impact on the nature and health of our body.

Organs and Tissues

The Liver

WESTERN MEDICAL PERSPECTIVE

The liver is a large triangular organ that rests in the upper part of the abdominal cavity, mostly on the right-hand side and mostly protected by the ribcage. Because of its many functions, it is an organ we cannot live without; no artificial organ can currently perform these functions. If you want to live, you have to have a liver.

Of the approximately 500 functions of the liver, the most important include synthesis of amino acids and cholesterol; metabolism of carbohydrates, proteins and fats; and the production of bile which assists digestion in the small intestine. The liver plays several roles in the regulation of the blood, breaks down insulin, breaks down toxic substances and allows them to be excreted. In short, the liver supports almost every other organ in the body.

CHINESE MEDICINE PERSPECTIVE

The Liver is the yin organ of the Wood Element. It manifests in the nails, opens into the eyes, controls tears and is affected by anger.[2] The main functions of the Liver are as follows:

- It stores Blood.

  The Liver is the most important organ for storing Blood.[3] It regulates the volume of Blood in the body at any one time and as such regulates menstruation. Blood moistens the sinews and so more Blood is needed at times of activity and less at times of rest. When the Liver is not doing this job adequately, there is not enough energy for activity and so a person becomes easily tired. For women, when the Liver is not regulating Blood optimally, it results in menstrual irregularities. A deficiency of Blood causes scanty or absent periods; an excess causes heavy periods; stagnant Blood causes painful periods with dark clotting. This regulation of the Blood also plays a part in maintaining resistance to external pathogens, thereby contributing to the body's immunity to disease.

- It ensures the smooth flow of Qi.

  Perhaps the most important function of the Liver is to promote the smooth flow and movement of Blood and Qi. The Liver's task is to send Qi everywhere in the body and to support the appropriate movement of Qi in all the other organs and meridians. Here we see a direct parallel with the Western view that the liver supports almost all the other organs of the body. When this quality of smoothness is absent, conditions of agitation, shaking and lack of coordination can result. This smooth flow of Qi extends also to the psycho-emotional level: a smoothly functioning Liver is essential to a balanced emotional state, as we will see later.

- It houses the Ethereal Soul.

  Each of the yin organs is considered to be the dwelling place of the 'spirit' associated with its Element. The spirit of the Wood Element is the *hun* or Ethereal Soul which dwells in the Liver. The *hun* is responsible for planning and finding a clear path through life. We will explore this more fully in the section 'The Spiritual Level of Wood'.

The Gall Bladder
WESTERN MEDICAL PERSPECTIVE
The gall bladder is a small organ that sits below the liver on the right side of the abdomen, just below the fixed ribs. Its primary function is to collect bile from the liver and to concentrate and store the bile. When ingested fat reaches the duodenum (upper intestine), the gall bladder contracts and secretes the concentrated bile into the duodenum to assist in the breakdown of fats. Recently it has been discovered that the gall bladder also contains pancreatic hormones including insulin.

CHINESE MEDICINE PERSPECTIVE
The Gall Bladder is the yang organ of Wood and as such is partner to the Liver. Its physical function is to collect, store and excrete bile. In this regard its function is identical to that in Western medicine. However, for the Chinese, there are two other important functions of the Gall Bladder:

- It controls the sinews.

    As with the Liver, the Gall Bladder controls the tendons, ligaments and cartilage, particularly in the limbs. The difference is that the Liver is responsible for nourishing the sinews with Blood while the Gall Bladder provides Qi to the sinews to provide for proper movement and flexibility. Healthy tendons and ligaments are necessary for the body to move quickly and efficiently into action. Thus, we can see how taking firm and decisive action requires a smoothly functioning Wood Element through both its yin and yang organs.

- It controls decisiveness.

    The Gall Bladder is not only responsible for decision-making, but is also the motivator for all the other 11 Officials which depend upon its decisions. 'The Gall Bladder is like an impartial judge from whom decisiveness emanates.'[4]

In Western medicine the gall bladder is often viewed as a disposable organ, much as the appendix is regarded, but as we have seen, the organ itself is involved in important physical as well as mental functions. Its malfunction is an indication of an imbalance that goes far beyond the organ itself.

Eyes

Earlier we talked about the importance of the Liver in relation to the eyes. The eyes are the sense organs of Wood and are directly related to this yin organ. The Liver moistens the eyes and thus plays a part in the production of tears. An imbalance in the Liver can result in dry, red or painful eyes and blurred vision.

The old saying 'The eyes are the windows of the soul' is particularly apt from the perspective of Chinese medicine. The ethereal soul or *hun*, which we will look at in more detail in the section 'The Spiritual Level of Wood', is housed in the Liver, which in turn opens to the eyes.

As we age, our vision tends to deteriorate as a result of damage to or degradation of the four major structures of the eye: the cornea, the lens, the retina and the optic nerve. From the Chinese perspective, this degradation relates directly to the health of the Liver and of the Wood Element.

The cornea is the transparent tissue at the front of the eye that admits light. Its surface is coated with a thin film of tears. Any breakdown in the production of tears compromises this tear film and results in degradation of the image. Consequences of this are blurred vision, dry eyes and inflammation of the eyes producing redness. An irregularly shaped cornea is what produces the condition of astigmatism, which produces a blurred image.

The lens of the eye is crystal clear at birth, but over the course of a lifetime it becomes increasingly cloudy (cataract), which means that the light coming into the eye has to travel through a distorted medium resulting in diminished vision. Another result of the ageing process is that the lens loses its pliability and thus its capacity to focus. This results in difficulty focusing on close images, a condition called presbyopia – literally 'old man's eye'.

The retina of the eye acts like the film in a camera that converts light into a neural signal that can be interpreted by the brain. The optic nerve transmits the neural signals and thus is an extension of the retina. Age does not deteriorate these structures like the cornea and lens, but conditions such as macular degeneration and glaucoma do. They are not uncommon and can produce serious loss of vision.

Also of significance in our vision is the role of the seven muscles that control the movement of the eye. Difficulty moving the eye in a certain direction results from a weakness or tightness in one or more of these muscles.[5]

Tendons and Ligaments

The tendons and ligaments of the body, sometimes called the sinews, are the tissues of Wood. The state of health of these tissues is closely related to the health of the Wood Element within us.

The ligaments are very strong, tough bands of connective tissue that connect bones together and support the joints. There are also ligaments that hold the internal organs in place. Ligaments have very little blood supply and only a little elasticity. This allows them to stretch a little as we move, while being strong enough to ensure joint stability and structural integrity.

The tendons are made up of similar tissue to ligaments except they have a greater blood supply and are more flexible. Their function is to attach muscles to bones so that when a muscle contracts, the resulting force is transferred to move the bone which articulates at the joint.

Tendon length appears to be genetically determined and in turn is a significant factor not only in flexibility but in potential muscle size. The longer the tendon, the smaller the potential muscle mass but the greater the range of movement.

When Wood is out of balance, the ligaments and tendons tend to be either too rigid or too flexible. Rigidity causes stiffness in the joints and limits movement, while over-flexibility causes joint instability and weakness. In both cases coordination and movement become affected.

Nails

The fingernails and toenails are said to be the external manifestation of the Liver and a by-product of the sinews.[6] One of the tasks of the Liver is to nourish the nails via the Blood. Their health will give an indication of the balance of Wood. Nails that are ridged or warped in some way, brittle, dry or overly soft, suggest an imbalance in the Wood Element and the Liver.

Movement

Of all the Elements, Wood likes most to move. In a way, movement is its natural state. The natural direction of Wood energy is upwards. Its energy is active, dynamic and irrepressible.

Imagine you are a runner getting ready for a sprint race. The starter calls you to the blocks and you steady yourself. The starter calls 'set' and you raise yourself up in readiness for the starting gun. In that few seconds between the set and the off, all your energy is gathered in coiled potential, like an arrow drawn and about to be loosed. Your body is poised at a tipping point, your mind is totally focused on the lane in front of you and on the impending starting sound. Feel into this energy if you can, and you are feeling the very Essence of Wood. This is the focused, gathered, thrusting strength that is behind all movement.

Now imagine that there is a holdup with the starter's gun going off. You are on your blocks, body raised and poised for release. Waiting, waiting…waiting… How might that feel, to be all ready and set to go, and you can't go? Tense? Frustrated? Angry? That's what happens when Wood is contained, held back, restrained from its natural tendency to move.

We humans need to move often. We don't move all the time, but we are rarely still for long. Even in our sleep we tend to move around. For 24 hours a day we are cycling between movement and rest.

What happens when this natural desire to move is checked? It can best be seen in children. Children who are told to sit still and behave quickly become restless and irritable, perhaps loud and rebellious. Wood just cannot be boxed in for long. If we do try to box in all that dynamic energy, a resistance builds up, creating a pressure that must be released in some way. If it is not channelled into movement and action, then it leaks out, manifesting in conditions such as restless legs or some other shaking condition, nervous habits like nail biting or hair pulling; or it might come out as angry attacks on others or snide, cutting remarks.

This is why many people go to the gym or run or do some other vigorous exercise in order to release the Wood energy that builds up from a sedentary job or stressful interpersonal relationships.

 Not getting enough movement? Why not look through the list below for some direction. Maybe try something you've never done before, or at least not for a while. But remember that the tendons and ligaments are the tissues of Wood and can be strained, especially when you're starting up in early spring after a hibernating winter. So do some stretching and warming up before leaping forth.

Abseiling	Dishwashing	Jumping
Aerobics	Diving	Kayaking
Ambling	Dusting	Kickboxing
Archery	Egg-and-spoon racing	Kite flying
Arm wrestling	Fencing	Leap frogging
Ballooning	Five rhythms	Limbo dancing
Baseball	Flying	Marbles
Basketball	Folk dancing	Netball
Biking	Football	Nosediving
Bouncing	Galloping	Orienteering
Bowling	Go-karting	Parachuting
Boxing	Hang gliding	Paragliding
Bushwalking	Hoola hooping	Perambulating
Canoeing	Hopping	Pilates
Cartwheeling	Horse riding	Polo
Chi gung	Ice skating	Quidditch
Climbing	Jitterbugging	Quoits
Cricket	Jiving	Racing
Dancing	Jogging	Raking
Digging	Juggling	Rambling

Riding	Swimming	Walking
Rowing	Table tennis	Weightlifting
Running	Tai chi	Wii
Shopping	Tennis	Windsurfing
Shot putting	Tightrope walking	Wu Tao
Skating	Trampolining	Xtreme sports
Skiing	Undulating	Yachting
Skipping	Vaccuuming	Yoga
Stretching	Volleyball	Zumba

Diet and Lifestyle
Foods That Support Wood

It is interesting to reflect that our parents never told us to eat our reds, blues or yellows, but they were insistent about the greens. As the colour of the Wood Element, green vegetables are particularly supportive of Wood and its organs of Liver and Gall Bladder. And in spring, leafy greens abound. Get to a farmers' market and load up on leafy greens, the darker the better. Kale, collards, chicory, spinach, rocket, mustard, bok choi, chard, endive, coriander, parsley…the list goes on. You can also eat the green tops of many vegetables such as beetroot and celery. Wild greens, such as nettles and thistles, are plentiful and free. (If chickens eat them, they're probably good for you too!) Lightly steamed or even raw, all of these veggies are really supportive of good liver health.

Besides the leafy kind, other green-coloured vegetables include avocado, asparagus, cucumber, broccoli, Brussels sprouts, green beans, leeks, peas, spring onions, green peppers and zucchini. Of all the vegetables, the humble and ubiquitous broccoli is perhaps the single most health-giving plant food available. It has cancer-fighting properties that probably come from its high sulphur content.[7]

Green fruits are less abundant than their vegetable cousins. Try green apples, grapes, kiwis, limes and honeydew melons.

Here are some suggestions to get more green food in your diet:

- Try a smoothie made with raw greens, fruit and almond milk.

- Snack on sugar snap peas.

- Make a delicious leek and potato soup for the cool spring evenings.

- Don't throw away leek tops: boil them for 30 minutes for a great stock.

- Chinese stir fries can take lots of greens: kale, bok choi, spring onions, peas and beans.

- Add peas to curries, stir fries or pasta dishes.

- Use collard leaves as a substitute for tortillas when making wraps.

- Green up your fruit salad with green grapes, kiwis and melon.

- Make homemade guacamole when avocadoes are in season.

The flavour of Wood is sour, so sour-tasting foods are also good for the Wood organs. The juice of half a lemon or lime in warm water first thing in the morning is a great way to start a spring day.[8] Organic apple cider vinegar is also cleansing for the liver. Drink this in warm water, or use it as a dressing for salads. Small quantities of sour pickled vegetables are also good. As with any flavour, avoid excessive consumption of sour foods. Too much of the sour flavour will impact the Spleen.

Gall Bladder Health

Most problems of the gall bladder are associated with the formation of gallstones. These pellets are accumulations of cholesterol and pigment and can block the flow of bile from the gall bladder through the common bile duct to the duodenum. They range from the size of a grain of sand to as large as a golf ball. Approximately 10% of people in Western countries have them and the incidence increases with age.[9] Ninety per cent of gallstones show no symptoms. When symptoms do appear, most common are nausea, vomiting and pain in the right upper abdomen, sometimes radiating to the back. Episodes last from one to three hours after which time symptoms subside. Pain lasting longer than this needs medical attention.

For those who are prone to this condition, eating a low-fat diet is important as well as avoiding foods that trigger attacks. Foods that are known to challenge a weak gall bladder are eggs, pork, onions, poultry, milk, coffee, oranges, corn, beans and nuts.[10]

Many sufferers opt for gall bladder surgery, though this does not always eliminate the symptoms. Another way of approaching the problem is the gall bladder flush. This is a dramatic and highly effective way of clearing out stagnant bile and gallstones from a sluggish gall bladder organ.

There are many different methods which can be readily researched on the Internet. All these ways involve the ingestion of substantial quantities of olive oil and citrus juice. The oil provokes the gall bladder into discharging bile, while the lemon juice acts as an astringent, contracting the organ. The combined effect of these actions is to pump out the contents of the gall bladder including any congested bile, gallstones and other deposits. These substances are then excreted.

This is a challenging procedure and should be done under the supervision of a naturopath or other health professional. Do not attempt this if you know you have large gallstones, as they can become lodged in the bile duct after being expelled.

'An apple a day keeps the doctor away.' Maybe you should have health insurance too, but this old adage recognises the many benefits of this humble fruit. Besides containing fibre and vitamin C, apples are supportive of the gall bladder. Anyone with a tendency to gallstones or gall bladder attacks would do well to eat an apple or two every day. The malic acid in apples is excellent for dissolving the stagnant bile accumulated in the liver and gall bladder.

Other ways to support the gall bladder are with peppermint oil capsules and apple juice. Eat more raw food and do not overeat.[11]

Liver Health
Because the liver has so many functions vital to health, keeping the liver healthy is really important. When the liver is malfunctioning, signs and symptoms can include digestive disorders, blood sugar problems, high cholesterol, poor fat absorption, sluggish metabolism and immune system impairment.

An ongoing diet that includes lots of fresh fruit and vegetables as well as some raw food is very supportive of liver health. In addition, a periodic liver cleanse will be of great benefit.

The purpose of the liver cleanse is to clear out toxins that have become lodged in the liver. Since one of the functions of the liver is to detoxify the blood, it is clear how toxins can build up there. This build-up is common in people who consume a lot of alcohol or drugs and in women taking hormone replacements. If the liver becomes very toxic, then the toxins end up being stored in other organs and tissues as well, affecting function and health at many levels. Spring is a great time to take care of your liver health.

While the gall bladder flush is done on one day, the liver cleanse is done over a prolonged period of weeks or months. This involves taking the kinds of supplements that were described above. Again, there are many approaches that can be researched. There are proprietary blends of herbs that can be purchased as a full program or you can buy your supplements singly and create your own program. Some programs involve fasting but most include reducing food intake to simple foods like juices, rice and vegetables.

It is always good to seek the advice of a health professional who can determine the best approach for you. If you are going it alone, beware of detoxifying too fast. Prolonged nausea means that the toxins in your body are being flushed out of the cells faster than your digestive system can eliminate them. While it is not life-threatening by any means, it's not good to put too much strain on the liver in this process. Usually, cutting back on the dosages does the trick, and as you proceed, the dosages can be gradually increased.[12]

Another way of detoxifying the liver is to use a castor oil pack. Soak a double layer of cotton cloth in organic castor oil and place over the area of the liver. Cover this with a plastic bag, then a hand towel, and finally put a heating pack on top. Lie down for 20–30 minutes. The toxins in the liver are drawn by osmosis to the oil in the cloth. Do not reuse the cloth. Wash the oil off the skin afterwards. Weekly castor oil packs are a great way to support the cleansing of the liver.

Besides following these dos, there are also some don'ts when it comes to supporting a healthy liver. Avoid overly fatty foods, especially deep fried food. In particular avoid the hydrogenated oils and fats that are often found in margarine, processed foods and commercially produced baked goods. Alcohol in large quantities is damaging to the liver, so keep intake to a minimum. Prescription and recreational drugs are also harmful to the liver, so try to avoid long-term consumption of them.

Western naturopathy knows many herbs that help to detoxify the body by cleansing the liver. The most commonly recommended are turmeric, milk thistle, artichoke and dandelion root. Also very useful are coriander, parsley, rosemary, kelp, spirulina, ginger, peppermint, nettle, yellow dock, rose hips, licorice and sarsaparilla. These herbs can be used variously in cooking, brewed as teas or taken as supplements. Once again, taking these herbs in springtime is more effective because they are empowered by the Wood energy that is all around us in nature.

Allergies

Many people suffer from allergies of various kinds. Some of us have respiratory allergic responses to things like pollens, dust and chemicals. For others the allergies affect the skin with rashes or eczema. Perhaps more common are food allergies, particularly to gluten, wheat and dairy products. From the perspective of Chinese medicine, all of these allergic responses stem from a weakness in the Liver.

Other organs may be implicated too – for example, the lungs and intestines – but the liver is more fundamental to the overall health of your immune system. If you suffer from allergies, and especially if you have multiple allergies, then paying attention to liver health is most important. Getting started on a liver cleanse is your best first step.

Spring in the Garden
Rapid Growth

Spring has to be about the best time in the garden. Warm days, warm soil, happy plants shooting out of the ground, all filling the gardener with visions of future produce. The qualities of Wood can be seen in every corner as the rapid uprising energy makes seedlings pop out of the ground. Some days you can see the rapidity as plants visibly grow during the course of a day. We wait for our seeds to germinate for days or even weeks, then suddenly – *POP* – there they are! And like the nature of Wood, growth is not always smooth and even. Plants will put on growth spurts, like young children. Some days nothing, others whoosh. But all around is the unmistakable feeling of things rushing upwards. You may even feel the resonance in your own body as the Qi rises up the Liver meridian to power your plans and activities.

Planning

One of the gifts of Wood which we've already looked at is planning. Spring is the best time to utilise this skill in laying out a vision for your garden, not just in the coming months but over the course of years.

Crop rotation is an indispensible part of organic gardening for a couple of reasons. First, different families of plants draw different nutrients from the soil, so rotation of crops is needed to balance this demand upon the soil. Second, rotation prevents the build-up of pests and diseases that can occur when the same crops are planted year after year.

So while throwing a few seeds in the soil to see what happens is one way of learning, planning is needed if we are to maintain a viable, ongoing plot. Pay attention to each of these steps:

1. Make a list of all the veggies you would like to grow in your garden.

2. Group the veggies together by one of the two methods below.

3. Draw a plan of your growing area and divide it into four sections.

4. Be flexible and adapt to unexpected changes of weather and conditions.

5. Keep records of what happened so you can adjust future planning.

METHOD 1: ROTATING FAMILIES OF VEGETABLES

Table 7.1 shows one plan for a four-year cool climate crop rotation. Next year, rotate the veggies clockwise around the table. If you live in a tropical area, just check the Internet for variations.

Table 7.1 Crop Rotation of Vegetable Families[13]

Plot 1	Plot 2
Solanaceae and *Cucurbitaceae* Manure in spring, then grow potatoes, tomatoes, zucchini. After harvest, plant overwintering onions, garlic, leeks.	*Apiaceae* and *Chenopdiaceae* Carrots, parsnips, celery, beetroot, spinach, chard, lettuce. Green manure crop over winter.
Plot 4	**Plot 3**
Alliaceae and *Papillionaceae* After harvesting onions, garlic and leeks from previous year, grow peas and beans, then a green manure crop over winter.	*Brassicaceae* Huge range including cabbage, cauliflower, collard, kale, kohl rabi, pak choi, radish, rocket, swede, turnip. Sow spring and autumn after manuring.

METHOD 2: ROTATING PARTS OF VEGETABLES

Rather than focus on families of plants (and all that Latin!), the method shown in Table 7.2 divides vegetables according to which parts are eaten. At the beginning of the cycle, enrich the soil with lots of compost and manure, and add potassium and phosphorus.

Table 7.2 Crop Rotation of Plant Parts[14]

Year 1	Year 2	Year 3	Year 4
Leaf crop	Fruit crop	Root crop	Legume crop
Lettuce, spinach, herbs, cabbage, broccoli	Tomatoes, zucchini, capsicum, cucumbers	Onions, radish, garlic, turnips, carrots	Peas, beans
Leaves love nitrogen	Fruits love phosphorus	Roots love potassium	Legumes restore nitrogen

Meridian Pathways

The Gall Bladder and Liver meridians are the energy pathways of the Wood Element. The yang partner is the Gall Bladder meridian which describes a complex pathway down the body (see Figure 7.2). It zigzags like the Chief of Staff riding back and forth across the battlefield.

The pathway begins at the outside of the eye, moves to the front of the ear, up into the temple, then around the back of the ear to the outside of the base of the skull, up over the top of the head to a point above the eyebrow, then back over the head to the base of the skull again, before moving down to the top of the shoulder. From here it zigzags down the side of the body, taking in the ribcage and the hip, before it finally straightens out down the outside of the leg, under the outer ankle to the outside of the fourth toe.

There are 44 points on this meridian and 20 of the them are in the head. As you can imagine, congestion in this channel often results in pressure in the head, frequently producing neck tension and pain, eye strain and headaches.

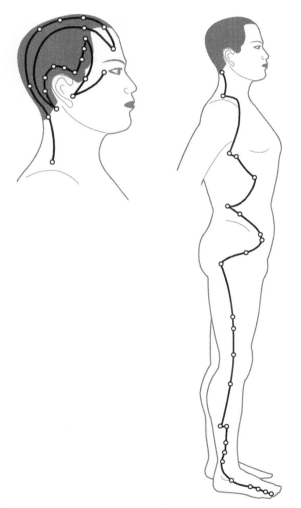

Figure 7.2 The pathway of the Gall Bladder meridian

The Liver meridian has a much simpler pathway. It begins at the outside corner of the big toe, moves up the inside of the leg and thigh and does a loop around the genitals before ending at a point in the ribcage below the breast.

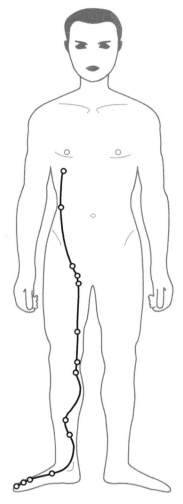

Figure 7.3 The pathway of the Liver meridian

If you feel pain, discomfort, congestion or other symptoms along these pathways, or if you have health conditions that relate to these organs, you can move the congested energy with this visualisation practice. Imagine a ball of green energy or light passing along the pathways of the meridians, first down the body along the Gall Bladder channel, then up the body along the Liver channel. You can use your breath to help move the energy. Try breathing out as you go down the body, breathing in as you come up the body. If you are more of a kinaesthetic person, you can use your fingers and hands to trace the pathways. Do this several times. If you find a place where it is difficult to move the energy through, stay there and focus your mind, hand and breath to help free the block.

Organ Awareness

After doing the meridian visualisation practice, you can then do the organ awareness practice for the liver and gall bladder organs. Place your right hand on the right side of your body where the ribcage ends. Place your left hand over the right. Spend some time tuning into your liver, that large organ of so many functions that is vital to your health, to your very life. Bring to mind the colour green. Maybe think of a forest or green fields. Allow this colour to infuse the liver with green. Acknowledge all the work it does for you in service of your life. Send it your love and gratitude for its work. Notice its response. Notice how you feel as you tune in.

Leaving your hands where they are, tune in now to the smaller organ of the gall bladder that lies tucked into the liver. While its function is simpler than that of the liver, it plays an important role is storing bile and eliminating toxins. Infuse it with a healthy green colour. Acknowledge it for its service, send your love and gratitude for its work.

Acupressure for Physical Health

After the meridian visualisation and organ awareness practices, you can focus specifically on the source points for each meridian. The source point heals the organ directly as well as balancing the meridian. They are powerful points while at the same time being very safe. They have the effect of tonifying the meridian if it is deficient, or sedating it if it is in excess. It is the balancing point par excellence.

Press and hold each point for 2–3 minutes. Start with the left foot, then the right. Use a level of pressure that is comfortable for you. Don't press so much that it hurts. Tune in to the point. Feel for the energetic pulse or wave. If you feel nothing, stay in tune and notice if things change.

After you've held each point singly, try holding both Liver 3 and Gall Bladder 40 in combination, again left foot first, then the right. Together, these points act synergistically and create an impact that is stronger than the points on their own.

LV 3 *Taichong* Great Rushing

The Liver source point lies between the first and second toes in a large depression halfway along the metatarsal bones (see Figure 7.4). There will probably be a sensitive spot. If the liver is very congested, the point itself may feel thick and swollen.

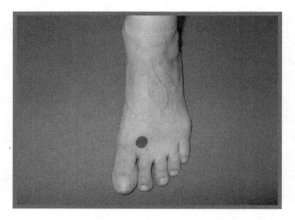

Figure 7.4 The Liver source point (LV 3 *Taichong* Great Rushing)

GB 40 *Qiuzu* Mound of Ruins

The Gall Bladder source point is found below and in front of the outer ankle bone in a large hollow (see Figure 7.5). Locate with the foot at a right angle to the leg.

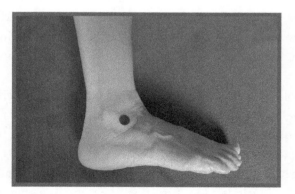

Figure 7.5 The Gall Bladder source point (GB 40 *Qiuzu* Mound of Ruins)

Headache Journal

I used to suffer from severe headaches. I was forever going to chiropractors and massage therapists trying to 'fix' my neck so it wouldn't tighten up and give me the headaches that would last for up to three days. In the early years, this treatment helped and I would get relief until the next round. But then even chiropractic adjustments wouldn't work and often made things worse. I had headaches several days a week.

Then in January 2003, inspired by the inquiry method of the Diamond Approach, I decided to keep a journal to track these headaches. I found a dun-coloured notebook someone had given me that seemed perfectly matched to the subject, and began to take notes.

I began to record details of frequency, duration, intensity and location of the pain as well as possible precursors such as what was happening in my life and my attitudes and feelings at the time. The very first entry, given below, began to reveal the causes.

Journal Entry: 5 January 2003

It began this morning as a stiffness. I lay down for an hour by which time my neck had seized up and the headache set in with increasing strength. Not severe but above average – perhaps a 6.5. While I may have slept on my stomach, the likely precursor was last night's emotional process. My restlessness has been very much up of late – anger which, it is becoming increasingly clear, is related to pre-memory infancy. Anyway, in the evening S asked if I was angry at her. I looked and did find something (I forget what) but in a short while, my neck adjusted and the headache began to recede. It was gone the next day.

Over the next few months the entries revealed a consistent pattern. What I discovered was that in *every* case the headache was associated with emotion. Either there was an emotion I was aware of that I was not expressing, or there was an emotion I was not aware of that became clear once I began to journal. And in most cases, that emotion was anger.

This discovery led quickly to a reduction in the frequency and duration of the headache pain. Over the course of a year, the headaches went from weekly, to monthly, to three-monthly. The final entry in this short journal is given below.

Journal Entry: 19 November 2004

A two dayer. Emotional stress over moving house and dealing with a big piece of process about the way I merge with others produced the first headache of note for eight months. What an improvement, eh?

My headaches have not gone away, and occasionally I resort to aspirin to help me over the worst ones. But I now see the pain differently. Rather than seeing it as something to be expelled and eradicated, or as some kind of enemy that has to be defeated, I regard it as a signal that my emotions are not flowing smoothly and so I begin to inquire into the underlying cause. This year I've noticed that they have returned with more frequency in the Spring which reminds me of my ongoing need to work with my Wood. I need to know more about who I am, what I want, what I stand for and how to assert this appropriately in the world. It is my life's work.

The Psycho-emotional Level of Wood

Having explored the ways in which Wood shapes us at the physical level, let's now look at the ways it shows up in our mental and emotional life. Thoughts and feelings are of a finer vibration than the body and so their energies are swifter and can change rapidly. But in another way, our emotional patterns, beliefs and attitudes can become fixed and entrenched. Here we will look at the ways in which the Wood Element can appear in us.

The Emotional Landscape of Wood

Anger

I once asked someone, 'What is your relationship to anger?' She replied, 'Oh, I don't get angry.' After a pause, she added, 'But I do get frustrated.'

Many of us are taught from a very young age that our anger is not acceptable. We grow up learning that anger is bad, that if we get angry we are bad and that 'nice' people don't get angry. We learn this first from our parents, later from teachers and society at large. Certainly as children we need to be 'civilised' so that we don't grow up to be unruly savages. We need to learn not to act out the destructive anger which is damaging to property, people and relationships. But often this civilising process also makes us afraid of anger; or it causes us to suppress it so deeply that we are not even aware we are angry; or we are aware of it but hold it in so tightly that it creates physical tension and pain. Often, anger becomes layered over by other emotions that are more acceptable.

These exhortations to be good, nice and not angry actually lead us to suppress and distort what is a natural and necessary human emotion. Many of us have learned to cram our anger into a narrow, acceptable range that includes frustration and irritation but excludes anger and rage.

The truth is that all of these are expressions of the same energy, just at different levels of intensity. There is a continuum of emotion that I call the *anger spectrum*. Along this spectrum the feelings all carry the same note, the same quality. At one end lie feelings such as annoyance, irritation and impatience. As we move along the continuum the feelings become stronger: things like resentment, aggravation, frustration, exasperation and intolerance. And as we move towards the other end of the spectrum we feel much stronger feelings like rage and fury.

But if we really feel into each of these feelings, which all of us have felt at some time, we notice that they all carry the same emotional affect and we notice the same kinds of sensations in our body. It's just that they are of different levels of intensity. They are like winds that range from breezes to gales.

Where do these powerful feelings come from and why do they arise?

As we have already seen, the energy of the Wood Element is an upward movement towards what we want and need. In nature we see this energetic force in the plants and trees whose leaves and branches move upwards and towards the light, and whose roots move towards water and nutrients in the soil. These are simply unstoppable forces of life. The same process occurs in humans. The dynamic energy of Wood helps us to get the goodies that the other Elements have to offer. So we gravitate towards that which feeds and nourishes us (Earth), we embrace those who love us (Fire), we hold on to that which makes us feel safe and secure (Water), and we reach for things that give value and meaning to life (Metal).

But when the movement towards these things is thwarted in some way and we do not get what we want and need, we begin to feel the energy that is behind this movement coming up against a boundary of limitations. Think of it like gas in a bottle that builds up pressure. It is this pressure that creates the feeling of anger. The gas represents our needs and desires, and the bottle represents the limitations or obstacles that lie in the way of getting what we need and want. As long as we have unmet needs and desires, there will be the tendency for anger to arise.

The origin of the word 'anger' gives some insight into the feelings and sensations that arise when we are angry. It is one of the oldest word roots in the Indo-European family of languages. *Angh* originally meant narrow, tight or painfully constricted.[15] This describes well some of the bodily sensations that arise when we feel angry as the forceful energy of what we want pushes through the narrow apertures that life presents. The breathing becomes constricted, the face reddens, the jaw tightens and overall there is a feeling of a powerful force rising upwards.

Depending on our constitutional Element, each of us will tend to get angry about a certain category of things. We tend to have our anger triggered more frequently when a particular need is frustrated.

For the Water type, anger arises more often when it seems that her survival is threatened. This can relate to physical safety – for example, getting furious at the other driver who almost caused an accident. It also applies to financial security, so anger arises if the money supply is threatened or employment is at risk.

For the Fire type, the main trigger derives from feeling unloved or unlovable. Anger can arise from feeling unwanted, abandoned or betrayed. Since the primary orientation of the Fire person is towards relationship, unmet relationship needs are more likely to trigger the emotion.

For the Earth type, the main source of anger comes from feeling she is not supported or gets no sympathy. For Earth people, feeling connected with others is of utmost importance. Disruption to this sense of connection will engender feelings of being alone and unsupported, which can prompt an anger reaction.

For the Metal type, the principal cause comes from feeling unseen, unrecognised, disrespected, unvalued or undervalued. There is a reaction to feeling that their value as a person is not respected. Often the anger of the Metal person is cold and cutting.

For Wood types, anger is the primary emotion of their life and 'lies at the heart of their suffering'.[16] The major source of this anger arises from a sense of personal injustice, that things are just not fair. Wood types have the most difficulty with the emotion of anger and their greatest challenge is to find a balanced, healthy way to deal with it that is neither explosive nor suppressive.

But for all of us, when it seems we are not getting the things to which we are rightfully entitled, the things we need, want and deserve, we get angry. This can range from small things like not getting the green light when we're driving or nice weather for our day out, to large things like not getting the relationship, the job or the house we want. In short, we are not getting the life we think we should have.

When our Wood is healthy, we know what we want and need, we set goals and make plans to get those things and we set out to achieve those ends. This is a natural, healthy assertion of ourselves in the world. Healthy assertion is the hallmark of a healthy Wood. When this healthy assertion meets obstacles and limitations, as it inevitably does, it tries to find a way past the block.

We live in a world of limitations; encountering limits is part of living a human life. The way we deal with these limitations shows us the health of our Wood Element. When the Wood Element is balanced, we are able to see the actual truth of the situation, recognise the limitations for what they are and see that they are seldom directed personally at us. We can adjust our direction with smoothness, flow and equanimity.

A plant growing from a crack in the footpath is a demonstration of the strength and flexibility of the dynamic power of Wood energy. Its irrepressible growth finds its way around and through obstacles as big as slabs of concrete. In our human lives, we are constantly meeting with slabs of concrete that block our forward progress. If our Wood is healthy, when we meet with constraints we look for another way. We can re-evaluate the situation and strategise another plan. The previously constrained energy becomes available to us to fuel our new way forward.

If our Wood is not so healthy, then we see these constraints and limitations as insurmountable obstacles and we react with frustration, anger and rage. If we are unable to use this energy to find a plan B, then our vision becomes clouded and we rage impotently against our situation. When this emotional state becomes habitual, the Liver Official is injured. The Liver is responsible for the smooth flow of Qi, of movement and of our life in general. When this Official is sick, our way forward looks like a rocky road.

If we find ourselves at this stage, what do we do with all this churning energy inside us? There are two directions that we can take. One way is to turn the anger outwards towards others. The alternative is to turn it inwards upon ourselves.

If we turn it outwards, it can be expressed by blaming others for our problems, by shouting and being very loud, by becoming physically violent, by becoming increasingly aggressive in the world to grab what we want. Or we can become passively aggressive, showing our anger while at the same time denying it.

If we turn it inwards upon ourselves, we develop a strong inner critic or judge who berates us constantly for doing the wrong thing, or we collapse under the weight of our anger and become depressed, resigned and apathetic.

While most of us can respond in either of these ways, we all tend to favour one response over the other. We'll look in detail now at these responses.

THE YANG RESPONSE: ANGER TURNED OUTWARD

Let us begin by examining the ways that anger is turned away from ourselves and projected onto others. This can be done by blaming others for our problems, becoming physically violent, aggressively pursuing our desires at the expense of others, and by resorting to passive aggression.

Blaming others. Blaming is the act of censuring, holding responsible or finding fault for an offence. In some cases, blaming someone else is appropriate in identifying responsibility for an action. But when blaming becomes a habitual shifting of responsibility from oneself to another, this becomes an example of outwardly directed anger.

Blaming then becomes a form of attack upon another person, however subtly it may be couched. We become frustrated that things don't seem to be going our way and we look for some other target to blame for the situation. When it comes out as inappropriate venting and blame fixing, it becomes harmful.

We can see blaming happening in many ways. The cliché of getting angry at our spouse for leaving the cap off the toothpaste is representative of the countless ways we blame others in our household and family. We blame our boss for our difficulties at work. We blame others in the community for not upholding community standards. Nations blame others for not respecting rights, borders and international law. Some people blame God for their problems.

In all cases, the anger at the world for not being 'as it should be' becomes fixed upon a target that is not ourselves. Just remember that when you point a finger at someone else, there are three fingers pointing back at you. A graphic reminder to us to examine our own responsibility in any situation.

Physical violence. When frustration escalates to the level of rage, the energy becomes very difficult to manage. When anger becomes uncontrollable, it can lead to actual violence that is destructive to property, to people and to relationships. People talk about 'seeing red' and 'blind fury'. Sometimes anger becomes so strong that it literally affects our vision and our eyes, the sense organs of Wood.

Other resonances of Wood are also affected by extreme anger. Think of all the Gifts of Wood we looked at earlier – for example, the ability to negotiate, the capacity for clarity and wise judgement. All of these gifts go out of the window once the anger has reached extreme proportions.

A lot of physical violence happens in conjunction with alcohol consumption. Here again we see a connection to the liver. Large amounts of alcohol in the blood must be processed by the liver. If it is under stress, then its capacities become impaired. Studies have shown about 40% of violent crimes involve alcohol and that reducing outlets of alcohol results in lower domestic and community violence.[17]

Aggressive need fulfilment. Another expression of outwardly directed anger is to find more and more aggressive ways of going after what we want. When our goal is thwarted, we aggressively find another way through. We won't take no for an answer and override others' feelings as we pursue our goals.

Many successful enterprises have been founded on this approach to life. The powerful drive to achieve at all costs can often result in commercial success and consequent riches. But it is bought at the cost of crushing others and violating their rights.

This can be seen in the playground bully who uses force to grab another child's lunch, the corporate executives who allow pollution in order to make greater profits, and the nation with the bigger army invading its neighbour for power and control.

Passive aggression. Another way that anger can be directed outwards but without being actively expressed is through passive aggression. This is obstructive behaviour that expresses aggression in subtle and indirect ways. It can be a personality trait or even a personality disorder, so some people behave habitually in this way.

Passive-aggressive behaviour tends to create frustration and anger in others and so can become a way to get others to act out our own unexpressed anger. Some of the ways this behaviour appears are repeatedly breaking agreements, being obstructive, being sullen and argumentative, dwelling on one's own misfortunes and speaking ambiguously so as to create insecurity in others. Usually this type of behaviour is unconscious and is motivated by a fear of direct assertion.[18]

All these kinds of harmful behaviour have led society at large to label anger as negative. But the truth is that it is not the anger itself that is harmful to others, but rather the aggression that arises from it. It is the automatic linkage between anger and aggression in many people's minds that has led to the belief that anger is a negative emotion and therefore needs to be controlled or suppressed.

THE YIN RESPONSE: ANGER TURNED INWARD
While outwardly directed anger tends to be blaming, inwardly directed anger is shaming. In order to cope with the huge amounts of unexpressed anger that build up, many people unwittingly direct the anger inwards upon themselves. Self-blame, self-criticism, low self-esteem and self-harm are all ways in which anger becomes self-inflicted.

Shame and guilt. There is no clear agreement about the meanings of the words 'shame' and 'guilt', or of the particular distinction between them.

According to cultural anthropologist Ruth Benedict, shame is a violation of cultural or social values while guilt feelings arise from violations of one's internal values. Thus, it is possible to feel ashamed of a thought or behaviour that no one knows about and to feel guilty about actions that gain the approval of others.[19]

Psychoanalyst Helen B. Lewis argues that 'The experience of shame is directly about the self, which is the focus of evaluation. In guilt, the self is not the central object of negative evaluation, but rather the thing done is the focus.'[20] Lewis also argues that shame really represents an entire family of emotions including feelings of humiliation, embarrassment, low self-esteem, belittlement and stigmatisation.

Whichever way we define these terms, they are expressions of anger turned inwards upon ourselves. While it may be argued that the attacks are coming from outside and from other people's ideas about our 'bad' behaviour, the point is that we believe them. We take them on, aiding and abetting the attacks upon ourselves. This happens because we have taken on a whole raft of beliefs about what is right and wrong behaviour from our parents, teachers, peers and society at large. These rules of right and wrong coalesce to form a structure in our mind known as the inner critic.

The inner critic. We all have an inner critic. It is also known as the judge or the superego. This is a normal development in the psychic structure and acts as a guide to what society considers appropriate action. It also acts as a restraint on destructive behaviour. It is a civilising part of our makeup. Without it there would be no possibility of an organised society, and even family relationships would be chaotic. It acts as a conscience that restrains us when we feel impulses arise. Without an inner critic, we'd end up in prison pretty quickly.

This inner critic is what Freud termed the superego.[21] Superego literally means 'over-I'. This is the part of us that watches over and controls the impulsive parts of us. The superego is believed to be the last piece of the ego structure to be formed and is complete around the age of five years, just in time for us to go to school. At this stage, the superego forms a list of dos and don'ts, shaped largely by our parents, which guide us in becoming an accepted part of civilised society. As we grow, this inner list of rights and wrongs is added to and subtly modified as we move through the various stages of development on our way to adulthood.

It is clear that this is a normal and necessary part of human development. Even if it were possible to have a superego-ectomy to remove the inner critic, it would not serve us because we would lose the civilising part of ourselves that allows us to function as a member of society.

But for many people, this structure assumes a disproportionate role. When this happens, we continually attack ourselves, beat ourselves up and judge ourselves with shoulds and shouldn'ts. We blame ourselves and feel ashamed and guilty.

For some of us, the critic is a voice in our head, as if there is another person leaning over our shoulder constantly monitoring our actions, speech and even our thoughts. We hear comments like 'They're going to think you're a terrible person for saying that', 'You ought to be ashamed of yourself for having that thought' or 'Everyone's going to think you're such an idiot for what you did at the party last night'.

The inner critic doesn't only punish us with verbal criticism. Attacks can come in the form of an inner feeling of being small, heavy and weighed down, as if the upward-rising dynamic energy of who we are is being crushed. We may have feelings like embarrassment where we want to hide, shame where we feel like covering ourselves up, or guilt where we feel like we've been caught out and need to repent. All of these feelings arise from the inner critic turning upon us.

In terms of the Five Element model, what we are doing here is taking the Wood energy that would otherwise fuel action and assertion in the world, and turning it upon ourselves. It is one of the primary limitations to being truly ourselves.

So how can we live with our inner critic in a way that takes note of the advice it has to offer us without taking it as a personal attack on how we live our life? See the exercise below for some suggestions on how we can work with this part of ourselves.

Depression. One of the most common outcomes of inwardly directed anger is depression. While not all depression is a result of suppressed anger, it is one of the most common causes. Turning this energy inward can result in collapse, leading to resignation, abdication and giving up on life.

While the causes of depression are complex and arise out of each person's personality, perspective and life circumstances, the result brings feelings of hopelessness, helplessness and pointlessness. Depression, as the very word itself suggests, represents a counter-flow of the natural upward-rising energy of the Wood Element. Our energy sinks, our spirits are lowered and we feel dejected and unhappy.

Most of us have had a period in our life when things seem so bad, so hard to cope with, that we sink under the weight of our difficulties. It seems that life has dealt us a knockout blow from which we can't get up. When this response becomes entrenched for a long period, depression is the result.

One way to counteract depression is through exercise. Studies have shown that regular exercise has at least as much of a positive effect on depression as antidepressants.[22] Even better, it is non-toxic. Exercise activates and invigorates the Wood energy.

Gall Bladder timidity. Not known in Western medicine, but recognised in China, is the condition known as 'small Gall Bladder' or 'Gall Bladder timidity'. In Chinese, the expression 'big Gall Bladder' means courageous, and 'small Gall Bladder' means timid or fearful. We've seen that the Gall Bladder Official is responsible for decision-making and for taking action. The capacity to be bold and take decisive action when necessary are hallmarks of a healthy Gall Bladder. When this Official is weak in us, the opposite happens. We vacillate, shrink from deciding and become afraid of taking initiative. This fear is not the fear of the Water Element but rather a timidity that stems from lack of courage to move forward.

While this condition is not exactly a turning inward of anger, it nonetheless represents a collapse of the natural upward-rising energy of Wood.

RETURNING TO BALANCE

We can work towards a healthier relationship with our anger by becoming as fully conscious as possible of our feelings in the anger spectrum. The more we are aware of our anger, the less likely we are to act it out in harmful ways. Unconscious anger gets expressed in ways that we may not even realise. It can come out as meanness, carping, cutting remarks, hurtful comments and biting jokes. Sometimes it takes someone else to tell us how mean and angry we are being before we realise what we are doing.

Depending on whether you tend to express your anger outwards or turn it inwards, there are different strategies you can employ.

If you are the kind of person who turns anger outwards towards others, when you feel the upward surge of emotion you can do the following:

- Breathe deeply and slowly. Take five long, slow breaths. This will help calm the upward surge.

- Feel your legs and feet on the ground. Anger rises up the Liver meridian from the big toe up to the chest. Bring your focus to your big toes. This will help bring the angry energy back down your body and make you more grounded.

- Relax your jaw, shoulders, arms and hands. These are the areas of the body that tighten when you get angry.

- Count to ten before you say anything. It's an old trick but a good one. You can do this while you're taking those five long breaths.

- Leave the room. If you find yourself moving into a state of rage while relating to someone, say something like, 'I need to talk about this later' and leave. I'm not saying you should repress your feelings, but rather suggesting a way to interrupt the pattern of turning the anger into aggression upon someone else.

You can do the following as an ongoing practice:

- Exercise regularly. You can recycle the energy behind the anger by moving vigorously. Exercise that engages the upper back, arms and shoulders will help free the musculature that tends to tighten when anger rises. Punching, boxing and rowing are good exercises for this.

- Meditate. Try a simple meditation practice of sitting down, closing your eyes and counting your breaths. Do this daily. Join a group. If you find sitting meditation too difficult, try walking meditation where your focus is on the slow movements of your body. Over time these practices will make you a calmer person, less inclined to fly off the handle.

- Anger management. Sometimes we need the help of others to work with these habitual patterns. There are many therapists and groups that can help.

Understanding the reasons behind the anger is crucial. Most of our personality patterns are rooted in our early history. Coming to understand why these angry parts of ourselves developed is key to softening and dissolving them. Imagine that your angry part is a separate person and engage in a dialogue with him. Find out what makes him tick. You may find that these parts are actually trying to help you, to protect you from something. Try to find out how Mister Angry thinks he is helping you.

This process is a deep one and usually needs the help of an experienced counsellor or therapist, but you can certainly begin the process in your journal.

We can begin by emulating that most flexible wood, the bamboo: to weather the storm, bend with the wind, and when the storm of anger passes, return to upright balance.

In modern psychological terms, we can try not to become identified with our anger, instead seeing it as a passing phenomenon and not who we really are.

If you are the kind of person who turns anger inwards towards yourself:

- The most important thing is to recognise that you are attacking yourself. It is necessary to identify when and how you are feeling ashamed, guilty, self-diminishing and of low worth. This is the first step in pushing back against the part of you that is crushing your uprising Wood energy. Once you see that this is happening, it is possible to take steps to fight back. (See 'Activity: Working with the Inner Critic' on how to take action to reclaim yourself.)

- Exercise regularly. Exercise helps lift depression and we feel better about ourselves afterwards. Exercises that work the muscles of the upper back, shoulders and arms are particularly effective in mobilising the stuck Wood energy in the upper body.

- Shout! Shout! Let it all out! While those who turn their anger outwards probably already do a lot of shouting, many of us who turn it inwards have swallowed our shout. Sometimes shouting is necessary to get attention or to express outrage at injustice. If you find it difficult or frightening to shout, then some exercising of the voice is needed. It's a good idea to do this when alone so as not to alarm others. Shouting in the car is a safe place. Or get together with others and have a group shout. Football matches are a great venue for acceptable shouting.

- Punching is another good activity to raise up a diminished Wood Element. Get a punching bag and begin mobilising the punching muscles in your upper back as well as your arms. There is a qigong exercise called Punching with Angry Eyes that is excellent for contacting suppressed Wood energy.[23]

- Understanding why we suppress our anger is a vital step to reclaiming our vitality. In our history there were good reasons not to get angry or show our anger. We developed protective parts that served us when we were young but which no longer do so. Uncovering and understanding these patterns shows us why we have behaviours that are holding us back in our life. Journaling is a great place to begin, and experienced counsellors and therapists can help us go further in this exploration.

BEING CONSCIOUS OF ANGER

All anger arises from things not going the way we want. Either we're not getting what we want or we're getting something we don't want. Either way, it amounts to a negative reaction to what is happening in our life. Consider these examples:

- I'm annoyed that the rain is ruining my plan for a hike.

- I'm disappointed that I didn't get the job I applied for.

- I'm frustrated that my cake sank in the middle.

- I'm angry at my partner for having a headache on our anniversary.

- I'm outraged at the way corporations are ruining our planet.

- I'm enraged at the driver who crashed into me.

Below is a list of words, not in any particular order, that reflect many of the points along the anger spectrum.

Resentful	Wrathful	Ruffled
Bitter	Irascible	Miffed
Indignant	Furious	Peeved
Frustrated	Testy	Crabby
Infuriated	Enraged	Ratty
Put out	Vexed	Tetchy
Cross	Annoyed	Livid
Exasperated	Pissed off	Grumpy
Impatient	Irritated	

Take the following steps with regard to this list:

1. In your Wood journal, arrange these words in order from lowest intensity to highest intensity. There is no right way to do this. It will be different for everyone depending on your personal history and your associations with the words. If some words don't make sense to you, leave them out of your list. Add in any other words you can think of.

2. Take the words one by one and write a sentence about when you might get this feeling. If your first word is grumpy, you might write: I get grumpy when my neighbour's dog wakes me up early in the morning.

    Do this for all of the words on your list. Leave a line between each statement. Take your time. I'm encouraging you to feel the feeling as fully as possible. This exercise might take you all day or even all spring!

3. Continue each sentence with 'because I imagine that…' So your sentence may now read: I get grumpy when my neighbour's dog wakes me up early in the morning because I imagine that my neighbour doesn't care a damn about other people.

4. When you've written all your sentences about all of these feelings, take some time to write about how the process was for you.

   Was it easy, challenging, enjoyable, painful, insightful? Do you feel differently now in relation to your anger? Remember, what we're trying to do here is to bring more conscious awareness to our anger so that it can be expressed and managed in healthy ways. Personally, I'd rather be sitting next to someone who knows he is angry than someone who doesn't.

Activity: Working with the Inner Critic

Identifying Critic Attacks

The first step in freeing ourselves from our inner critic or superego is to become aware of when we are being attacked by this part of ourselves. We need to distinguish between the useful information that it is providing, and an attack that belittles or diminishes us in some way. For example, your critic might say something like, 'You're a crazy idiot for crossing the road against the red light.' It's actually good safety advice, but it comes with an attack on our mental state.

Sometimes the attack doesn't come in the form of words, but of a feeling of being small, humiliated, squashed or worthless. When you feel these kinds of feelings, try to put words to them. It can help to bring the attack more into conscious awareness. For example, a sinking in the stomach and a feeling of weakness might be expressing, 'You're really a worthless sort of person.'

If this is the first time you've worked with the inner critic in this way, spend some days or weeks identifying the times that you experience these attacks. You might carry a notebook or voice recorder around with you and note each one. You'll probably be surprised at the frequency of these self-attacks.[24]

Defending Against Attack

Superego attacks that belittle, humiliate, blame and shame us are almost always suppressing our natural, alive, dynamic Wood energy. The effect is to limit us by making us small. One way we can defend against these attacks is to summon the uprising energy of Wood and fight back. Say to your critic, 'Leave me alone you bully!' or 'Don't treat me like that, I won't stand for it' or just 'Go away' or simply 'No!' Use strong language and be forceful.

Imagine you were in the street and saw a parent berating her child in the kinds of ways you beat yourself up. You'd probably be outraged and want to come to the aid of the poor child. Well, summon up that sense of outrage and defend yourself against the attacks of your critic.

You might also try defending with humour or exaggeration. For example, your critic might say to you, 'You forgot your keys again, you idiot.' You could retort with, 'You're right, I must have dementia. I should check myself into an old people's home.' Sometimes this kind of approach pops the judge's authority quickly.

An important thing to keep in mind is not to engage in a dialogue with the critic. Don't give excuses or try to argue rationally. The important thing is not to engage at all, but to disengage and to free ourselves from this self-limiting part of our mind.

Understanding the Critic

While defending against attack in the moment is a good way of maintaining a healthy sense of self-worth, we also need to understand what this part of ourselves is trying to do for us. At its core is an intention to protect us.

These self-critical and attacking parts of our mind were created in early childhood. They were created to keep us safe. We needed to internalise our parents' and teachers' rules in order to survive in the world, as well as to keep their love and care. The trouble is that these internalised messages are somewhat out of date and we're acting as if we're five years old being scolded by mother.

While everyone has this structure as part of their personality, we all attack ourselves in different ways and for different reasons because of our particular history. We need to understand the reasons we do this if we are ultimately to break free of these old patterns. It is also most important to bring compassion to these parts of ourselves and to recognise their good intentions for us.

In short, we need to defend ourselves at the moment of attack, but in the longer term come to a deeper understanding of what is happening within us and why.

Boundaries and Individuation

When we are born, we are still very close to the state of Oneness from which we emerged. At this stage we are also still totally merged with our mother, open and porous with no sense of self. This state has been called the Dual Unity where we are at one with this field of mother and baby.[25]

As we grow we begin to see a world outside us. We learn to move through the world, first crawling, then walking. At some point, with the help of others, we begin to realise we are a separate individual interacting with other separate individuals. Then comes a stage where we start to move away from mother while making sure she's still there. We go through our 'terrible twos' as we explore our emerging boundaries by saying 'No' to everything, learning who we are and who we are not. By the time we are four or five years old, this sense of self has become complete and we know ourselves as a Johnny or Mary, separate from everyone else. We have individuated and our separation from the Oneness is complete. What is more, this separation is encouraged and celebrated by everyone around us.

Another significant stage of individuation occurs at puberty – what we might call the 'Fuck you' stage. As adolescents, we push our parents away in a more forceful way, pushing against boundaries to find out more and more about who we are.

I well remember my days as a high school teacher where at the start of each school year, students set out to find the limits of what they could get away with in the classroom. These young adolescents were really just expressing their Wood energy, sending out roots and shoots to see how much they could get and where they could get it, and what the limits and boundaries were. Once these limits were established between teacher and students, there would be a status quo, with the occasional retesting of the boundaries by the most assertive students.

This is the normal and necessary development of a human personality. For some of us, these stages of individuation were not completed. Maybe we didn't get to go through our 'No!' stage when we were two years old. Perhaps we were treated with severe strictness and were boxed in, prevented from expanding into ourselves. Or maybe we were given too much freedom and never got to understand that we live in a world of limitations.

When the questions of boundaries and limits are major issues in a person's life, we find that the Wood energy tends to move out of balance easily. Moreover, these issues will tend to be reflected in other levels of a person's being. At the physical level, there may be concerns with the gall bladder and liver, the eyes, the tendons and ligaments, and the nails. At the emotional level there will probably be issues of anger being either overblown or suppressed. And at the spiritual level, there may well be struggle finding one's true path in life.

They say that it's never too late to have a happy childhood. I'd say it's never too late to be a healthily assertive two-year-old or an angry young adolescent.

Knowing What You Want

What do you want? If you struggle with this question, then it is likely your Wood is wobbly. For a person of Wood constitution, this is often a difficult question to answer.

We have already seen that the Gall Bladder Official is responsible for decision-making and that a weak Gall Bladder will bring uncertainty, indecision and vacillation. This struggle to decide will reveal itself in matters large and small. It can show up in something as simple as choosing a dish from a restaurant menu and in something as significant as which college to attend or who to marry.

What lies behind this indecisiveness is a lack of clarity about what we want. If we don't know what we want, of course it's going to be impossible to make a decision that makes any sense. People with this configuration in their personality will tend to let others who do know what *they* want make the decisions for them.

There is something still deeper beneath this psychological pattern. If we consider the process of individuation which we discussed above, we can see that if there is not a clearly defined sense of a separate self, then there isn't a definite person there to really want and desire. When the boundaries of the self are loose and porous, there is a tendency to merge with others and it becomes quite difficult to distinguish between what others want and what the individual wants.

As a result, such people usually need lots of time alone in which to become clearer about who they are, what they want and where they're going.

If you find yourself described here, first, don't attack yourself about it. It's simply one of the patterns that shows up in human beings. We all have patterns. We all have some work to do in our development. If you are beating yourself up, defend yourself now (see 'Activity: Working with the Inner Critic').

Second, you can begin to explore these issues by journaling. Make a list of all the things you want. Don't bother about whether they are realistic or likely to happen in this lifetime. Just dream! If you have trouble knowing what you want, try looking at what you don't want. This might be an easier way in. Now pick one of the simpler things you've described and make another list of the things you could do to move in this direction. For example, if you've chosen 'I want more friends', make a list of the things you might do to move in this direction. Again, don't worry if it is in fantasyland; just brainstorm.

After you have become clearer in your mind about what you want and how you might get it, perhaps talk to someone to get some feedback. There are lots of life coaches around these days who can be very good at motivating. Now *there's* another good Wood word. Motivation.

Write a list of all the things you want. Be as outrageous as you like. Choose one and list the things that will move you in this direction.

Acupressure for Psycho-emotional Health

The points I've chosen to support psycho-emotional health are known as the front mu points or alarm points of the Wood meridians.

LV 14 *Qimen* Gate of Hope

LV 14 *Qimen* Gate of Hope is a great point for releasing held in emotion, for accessing and recycling suppressed anger and for raising the Wood energy when it has become depressed. It supports creativity and vision, expanding the horizons of possibility in your life. This point can be held on its own or in conjunction with the source point LV 3, which we learned in the section 'Acupressure for Physical Health' above.

LV 14 is located in the ribs, on the nipple line and just above the xiphoid process (see Figure 7.6). The point lies in the sixth intercostal space and is often tender to pressure.

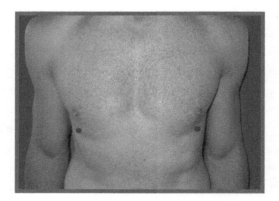

Figure 7.6 LV 14 *Qimen* Gate of Hope, the alarm point of the Liver meridian

GB 24 *Riyue* Sun and Moon

GB 24 *Riyue* Sun and Moon also supports clarity and vision. The Sun was considered to be the left eye, the Moon the right, so this point relates to the sense organs of the Wood and balances yin and yang. The point supports decision-making and helps strengthen a 'small gall bladder'. It softens rigidity of the Wood, easing frustration and resentment. This point can be held alone or in conjunction with source point GB 40.

GB 24 Sun and Moon is also located in the ribs, on the nipple line and just below the xiphoid process (see Figure 7.7). The point lies in the seventh intercostal space.

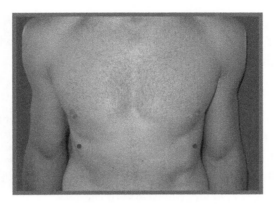

Figure 7.7 GB 24 *Riyue* Sun and Moon, the alarm point of the Gall Bladder meridian

The Spiritual Level of Wood

Our spiritual nature is that which is not our body, thoughts, emotions or personality. If there is anything that remains of us when we die, it is this. Let us look at how the Wood Element influences our spiritual life.

The Spirit of Wood: Hun

The Chinese character *hun* is made up of two parts, one meaning clouds, the other meaning ghost. Clouds are vaporous, light, constantly moving and changing shape. They reside high above the earth but they relate to the earth through the water cycle of evaporation and condensation. So too the *hun* is lighter than earth but contains enough density to keep it near the earth and not fly away to heaven.

In a sense, the *hun* is the intermediary between heaven and earth. If we look at the generation cycle (see Figure 2.1), we see that the Wood Element lies between Water and Fire, and is therefore a link between those two Elements. Therefore, it is the *hun*, spirit of the Wood Element, which regulates the smooth flow of Qi between Fire (heaven) and Water (earth).[26]

Of all the five spirits, the *hun* is closest to the Western concept of the soul.[27] In fact, the character *hun* is usually translated as ethereal soul. The *hun* enters the body after birth and at death it leaves through the top of the head. It then ascends to the stars whereupon 'it reports to the spirits that preside over destiny on the degree to which each of us has cultivated virtue during our lifetime'.[28]

During our lifetime, it is the *hun* which bestows the Gifts of Wood upon us. A healthy *hun* allows us to be clear about our purpose in life, find our path, know where we are going and orient ourselves in that direction. It is what helps us to navigate the rapids of life. The *hun* is like the map and compass of our soul.

It is said that during the day the *hun* resides in the eyes to help us to see how we can act in ways that best serve our life purpose.[29] At night when we sleep, the *hun* descends to the liver where it organises our dreams. Just as the *hun* acts as an intermediary between our Water and Fire, so too it mediates our waking and sleeping states.

If the *hun* is imbalanced, then our sleeping and dreaming may be disrupted. We might suffer from sleep disturbances, sleepwalking, intense dreaming or no dreams at all. In extreme cases we may find it difficult to distinguish between dreams and reality. Out-of-body experiences, near-death experiences as well as seeing ghosts and spirits are all associations of the *hun*.

The classics say that the Liver houses the *hun*;[30] therefore, anything that damages the Liver also injures the *hun*. Anger that does not flow freely and gets stuck in the body will damage the Liver. It is also easily upset by alcohol and drugs. Marijuana is particularly harmful to the *hun*. While it might seem to endow us with cleverness, creativity and vision when we are intoxicated, over time these very qualities are eroded and we lose both purpose and vitality.

The *hun* can also be injured by psychological scarring. In childhood the *hun* needs psychological support. If a child is severely constrained in his freedom, constantly criticised for his actions or emotionally deprived, the *hun* cannot develop freely. If there is alcoholism or abuse in the home, the development of the *hun* is harmed. In later life too, overwhelming emotional experiences can disturb the *hun*.[31]

The *hun* spirit needs a healthy liver to be invited to stay in our body. We have seen that *hun's* nature is to wander like a cloud. When its home in our body is unhealthy and uninviting, it will tend to fly away, leaving us bereft of its capacities of clarity, vision and purpose.

To understand more about the way the *hun* is tethered to our body, we must look at it in relationship to another of the spirits, the *po*. *Po*, the spirit of the Metal Element, is known as the Corporeal Soul. The *hun* and *po* are poles of the same phenomenon[32] and our soul comprises both our ethereal and our corporeal nature.

The *hun* and *po* are therefore bound together in a relationship in which the former's propensity to wander and fly is constrained by the latter's grounding in the physical body. Jarrett has a wonderful metaphor for this: the jack-in-the-box.

The *hun* is the jack which wants to bounce out and fly free; the *po* is the box which attempts to anchor the jack in the present.[33]

The *hun* spirit is what allows us to bring our Heavenly nature into earthly form and manifestation. When in balance, it is the source of our dreams and visions, our aims and projects, our creativity and ideas,[34] all of which can find expression in physical form in life on earth. A healthy *hun* is what we need to live a conscious and effective life as a being of spirit in a physical body.

Is life worth living? It all depends on the liver.

WILLIAM JAMES

The Virtue of Wood: Benevolence

The Taoist classics say that benevolence is the virtue of Wood. Benevolence is 'that which empowers the unconstrained evolutionary journey of all things from earth towards heaven'.[35] If we consider once again Wood's place in the generational cycle, it can be viewed as the vehicle for the transformation of the potential of Water into the realised fruition of Fire. This realisation is not just of our own development, but of the development of all of humanity, of the Tao itself. Our spiritual evolution does not belong to us, though our ego self may believe otherwise. Our evolution is the evolution of True Nature. We are no less than the arms and legs of the Tao, each of us contributing to its endless unfolding.

When we fall from the virtue of benevolence, we lose sight of this greater purpose. We see only the rocks in the path of our own life, our own small plan. In short, we cannot see the wood for the trees. Anger is then the response to the perception that our forward movement is being frustrated or thwarted. The anger response can be outwardly directed as rage, or inwardly directed as collapse, but both states indicate the fall from our true path.

Finding our own particular, unique path in this life and aligning with it brings us closer to the virtue of benevolence. It also begins to free us from the turbulent effects of anger. When anger does arise, it can become a reminder to us to consider and inquire into the ways in which our vision has become distorted, our direction misguided and our path lost.

The Spiritual Issue of Wood: Finding True Path

Where am I going? What is the point of being here? Existential questions such as these point to the spiritual issue of Wood, that of finding a path through life that best expresses and unfolds the individual soul. The issue of Wood is concerned with the fundamental orientation of our life, our direction and trajectory.

It is difficult to talk about path without talking about purpose. We tend to link goals with the achievement of those goals. We must distinguish here between the path through life and the purpose of life, between the goals we have and the realisation of those goals. The manifestation that arises when goals are met, the fruits of our labours, relates to the spiritual issue of the Earth Element. Here we are focusing on the direction that our life takes, not its destination. If Earth is concerned with the destination, Wood is about the journey itself.

Adolescence is the stage of life that relates to the Wood Element, a time when we are called upon to clarify our direction in life. Teenagers are faced with the challenge of discovering their life path and a set of principles to guide them. Many teens adopt idealistic positions, taking on a ready-made philosophy to guide them because they have not had enough life experience to mould their own. As teenagers grow to adulthood, they develop a more nuanced philosophy of life to guide them. But for some the issue of finding the most appropriate path to follow remains a struggle.

People of Wood constitution are often challenged in finding and maintaining a steady course. They may continually look to others to help them find their way. The pattern of confusion that such people have about finding a direction in life derives from not knowing what they want. They need help in finding out what it is that they want. We move naturally towards that which we desire, but if we are unclear about what we desire, there is no impulse to move in a particular direction.

What are the physical and metaphysical goals of your life? What is the right direction, the true path? In pondering these questions, I invite you to be specific to your own life. Certainly the overarching purpose of human life is to evolve towards Heaven. But how is this evolution happening in your particular life? How are your gifts bringing this about? We are all unique individuals, an infinite variety of expressions of the Tao. Therefore, there are an infinite number of paths that this evolution can take. How is it happening in your location?

We have seen that the *hun* spirit is linked to our nightly dreams. It is also responsible for the dreams we have for our life. A healthy *hun* dreams for our future and helps steer us along the path towards those dreams. It is the map and compass of life's journey. If your map is sketchy or even non-existent and if your compass needle is unsteady, working with Wood at all levels will help you illuminate the direction and trajectory of your soul's evolution.

 Where does your inner compass point to? What are the guiding principles that steer your life?

The purpose of my life is to get closer and closer to who I really am. The closer I get to my True Nature, the less I'm interested in things like purpose or meaning. I'm just living.

P.M.

Guidance

The deepest Essence of Wood provides us with guidance for our life. When our Wood is in healthy balance, its gifts of vision, clarity and perspective provide us with the tools to know our direction and purpose. The guidance comes as a simple knowing. When we drop into that still place inside us, the way forward becomes clear.

However, when our Wood is clouded and our inner vision is obscured, we can feel lost, without direction, rudderless, becalmed and bewildered by life. We might have trouble even seeing what are the possible roads forward in our life. Or we may see possibilities but be unable to decide which path to take, succumbing to paralysed inaction.

When faced with difficult decisions, or even having no clue as to what to do or where to go, many of us seek guidance from outside. While it is good to get the opinion of others and gather information that is important to our decision-making, if we continually rely on others to make our choices for us, it indicates that our own Wood is unstable.

Some people make use of divination to guide their lives, seeking out psychics and clairvoyants, astrologers and tarot readers. Of course, these methods have a place and can help provide insights into our path in life. The Dalai Lama himself used the Tibetan Mo divination to help him decide when to flee Tibet in 1959.[36]

But if we are continually using outside sources to make our decisions for us, it is because our own inner map and compass have been lost. Then, each time we rely on another to make our decision, we disempower ourselves and actually weaken still further our own capacity to decide.

If you are struggling with making a decision or finding your way forward in life, try this:

Frame a question for yourself. Maybe it's 'Is this a good time to sell my house?' or 'Is it good for me to get into relationship with Fred?' or 'Will this job provide me with satisfaction?' Keep it simple and specific. Don't ask either/or questions.

Once you've framed your question, write it down and let it go from your mind. Sit in quiet meditation for a time until you feel as though you have found your centre and disconnected somewhat from the thought stream. Then, when you feel ready, read aloud the question you've framed. Imagine you are dropping the question into your quiet centre like dropping a pebble into a pond. What do you notice happening as the ripples fan out from the question you've just dropped? Pay attention to the feelings both in your body and in your emotions. These responses can guide you in your choices.

Do not do this lightly, but rather treat it as a ritual. The more gravity you bring to the process, the more meaningful will be the results. By calling upon the Essence of your own Wood Element for guidance, you will be cultivating and strengthening that guidance.

Ultimately, the guidance is not ours. Nothing is. Our ego thinks it is in charge of the show, but what is really happening is True Nature unfolding moment by moment. Each moment is unfolding into the next moment. And since True Nature and our true nature are the same, then we ourselves are unfolding moment by moment.

True Guidance is the intelligence of the Tao guiding our personal unfoldment in a human life.

The Diamond Approach
Strength
All anger arises from resisting the way things are unfolding in our lives. The more we resist what is happening, the greater is the emotional impact. We make a judgement that this event, this development, this state of affairs is not right. We resist the way things are. We want things to be another way.

In this world of form there are always limitations. If we have judgements about those limitations, we develop resistance. This resistance causes frustration and anger. We act like little kids, throwing tantrums because things are not going our way and we are not getting what we want.

We have a plan about where we are going and how our life should look. When we rage against the way things are going, we are saying, 'This isn't how my life is supposed to be.' We are rejecting our life as it is. We are railing against Heaven. We think our plan is superior to the plan of unfolding Tao. Ultimately, we are angry at God.

From the perspective of the Diamond Approach, anger is a distortion of an Essential Aspect called True Strength. Essential Aspects are qualities of True Nature that manifest in us and can be directly perceived at a subtle level. These Essential Aspects are mimicked by the ego but become distorted in the process. What happens when the ego mimics True Strength is that it becomes the emotion of anger. Therefore, we get to feel the qualities of True Strength – its expansiveness, aliveness and vitality – as we express our anger. The anger is not actually real in the way True Strength is, but rather is an expression of our ego state.

While anger is a distortion of True Strength, it is also a portal to that Strength. If we stay with our feelings of anger, neither rejecting them, nor suppressing them, nor expressing them, and we inquire into and explore the nature of that anger, its sensations and feelings, its history and origins, we eventually find that the anger dissolves and transforms into True Strength within us. From that place, the feelings of fullness, expansiveness and aliveness come through us as we discover more and more of our True Nature. We become aware that we are not just feeling Strength, but that we *are* Strength.

> It is as if your whole body were full of robust blood, pervaded with a pulsing, alive, dynamic quality. You feel as if your blood has a lot of haemoglobin in it, a lot of pure oxygen, and you feel vibrant, vital and capable.[37]

Dynamism

Throughout this chapter I have been referring to Wood as an irrepressible, uprising energy that seeks expression in the world. From the perspective of the Diamond Approach, this is the dynamism of Being. Dynamism is the spontaneous and natural flow of Presence.

> In the human soul the Presence functions as the inspiring and motivating centre of initiative, action and creativity, and its intrinsic patterning functions as the guidance that directs that activity. This activity is totally spontaneous and free from the constricting influence of psychic structure.[38]

It is therefore possible, at higher levels of realisation, to directly perceive that the actions of all human beings are really the dynamic unfolding of the universe, with no inherent relationship to human ego.

If we bring this teaching back to the Five Elements, we could say that one of the highest spiritual Gifts of the Wood Element is to realise that all doing happens from the dynamic unfolding of Being. Thus, all of the gifts of Wood – the vision, planning, judging, deciding and acting – are not arising from us as separate individuals but as part of the unfolding of the whole universe.

Autonomy

Earlier we saw that individuation and healthy boundaries are essential to the development of a healthy Wood Element. They are also necessary for the development of a healthy ego structure. This is a normal and necessary part of human life. When we enter the spiritual path, we begin to realise that the ego perspective of the world becomes an obstacle to our realisation. It is not that the ego needs to be destroyed but that its perspective needs to be unmasked.

As we have said, the ego is never original and all its characteristics are distortions of something real and essential. Boundaries and individuation at the ego level, while they are a necessary part of human development, are nevertheless distortions of True Autonomy.

> From the perspective of the man of spirit, however, one is actually a Being independent from mind, existing outside the field of memory. From this perspective, the accomplishment of ego autonomy is ultimately a prison. In identifying with the self-image constructed through the process of ego development, we cage ourselves. How can this be autonomy, this bondage which is the primary source of human suffering?[39]

Almaas teaches that True Autonomy comes from expressing the fullness of Being through one's Personal Essence. This Personal Essence is actually Presence operating as a person, but in a way that is independent of the person's personal history. True Nature acts through our particular location as the Personal Essence which is not related to our ego structure. 'The sense of freedom, independence, autonomy and individuation is experienced at such times as a very clear, precise and certain fact. There is no vagueness or uncertainty about autonomy when one recognizes the Personal Essence as one's true being.'[40]

If you want to make God laugh, make plans.

ANONYMOUS

Activity: Taking an Aim

One of the greatest difficulties of any practice, be it a spiritual practice such as meditation, or a more mundane practice like exercising, is maintaining a consistent practice over time. This requires discipline and commitment, both of which are very difficult to maintain on our own without the support of others. This is why so many people practise in groups: meditation groups, yoga classes, fitness training groups, Weight Watchers, 12-Step programs.

Remember all the New Year's resolutions you have made over the years? How many of those have you maintained? Often these resolutions are made with hope but without real commitment. Mostly they are unrealistic goals and are made without thought for how much support is going to be needed to carry them through.

The practice of taking an aim is a bit like a New Year's resolution, but with more consciousness. We can utilise many of the Gifts of Wood in this practice: clarity, vision, planning and wise judgement.

There are a number of things to consider when framing an aim:

- Be as specific as you can.

  Be very clear about the specific details of your aim. Rather than, 'I'm going to start exercising tomorrow,' you might specify, 'I'm going to go to the gym three times a week and do my 30-minute training program followed by a 30-minute swim.'

  Why do you need to be so precise? Because after a while the part of you who doesn't want to exercise will try to wriggle out of the agreement. Having specific tasks, times and frequencies makes it harder for the part who doesn't want to exercise to argue her way out of it.

- Is this a realistic goal?

  Let's say you want to firm up your meditation practice, so you take an aim to meditate every morning for 30 minutes. How realistic is that? What happens when you don't sleep well one night and are too tired to be bothered going to the cushion? Or you have a six o'clock plane to catch and simply don't have the time that day. Maybe it would be more realistic to say, 'I will meditate at least five mornings a week.' And is 30 minutes realistic for you? Maybe that's what your teacher suggested and what your friends do, but is it right for you? Perhaps starting with 20 or even ten minutes is more achievable at first. You can always take another aim later to increase your commitment.

  Another important question is how long are you going to have this aim? It's probably not realistic to think you will have this practice forever. Our lives change after all. So setting a time frame for the aim is both realistic and trackable. For example, 'I am going to go to the yoga class in town twice a week for the next month.' Remember you can always renew your aim at the end of that time.

- Who's going to check on you?

  Aims taken by ourselves do not have the strength of those made in the presence of others. Frame your aim in the presence of at least one other friend. You are making a public commitment. You are taking a vow so you need a witness to your commitment. This person then has the responsibility of checking in with you from time to time as to how your aim is going, and you know that you will be accountable to that person.

Another very important role for your witness is that she can help you to frame an aim that is specific and realistic. Your friend will know you well enough to know whether you are likely to be able to keep your commitment. For example, you decide to give up chocolate altogether because you're putting on too much weight. Your friend just knows you will relapse on that so she persuades you to begin by taking the aim of not having chocolate on weekdays.

• The importance of succeeding.

This is the ultimate reason for all of the above. We need to be specific, realistic and have support so that we will succeed in our aim. Success increases our sense of strength, our self-esteem, our capacity to carry through on our commitment. Succeeding in one aim makes us more likely to succeed in other aims in future, whereas failing in an aim can lead to a diminishment of these qualities.

Think of it like a high-jump competition. Start with the bar at a low enough level that you are pretty confident you can succeed. Afterwards, you can raise the bar so that the aim becomes more challenging, but you have the confidence to try based on your previous successes.

And finally, celebrate your success!

May all your problems be as short lived as your New Year's resolutions.

ANONYMOUS

Acupressure for Spiritual Health

In the first section on the physical level of Wood, we learned the source points of the Gall Bladder and Liver meridians. The source points are very useful for healing the organs themselves. Here we look at the outer shu point of the Liver. Located on the back, along the Bladder meridian, this point heals our Wood at the level of mind and spirit. It is even more powerful when held in combination with the source point LV 3.

BL 47 *Hunmen* Spiritual Soul Gate

BL 47 *Hunmen* Spiritual Soul Gate is located about two fingers' width below the bottom of the shoulder blade and four fingers' width out from the spine. It is level with the space between the ninth and tenth thoracic vertebrae.

Hun, as in the point name, is the spirit of the Wood Element, our spiritual or ethereal soul. It is the spirit that offers us the gifts of creativity, imagination, clarity, vision, planning, decision-making and good judgement. Moreover, it reveals our true path in life, and gives us the motivation and clear sight to follow that path.

When the *hun* is sick, these qualities are less available to us and we may become cloudy, confused, frustrated, directionless, indecisive or depressed. In short, our Wood becomes unrooted. We lose our way in the world. Things look pointless and hopeless, and we may sink into lethargic inertia.

At the physical level, an imbalance in the *hun* impacts the liver organ; conversely, damage to the liver impacts the *hun*. One of the functions of the liver is to purify the blood of toxins. Toxicity resulting from drugs, alcohol, medication or chemicals not only affects the organ of the liver but the gifts associated with a healthy *hun*. Thus, drugs and contaminants affect our ability to see clearly, make good judgements and decisions, know what is fair and just, and act decisively.

Hunmen is a great point for cleansing the liver organ, treating addictions and supporting the healthy functioning of the spirit of Wood. By clearing away this stagnation in the Liver Qi, *Hunmen* can resurrect the spirit and activate the core of a person's being.

This point also treats sleep disturbances and insomnia by settling the *hun* spirit during the time of sleep and allowing us to access the wisdom of dreams as they pertain to our life purpose.

When anger and resentment have solidified and been turned inward upon oneself, *Hunmen* can be used to release and mobilise this energy into the service of taking action. Wood that has become rigid and inert can become supple and active, providing the means to express the uniqueness of our individual self in the world.

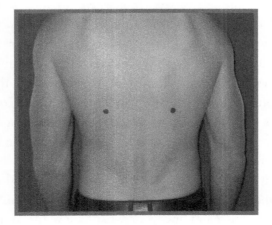

Figure 7.8 The outer shu point of the Liver
(BL 47 *Hunmen* Spiritual Soul Gate)

Meditation: Sensing Arms and Legs

When we meditate, we often come to a place of quiet stillness as we unhook from the thought stream of our ego mind. Even if we don't come to the quiet place, we usually have a deeper awareness of what is going on in our mind. But it is a great challenge to take this contactful awareness with us once we get up from our chair or cushion. This is because our ego is completely entwined with our body. We tend to view our body as the basis of who we are and identify with it thoroughly. Therefore, we also take the actions of our body to be who we are. As soon as we begin to move into action, even just standing up from our chair, let alone cooking breakfast, driving to work and doing a job, we tend immediately to lose contact with our true self and drop straight back into the small, separate, ego self.

It is said that functioning as Being rather than from ego is a very advanced state of self-realisation, so we shouldn't be hard on ourselves if we are not able to be our true selves in our doing. Even Sufi masters with a high level of self-realisation have observed that they still had not yet reached this stage of development.

The practice below brings greater awareness to the primary tools of functioning, our arms and legs. Continued dedication to this practice helps us to take the awareness we have in our sitting meditation into our functioning life so that our doing can gradually become a part of our being.

The Practice[41]

Find a comfortable position in a chair with your feet on the floor, sitting upright and relaxed. Feel your bottom in the seat of the chair. Rest your hands on your thighs. Take a few breaths down into your belly centre.

Now, bring your attention to your right foot and notice the sensations there. Feel the sensations in the sole of your foot where it contacts the floor, feel the arch of your foot, top of your foot and your ankle. Now allow the awareness to flow upwards into your lower leg, feeling the sensations in your calf muscles, your shin muscles and your knee. Allow the awareness to move up into your upper leg and notice the physical sensations in your hamstrings where they're contacting your chair, and your quads where your hands are resting. Become aware of the physical sensations in your upper leg, and now your hip joint and the sit bone where your weight presses into the chair. So now you have an awareness of the sensations in the whole of your right leg.

Without losing contact with this awareness of your leg, shift your focus to your right hand where it rests on your leg. Feel the sensation in your palm, your fingers, the back of your hand and your wrist. Allow the awareness to spread upwards into your forearm and into the elbow. Now you feel the sensations in your upper arm, the biceps and triceps muscles. And now the shoulder joint enters your field of awareness so that you are now aware of the sensations in the whole of your right arm and right leg.

Without losing contact with these sensations, move your attention now to the left shoulder and notice the sensations there, and the left upper arm. It is as if your awareness is flowing and spreading down the arm, through the elbow, the forearm and into the hand and fingers.

The awareness now flows into your left hip socket, down into your upper leg where you feel the sensations of your leg on the chair and your hand on your leg. The awareness flows gradually into the knee joint, down into the lower leg, the calves and shins, the ankle, and finally into the foot: the arch, the top of the foot, the sole on the floor and the toes.

You are now holding all of your limbs in your field of awareness of sensation: both arms, both legs.

Now bring your attention to your hearing, adding a new sense of awareness. Become aware of the sounds in the room and outside.

And finally, without losing contact with the sensations in your limbs, add the sense of looking to your awareness as you open your eyes.

Imagine as you get up from your chair that you are taking this sense of awareness out into the world as you move into doing.

Transition from Wood to Fire

As spring transitions to summer there is a qualitative change in the way nature looks and feels. The rapid, uprising, often erratic and unpredictable energy of Wood begins to level out. Nature has gone through its most rapid growth from tender sprout to fully grown plant, and the speed of growth begins to slow down. Likewise, the rapid acceleration in the length of the daylight hours also begins to slow. In ourselves, the sense of strongly uprising Qi may be replaced by a feeling of outward expansiveness.

The sun rises quite early now and tries to coax us out of bed earlier than in spring. The days are much longer and the increasing warmth persuades us to shed layers of clothing, to wear lighter and brighter-coloured garments. The temperatures are no longer simply warm but hot. The strength of the sun is noticeably more intense, encouraging us to wear hats and sunscreen. The night comes later, especially if there is daylight saving, encouraging us to stay outdoors and enjoy the lengthening days. Evenings are warm, and there are no longer the cool nights of spring.

In this transition, nature offers us an invitation to come out, to be outdoors more, to be more expansive, both physically and emotionally. This sense of expansiveness leads naturally to a desire to spend more time with others. The start of summer marks the beginning of the barbecue season, street parties, garage sales and get-togethers of all kinds. Calendars begin to fill up as invitations to social activities surge.

As the energy of Fire begins to replace that of Wood, we may notice more activity in the heart centre, prompting us to seek more human contact and to have more fun in the process.

After spending these months exploring the qualities of the Wood Element within you, you have been developing a healthier Wood, healing the gnarled and creaky places in yourself. A healthy Wood Element gives birth to a healthy Fire Element. The work you have done in the spring season will serve as a platform for continued exploration, growth and healing in the summer. As the season transitions to summer and the Fire phase, you will be much better equipped to move into the expansive, loving, heart-oriented Element of Fire.

Ready to fly?

Chapter 8 _____

Fire

The Nature of Fire

The movement of Fire is outwards.

The archetypal image of this Element is the hearth fire. In prehistoric times the human discovery of fire provided a central source of warmth and light, a place for cooking and a means of protection. The tribe gathered around the fire which engendered community and social contact. Even when humans began to settle in villages and live in houses, the hearth fire became the central focus of the home, a place not just for physical heat but for human warmth. Today few people have indoor fires, but campfires and bonfires remain an irresistible draw.

Ultimately, all fire originates from the sun, the biggest, brightest and hottest fire in our world. All fuel for earthly fires originates from the energy of the sun, trapped and stored in the trees.

The various ways that flames and fires behave offer illustrations of the qualities of the Fire Element. As the most yang of the Elements, Fire most exhibits the qualities of yang: hot, bright, expansive, active. To begin with, flames dart and leap out in unexpected ways and they go out in all directions. Fire is hot and bright. It can be explosive and bursting like a firework and as overwhelming as a raging bushfire. It can be a fast-burning grassfire that burns itself out quickly, or the slow quiet heat of embers. When fire goes out it leaves cold grey ashes.

The Chinese character for Fire is *huo* (see Figure 8.1). It represents ascending flames.[1] The flames go out in all directions, a reminder that the fundamental nature of Fire is to move outwards. When I look at this symbol I see a childlike stick figure of a person running with arms outstretched, fully open to the world.

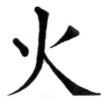

Figure 8.1 The Chinese character for Fire

The Resonances of Fire

The Season: Summer

The Fire Element is most easily observed in nature as the season of summer. Following the rapid upward growth of spring, it is as if nature is now reaching outwards to fill as much space as it can. Like a ball tossed in the air which reaches its apogee before descending, summer is the highest peak of growth when things can grow no further and seem to hang in mid-air for a time, celebrating the fullness of expansion.

Summer is the hottest time of the year because at this time the sun's rays hit the earth at a steep angle. The light does not spread out as much, thus increasing the amount of energy hitting any given spot. Also, the long daylight hours allow the earth plenty of time to reach warm temperatures. Likewise, it is the brightest time of the year, with the sun at its highest elevation. Heat and light. Hot and bright. These are intrinsic qualities of summer and of Fire.

When does summer begin? This depends on your latitude and climate. In temperate climates you can expect to feel the beginnings of summer in early May or early November depending on your hemisphere. This is a month earlier than what is usually considered to be the start of summer, but the first hints of a season are often the most potent in their effects upon us. The transition between spring and summer can be a challenge for some people, an indication of imbalances in Fire.

The cross-quarter days were celebrated in European traditions. May Day, the first day of that month, was celebrated with maypole dancing. It lies roughly halfway between the spring equinox and the summer solstice and was celebrated in pre-Christian Europe as the start of summer. This accords with the traditional Chinese almanac, the *Tong Shu*. This cross-quarter day marks the beginning of a deceleration in the lengthening of the daylight hours.

If you live closer to the equator, summer will come earlier, while if you live closer to the poles, your summer will be later. You can look for the signs of summer within yourself. As the days become warmer, you will wear fewer clothes, and this makes for a feeling of relaxed expansiveness. You will probably find your social calendar gets busier as invitations to summer parties and events jostle with one another for attention. Like the natural movement of Fire, your view tends to turn outwards to relationship and community.

The Sense: Speech (Touch)

It is becoming clear that the Fire Element is strongly connected to relationships with others. Perhaps the most direct vehicle for humans to connect with one another is through language and speech. The tongue is vital to this process of communication. Speech is therefore the sense of the Fire Element and the tongue its sense organ.[2] This refers not to the tongue as it is used for tasting, but its power to enable speaking. Words communicate the feelings of the heart and the content of the mind. We will see later that, to the ancients, heart and mind are one and the same.

In the West we speak of the five senses of hearing, sight, taste, smell and touch. While the first four of these align neatly with the Elements of Water, Wood, Earth and Metal respectively, it is the sense of speech that is allocated to Fire and touch is not included. Nonetheless, the sense of touch is dependent on the heartmind[3] as this is responsible for the cognition and organisation of external stimuli sensations.[4]

Touch is certainly in vibrational alignment with the Fire Element. It is a primary component of most relationships, from the handshake to the hug to the tender embrace. It is no accident that all of the Fire meridians travel along the arms and hands, providing a medium for sensing the world and communicating the feelings of the heart.

Summer brings with it an increase in group events, and consequently our communication increases. We tend to be more outgoing and have more opportunities to talk. With the increase in daylight hours we are likely to stay up later and spend more time interacting. While winter draws our attention inward and spring brings our focus to action, summer invites us to move outwards towards others. The ambient energy of the summer season is supportive of connecting though speech.

When the Fire Element is out of balance, one of the ways it can show up is in speech disorders. This can be a physical anomaly such as tongue tie which decreases the mobility of the tongue or lisping that comes from an oral deformity or medical condition. Many speech disorders have a psychological origin. Stuttering affects about 1% of the population. It is characterised by involuntary repetition or prolongation of words, hesitation or silent pauses that affect the flow of speech. Causes of this are anxiety, stress, shock or trauma. From the Chinese medicine perspective, all of these are manifestations of imbalance in the Heart.

The film *The King's Speech* (2010) brought to light the impact that childhood events can have on speech. King George VI stuttered badly when making public speeches. The roots of this speech disorder included his relationship with his overbearing father.

At the other end of the spectrum, Fire imbalance can reveal itself as an overabundance of speech. Not only are there a lot of words but they are delivered at breakneck speed. The speaker bounces around from subject to subject in a chaotic fashion that can be quite exhausting for the listener.

The Colour: Red

While the nature of the Fire Element is to proliferate, it might be surprising to consider that its colour, red, is one of the rarer colours in nature. Perhaps it appears so sparingly because it is such an intense colour. Yet its rarity is more than compensated by its vivid visibility. A red sunset captivates us. Flashes of red on birds' wings grab our attention. Red fruits, such as strawberries, raspberries and red apples, leap out from bushes or trees. Red flowers, such as red roses, bottlebrush, poinsettia and hibiscus all stand out strikingly.

Red sports cars are highly noticeable, especially to the police. People with red hair stand out because of their rarity (1–2%) and are stereotypically famous for their fiery nature. Red is the colour of our blood. It is the colour most commonly associated with joy, love, warmth, passion and sexuality, all of which are associations of the Fire Element. Because of its attention-getting qualities, red is universally used as a warning colour, something which can be traced back to Roman times.

How do you feel when you wear red? If you are always wearing red or hate wearing the colour, it may indicate an imbalance in your Fire. Is there any red in your home? A lot of red can be overpowering, but some red within the house brings Fire into your life. According to feng shui principles, it is good to have some red on the Fire wall of a room, the one facing you as you enter.

In Five Element Acupuncture diagnosis, the colour red at the sides of the eyes indicates a Fire Constitution. However, much more commonly seen is a 'lack of red', a kind of grey, ashen colour that is more usually diagnostic of a Fire type of person.

The Sound: Laughing

Whether it is a chuckle, a giggle, a guffaw or a good belly laugh, the sound of Fire is laughter which emanates from the heart. Consistent with the nature of the Element, laughter fizzes up like champagne bubbles rising to the surface and popping, or bursts out unexpectedly and explosively. Laughter is a universal language. While there are thousands of languages and dialects, the way all humans laugh is remarkably similar.

Laughter is used as a signal for being part of a group, indicating acceptance and positive interactions with others. Laughter is sometimes seen as contagious, and the laughter of one person can itself provoke laughter from others, creating a positive feedback loop.

Children laugh much more frequently than adults; adulthood is often seen as being a much more serious business. Interestingly, many Fire types look younger than their years, as if the tendency to laughter keeps them more connected to a childlike state.

The sound of someone's voice is diagnostic of their Constitutional Element. The laughing voice carries the emotion of joy. A person of Fire constitution has a laughing voice. Sometimes it sounds as if the person is being tickled and is about to burst into laughter. The voice can seem to be rising up, as if lighter than air. These qualities will be present even when the person is not talking about something enjoyable or funny.

Sometimes a Fire person will have an overall flat voice, as if the joy has gone out of their life. In this case, the voice will have a conspicuous absence of laughter and sound like a flat monotone with no sense of enjoyment of life.

The Odour: Scorched

The resonance of odour is the third of the diagnostic tools in determining a person's Constitutional Element. People of a Fire constitution have a scorched odour emanating from their skin. When the person is in good health, this odour is faint and light, like the smell of dry grass in summer. When there is imbalance in the person's health, the odour becomes stronger, like a garment scorched by an iron, or even like burnt toast. The scorched odour is the lightest of the five odours and often the most difficult to catch.

The odour arises from the organs of the Element not doing their job optimally. In this case the Heart Protector and Triple Heater are the 'organs' that are under stress, producing an imbalance in the heating system of the body and thus the smell of something burning.

The Emotion: Joy

The movement of Fire is outwards, so it is natural that its emotion will be expansive. The Fire Element is the highest point of the cycle, so you would expect its emotion to be 'out there'. We speak of bursting with joy and jumping for joy. It is associated with music, dance and parties, all outward moving expressions of an inner feeling of well-being.

Many people, when they come to the Five Element model for the first time, see joy as a positive emotion compared with emotions like anger (Wood) and fear (Water) which are considered negative. Many people feel they would rather be identified as Fire types. But this misunderstands the fact that the predominant emotion indicates where someone is most challenged. For the Fire type, there is a fundamental challenge around joy. Either there is a tendency to seek joy most of the time, avoiding thinking or talking about things that bring the mood down, or there is a tendency for joy to be absent, even when it would be appropriate and expected.

The resonance of emotion is the fourth of the diagnostic tools of the Five Element practitioner. When there is a sense of something being not quite right or off-note in the area of a person's joy, this suggests a Fire constitution.

When we are in a situation which engenders happiness or pleasure, we tend to smile and laugh and our voice becomes animated. When the situation changes, these responses also change to be congruent with what is happening. But when the joy continually goes out of control and turns into overexcitement or even hysteria, the practitioner notices an incongruence or inappropriateness in the joy. Likewise, an off-note can be observed in a flat joylessness that pervades the person's life. We will look at this in more detail in the section 'The Emotional Landscape of Fire'.

The Gifts of Fire

The Gifts of an Element are those qualities which are available when that Element is in harmony and balance within us. When the Element is out of balance, these qualities become less available or distorted. The Gifts of Fire are quite varied in their expression. This comes from the fact that Fire has four meridians instead of the usual two, and its four Officials provide a broad range of capacities.

As you read about these qualities, consider how much you are in touch with them in your own life and where you might have room for expansion.

Love

Perhaps more words have been written and spoken about love than any other subject. Certainly it is a major focus in books and music. There is no simple definition of love because it has different meanings in different contexts. There are many kinds of love.

We can say we love certain foods, like ice cream or chocolate, we love our hobbies or our work, we love our pets, we love our neighbours, we love our family, we love our partner, we love the earth, we love God. Maybe it is because the word 'love' is used in so many different contexts that confusion arises. We are actually talking about different things.

What unites all of these different kinds of love is the fact that the more you love something, the more you want to know about it and the more you want to be with it. Whether it be ice cream, surfing, your dog, your job or your lover, you love something when you want to be wrapped (or rapt) in it.

Whichever culture or system you look at, there seems to be universal agreement that love is associated with the heart. Whatever kind of love we are talking about, it is a state that is perceived by and expressed through the heart centre. Love is often experienced as a warmth or expansive feeling in the chest. This is a direct experience of the fact that the heart is the primary organ of the Fire Element. The extent to which we are able to feel love, receive love, give love or express love indicates the health of our Fire. We will be revisiting this crucial topic in later sections.

How easy is it for you to give love and receive love? What gets in the way of giving and receiving love?

Relationship

There is no doubt that humans are social beings. Very few people are comfortable being totally solitary. Almost everyone has a need for social interaction. This means relating to others in some way, making connections and forming relationships. These activities are the province of the Fire Element and the ease or difficulty we have in this area of life tells us a lot about the health of our Fire.

There are many levels of relationship. We form relationships with people like shopkeepers, our barista, hairdresser or postman. These are people we don't know all that well but whom we see fairly often. There are relationships with work colleagues, people we do not really choose but with whom we must interact. We have friends of various kinds: neighbours, peripheral friends, close friends, best friends. We have relationships with family: parents, grandparents, children, grandchildren, siblings, aunts, uncles and cousins. And there is relationship with a partner that usually involves close physical intimacy and long-term commitment.

All relationships provide us with something we need whether it is the simple pleasure of interacting with a stranger, the feeling of connection and belonging to a family or social group, the deep joy of birthing and raising children, the bliss of sexual union or the deep bonds of a long-term partnership.

Yet relationships at all these levels are often difficult. There is an old saying: 'Can't live with them, can't live without them.' Why is this so? While we still have an ego, and that includes most of us, we will continue to project onto others all kinds of assumptions and beliefs. We see others not for who they are but through a distorted lens created by our history. We love one person because they remind us of a good parent, we hate another because they look like a bad parent. It is impossible to see others for who they really are while we have these obscurations of the past distorting our view. When we begin to interact with another, we have all kinds of reactions to how they are, what they are saying and doing that are all based on our history and self-images. Relationship from ego is a chaos of interacting histories.

You may be wondering, 'How is this a gift?' Relationships are the crucible in which humans can work out the still unconscious and unexplored parts of themselves. Every reaction you have to someone else is a clue to what is still unclarified in you. Whether it is getting irritated because hubby leaves the toilet seat up, or sad that a friend dumped you, or afraid that you won't be liked as you get older, all these reactions are nothing to do with the other person, but are all about you. They provide doorways to self-understanding and inner peace.

Ultimately, the way through all the difficulties of relating is through our heart. The heart knows how to simply be, and in that place of being there are no veils distorting the truth of ourselves or others.

 What is the right amount of relational contact for you? Do you tend to move towards others or away from others in relationships?

Intimacy

Intimacy is a quality that arises in relationships. It means different things to different people, and it means different things in different relationships. Intimacy with a good friend is expressed and felt quite differently from intimacy with a lover.

There is physical intimacy which involves touch and physical contact and often sexual interaction. There is emotional intimacy which involves a sharing of deep thoughts and feelings. There can be intellectual intimacy which involves close connection at a mental level, seen commonly in friendships. There can be spiritual intimacy in groups of like-minded followers of a religion or spiritual path.

What unites all of these expressions of intimacy is closeness and openness. There is both the choice to be intimate and the capacity to be intimate. Closeness can arise when there are feelings of trust and safety. You feel you can trust the other person to be respectful of your feelings and what you are choosing to share. Openness includes being vulnerable and self-disclosing. For intimacy to arise, there must be reciprocity. Both partners in the relationship must be willing to be mutually self-disclosing and vulnerable. The holding of secrets is generally inimical to intimacy in a committed relationship. The more trust, safety, candour and vulnerability there is in a relationship, the deeper the intimacy.

For there to be real intimacy, we first need to know ourselves. The more understanding we have of ourselves and the more we have developed a clear sense of who we are, the more able we are to share ourselves. Without this sense of self and the boundaries of self, the less able we are to bring that self to relationship. If we don't know who we are, then who is it who is in relationship?

The more we know about ourselves, the more we can be our authentic self in relationship, and the deeper the intimacy that is possible. The extent to which we are intimate with ourselves, we can be intimate with others.

Intimacy is often defined in terms of passion, and sexual intimacy means getting naked. While sex is one of the great delights of living in a human body, it is not by itself true intimacy. It is a physical expression of a much deeper intimacy that it is possible to experience. Real intimacy involves vulnerability, openness, closeness, contact, transparency and honesty, all of which make us naked on the inside. At this level of realness, we can be truly naked with all our clothes on.

What does it mean to you to be intimate? What are your limits to being intimate?

Sociability

So far we have been looking at close relationships. But also important in life are relationships with groups and the wider world. We are continually relating to groups of people, whether it is standing in line at the supermarket, activities with clubs, having dinner with friends, going to parties or having business meetings.

Some people are more comfortable in relating to one person, less so with groups. Others are happiest when interacting with groups. Why is this so? It is partly to do with the circumstances in which we grew up, whether there was good modelling for how to interact socially, and whether it was encouraged and supported by our family of origin. Culture also influences the ways people socialise. And there is the fact that some people are born socialisers for whom mixing with people is a prime focus of their lives. The Enneagram system, for example, recognises that there is a social subtype whose primary drive is towards the satisfaction of the social instinct.[5]

Whatever your personal history or culture, the ease or otherwise of interacting in groups is closely related to the health of the Fire Element, in particular what might be called the Outer Fire.[6] We will learn more later about the way the Triple Heater Official is responsible for mediating social relationships.

When this aspect of Fire is in balance and harmony, there is ease in social settings. There is the capacity to be friendly, warm and open in groups, a sense of relaxation and comfort without anxiety or defensiveness. At the same time there is an awareness of social propriety, of what is appropriate in the particular social and cultural context, and there are well-defined boundaries. This includes knowing the difference between how to act at a card night with the boys, a work social and a formal wedding reception. This means understanding how the relationships in these different settings require different sets of behaviours and interactions.

 Where are you on the sociability spectrum between recluse and socialite? How do you feel about being in groups of three, seven, 20, 100?

Discrimination
One of the capacities of Fire is to know what is good for you, what is not good for you and to make choices that reflect that knowledge. It also includes knowing that choice is both possible and necessary. This capacity derives from the Small Intestine Official whose task is to separate the pure from the impure, letting in what is good for the person and excluding what is bad.

This capacity of discrimination extends to all areas of life. At a physical level it appears as the ability to make good dietary and lifestyle choices that will nourish the body and are non-harmful. It also reflects in the choice of a place to live that is supportive and homely. In the sphere of work it manifests in the choice of occupation and workplace. The capacity to choose with discrimination is particularly important in the realm of relationships, from the friends we choose to spend time with, to the partner with whom we choose to spend our life. In the spiritual realm, it extends to choosing among various paths that support our quest for truth.

In the modern world we are literally spoiled for choice, in the food we eat, the clothes we wear, the car we drive, the events we attend, the bargains we buy. More recently we have become increasingly bombarded with information via the Internet and social media, and with Googling and blogging, texting and tweeting, inboxing and snapchatting, friending and unfriending, the need to make discriminating choices now multiplies dramatically.

The important thing to realise is that this ability to make good choices is necessary to protect the Heart. When the capacity to sort the good from the bad is challenged and harmful influences are let in, it is the Heart that suffers at all levels. Whether it is a plate of food that does not suit us, a person whose influence is bad or a habit that is destructive, when harmful things are let through to the Heart, the ruler of our inner kingdom is hurt in some way. A good discriminating mind is essential to protect our whole realm.

How easy is it to know what is good for you? How would you rate your sorting skill?

Communication

A healthy Fire imbues us with ease and skill in communicating with others. When Fire is in balance, its sense organ, the tongue, moves smoothly and effortlessly to convey our thoughts through words and sounds. Communication comes easily from the heartmind to be received by the heartmind of the listener. The flow of words is appropriate for the listener, neither too rapid nor too slow. There is an attuned awareness of the other's capacity to receive the communication. At the same time the expression is a reflection of the speaker's uniqueness. There is a free expression of truth while at the same time being attuned to the truth of the other.

Communication occurs not only through words. When the words come from the heart, the tone of voice carries the feelings behind the words and there is awareness of the feelings being communicated. The eyes express emotions too and are another vehicle of communication.

Other non-verbal communication happens through touch, especially as it is conveyed through the arms, hands and fingers. We reveal much about ourselves in a simple handshake, even more in the ways we hug other people. A gentle touch on the arm can communicate caring and compassion. A holding embrace can demonstrate support. A long embrace might show love or desire.

All of these different ways of communicating are the province of the Fire Element, the Heart and its attendant Officials. When they are in healthy balance, communication is aware, adept and alive.

Which is your best channel in communicating with others – words, touch or looks? In what way do you like to receive communication?

Intuition

It has already been mentioned that Fire is the most yang of the Elements. This means it is the most ethereal, the lightest, fastest and brightest of all. Like lightning, it moves with rapid brilliancy. It can connect dots with great speed. It has great awareness of all that is.

Intuition is the capacity to understand something immediately without conscious reasoning. This is not to say there is no rational component, but the reasoning happens so fast that it is below consciousness. Deductions are made and conclusions reached without there having been an awareness of thinking.

Insight is a similar quality, the ability to apprehend the true meaning and nature of something whether it is a person, an idea or a situation. The ancient Greek philosophers used the word *nous* to denote this quality. Insight, like intuition, appears fully formed without a conscious reasoning process. It is the caricature of the light bulb above a person's head, the 'a-ha' moment, the 'Eureka!'. The expression, 'a flash of insight' gives a clue to its Fire-like nature.

People of a Fire constitution, when they are functioning at their best, have access to these qualities in a way that can make them seem highly intuitive or even psychic. Since relationship is a major focus of attention for Fire types, they can bring these capacities to interpersonal interactions in a way that can sometimes seem as if they know what you are thinking. Maybe they do, for the gifts of Fire offer access to the nature of Heaven itself.

These gifts are not the monopoly of Fire people, however. For everyone, when Fire is in perfect balance and harmony, there is the potential to apprehend the nature of all things.

In what areas of life are you intuitive and insightful? What gets in the way of your intuition?

And More…

The gifts we have looked at here are just a few of the many qualities that the Fire Element has to offer. Here are more to consider. Think or write about how much these qualities show up in your life and how much they are available to you.

Awareness	Connection	Desire
Community	Delight	Enthusiasm

Expression	Inspiration	Sexuality
Fun	Optimism	Spontaneity
Harmony	Partnership	Touch
Humour	Passion	Warmth

Journal Entry: 1 December 2011

Tadpoles

What a delight to discover a teeming of tadpoles in the top pond! Today, passing by the fishponds, I noticed a lot of bubbles in the water and stopped to investigate. There were dozens, no wait, scores, no hang on, *hundreds* of tadpoles. Seeing the water level was low, I filled the pond with water from the rain tank to give them more room to swim about. In their reaction, they ringed the edge of the pond, wriggling in a vain attempt to get out. So many were there that they stacked shoulder to shoulder right around the perimeter.

Googling revealed they like fish food and lettuce. Experiments showed that they are partial to the dust from the chicken food pellets. When I fed them, hundreds of tiny mouths broke the surface, gulping down my offerings.

Why am I so delighted with my new pets? A childhood pastime I never had: no playing in the creek for little Johnny.

So now I get to have my childhood pleasure, fresh and clear as an early summer's day, full of joy and playfulness and delight at the teeming creation of Heaven.

The Physical Level of Fire

Now that we have a sense of the resonances and qualities of the Fire Element, let us look at the ways they manifest themselves in the physical body. The ways in which we respond to the vibrations of the Fire Element will influence the ways in which it materialises in our organs and tissues.

The Fire Element is unique in that there are four organs and meridians associated with it instead of the usual two. This accords with Fire's burgeoning nature. It is also because the Heart, the most important organ in the body, needs more support and protection from its partner organs. The ancients saw the Heart as the emperor of the kingdom with the other three organs providing successive levels of defence and protection.

Organs and Tissues

The Heart

WESTERN MEDICAL PERSPECTIVE

The heart is an organ about twice the size of a fist. It is composed of cardiac muscle and connective tissue and lies in the chest between the vertebrae and the sternum. Its function is to pump blood around the circulatory system by regular contractions in order to provide oxygen and nutrients to all the cells of the body. The simplicity of this description belies its immense significance to the human body. While many other organs are vital to our health, the heart is indispensable. On average it beats 70 times a minute which means it will beat about three billion times over the life of someone who reaches their eighties. Any interruption to this steady beat is dangerous to health. And if the heart stops for more than a few minutes, our life is over.

The importance of this organ to the body and to life makes it a primary concern in medical practice. A heart attack occurs when there is an interruption to the blood supply to the heart. Deaths from coronary heart disease are dropping, with increases in survival rates among older people, but it is still the most common cause of death.[7]

The heart is a part of the cardiovascular system, which also includes the blood vessels, specifically the arteries, veins and capillaries. The health of these vessels through which the blood is pumped by the heart is no less important to health. A hardening or narrowing of the arteries by plaque build-up (arteriosclerosis) increases the risk of both heart attack and stroke. High blood pressure (hypertension) also increases these risks.

CHINESE MEDICINE PERSPECTIVE

The Heart is the yin organ of the Fire Element. The Chinese character for the Heart is *xin*. Unlike the characters for all the other organs, it does not contain the radical meaning 'flesh'.[8] The ancient Chinese understood that the Heart governs the Blood and the blood vessels, but more importantly for them the Heart was a space in which resides the *shen*, that which is both spirit and mind. Other functions of the Heart are that it manifests in the complexion, opens into the tongue, controls the sweat and is affected by excessive joy, hyper-excitement or shock.[9]

Governs Blood and blood vessels. As in Western medicine, the Heart is responsible for the circulation of Blood throughout the tissues of the body. In addition, the state of the Heart and the Blood determine the strength of a person's constitution. A weakness in the Heart sometimes shows as a long, shallow crack in the midline of the tongue.

The condition of the Heart also directly influences the condition of the blood vessels; therefore, the condition of the blood vessels reveals the state of the Heart.

Houses the shen. The classics likened the Heart to a benevolent monarch or emperor ruling over the other organs. 'The Heart holds the office of lord and sovereign. The radiance of the spirits stems from it.'[10] When the sovereign is healthy and rules well, all other Officials and organs can do their jobs properly. But when the sovereign is not well, the functioning of the whole court or body is impaired.

Radiates virtue. Another important feature of the Heart as sovereign is that it does not actively do anything. Rather, it radiates virtue by simply being itself. Thus, the nature of the Heart is simply to *be* rather than to *do*. 'A healthy Heart with no obstructions does nothing other than allow our sprit to rest peacefully within it.'[11] *Shen* is the spirit of the Fire Element. As the most yang of the spirits, it is the one closest to Heaven. Indeed, it is the Heavenly light of awareness and consciousness residing in the heart of each one of us. When the heart is healthy, it provides a place for the *shen* to rest. But when the heart is unhealthy, disturbed and unsettled, the *shen* flies away like a flock of birds startled by a commotion. We will look more closely at the *shen* in the section 'The Spiritual Level of Fire'.

Small Intestine

WESTERN MEDICAL PERSPECTIVE

The small intestine is the part of the digestive tract that comes after the stomach and before the large intestine. Its primary function is the absorption of nutrients from food. The 'small' refers to the diameter of the intestine, 2.5 cm (1 in), rather than its length, for it averages 6.4 m (21 ft) in length and lies coiled in the abdominal cavity.[12]

It consists of three parts: the duodenum, the jejunum and the ileum. The duodenum is the first 25 cm (10 in) of the small intestine where food is broken down by enzymes. The jejunum is about 2.5 m (8 ft) in length and has a special lining which allows the absorption of carbohydrate and protein after their breakdown in the duodenum. The final portion is the ileum, about 3.6 m (12 ft) and joins the large intestine at the ileocaecal valve. Its job is to absorb vitamin

B12 and complete the process of absorption of remaining nutrients in the food. The waste matter then passes into the large intestine.

CHINESE MEDICINE PERSPECTIVE
The Small Intestine is the yang organ of Fire and so is partner to the Heart. At the physical level, the Chinese perspective is similar to the Western. The Small Intestine receives food and drink from the Stomach, which it separates into a 'clean' part and a 'dirty' part. The clean part is transported by the Spleen to nourish all tissues in the body while the dirty part is transferred to the Bladder and Large Intestine for excretion.[13] Therefore, the primary functions are receiving, sorting or separating, and transforming.

Of all the yin/yang organ pairings, the one between Heart and Small Intestine is the most tenuous at the physical level, though there is a growing body of evidence which links poor absorption of nutrients with some mental disorders including depression and schizophrenia.[14]

Sorting. The capacity of the Small Intestine Official to separate the pure from the impure at the physiological level also extends to the psychological level. It is this Official, sometimes called the Sorter, which is responsible for sorting out what is good for us and what is not good at many levels. In our modern world we are constantly subjected to barrages of information and stimuli which we need to sort through or risk becoming overwhelmed. The Small Intestine Official is responsible for this process of discrimination. Not only does it have the ability to make choices, but it has the knowledge that choice is necessary.

This process of choosing what to let in and what to screen out by making discriminating choices applies to many areas of life: dietary choices, the friends we choose to spend time with, the person we choose as a partner, how we spend our time, how we arrange our surroundings and how we manage our online presence. It is a kind of gatekeeper which filters out things that are harmful to our health and well-being. Without a healthy Sorter, we lose the ability to choose what is good for us and we let in things which are harmful to our Heart. In extreme cases, when the Sorter lets everything through, the resulting chaos can be overwhelming.

If you have read about the functions of the Gall Bladder Official in the Wood chapter, you may be wondering how the Gall Bladder's function of deciding differs from the Small Intestine's function of choosing. The Gall Bladder gives us the courage to decide between known options, while the Small Intestine allows us to have clarity of mind and an awareness of the choices available to us.[15]

Heart Protector (Pericardium)

WESTERN MEDICAL PERSPECTIVE

The pericardium is not an organ, but rather a structure, in Western anatomy. It is a double-walled sac which surrounds and protects the heart. Between its walls lies a fluid which acts as a shock absorber, protecting the heart from jolts, jerks and shocks. Another protective function is to prevent infections spreading from other organs, such as the lungs. The pericardium also anchors the heart in place and prevents it from overfilling with blood.

CHINESE MEDICINE PERSPECTIVE

The Heart Protector (also known as the Pericardium) and the Triple Heater are not organs in the usual sense and are often referred to as the functions of the Fire Element to distinguish them from the organs of Heart and Small Intestine. The Heart Protector is the yin organ/function and its capacities are closely related to those of the Heart. The term 'Heart Protector' describes its primary role.

At a physical level, the Heart Protector has a strong influence over the chest and in women has a relationship to the uterus and menstrual function. J.R. Worsley referred to it as the circulation/sex meridian, reflecting its role in circulating Blood and expressing the loving feelings associated with sexuality. Perhaps most significant is its role at the psycho-emotional level in protecting the emotional heart.

Guardian of the Heart. In the classics, the Heart Protector Official is described as the ambassador of the Heart, and joy and pleasure arise when it is functioning well.[16] Other interpretations describe it as a gatekeeper in charge of a pair of doors, or a drawbridge to a castle. There is an acupoint on the forearm (HP 6) called Inner Frontier Gate which graphically describes this role.

From these analogies we can see that the Heart Protector protects the Heart by regulating the level of intimacy in various relationships. It manages the degree to which the doors of the Heart are open in different interactions. For example, we open ourselves to our close friends in ways we are not open with shopkeepers, and we open our heart to our lover in ways we do not open it to our friends.

When the Heart Protector is healthy and the doors are operating smoothly, then there is open-heartedness at a level appropriate to each relationship contact. When there is an imbalance, the doors can become stuck closed or jammed open. When the Heart Protector is too closed, the person seems to lack warmth or is hard to reach emotionally. This state is often the result of very painful relationship experiences, betrayal or abuse. The doors close tight to avoid risking such pain again. When the Heart Protector is too open, the person is very sensitive and easily hurt or rejected. The expression 'wearing your heart on your sleeve' describes this oversensitivity. This approach to life derives from a great need to feel loved, and intimacy is sought at any opportunity. While open-heartedness may be a fine goal, in practice it can lead to a letting in of influences that are harmful to the Heart.

Triple Heater
WESTERN MEDICAL PERSPECTIVE
There is nothing in Western medicine that corresponds to the function of the Triple Heater. The concept that most closely approaches this organ/function is that of homeostasis. This is the capacity of the body to regulate its internal environment and to maintain a stable, relatively constant condition of properties such as temperature and pH.

CHINESE MEDICINE PERSPECTIVE
The Triple Heater is the yang organ/function of Fire and as such is partner to the Heart Protector. The Chinese term for this is *sanjiao* which is translated variously as Triple Heater, Triple Warmer, Triple Burner, Three Heater or Three Burning Spaces. The nature of the Triple Heater has been the subject of much controversy and debate over centuries. While it is included among the yang organs in the classical texts, there is no place you can point to and say, 'There is the Triple Heater.' Here we look at some of the main properties of this elusive 'organ'.

The Three Burning Spaces. The concept of a burning space comes from the idea of a transforming process like cooking. Indeed, part of the character for the Triple Heater is a chicken roasting over flames.[17] The burners are responsible for receiving, transforming and distributing air and food. The upper burner is located in the chest above the diaphragm and contains the Heart, Heart Protector and Lungs. Its main physiological process is the distribution of fluids by the Lungs. The middle burner is in the upper abdomen and contains the Liver, Gall Bladder, Stomach and Spleen.[18] Its main process is that of digestion, the extraction of nourishment and the distribution of its energy throughout the body. The lower burner lies in the lower abdomen and contains the Small Intestine, Large Intestine, Bladder and Kidneys. Its main process is the separation of pure from impure, absorption of the pure and excretion of the impure.

These three burning spaces are like three interconnecting and mutually supporting chambers. For there to be health and balance, all three must be operating optimally. One way to ascertain whether they are in harmony is to place a hand on each area of the body in turn. The relative temperature and the level of energetic activity in each burner will quickly determine if there is an imbalance. (See 'Triple Heater Visualisation' below.)

Minister of Balance and Harmony. The Official of the Triple Heater has a crucial role in coordinating all of the other Officials so that they are operating in harmony. It does this by regulating the smooth flow of fluids and Qi throughout the three burning spaces. It also acts as the body's thermostat, keeping body temperature within a comfortable range.

Another important function of this Official is to mobilise the *yuan Qi* (original or prenatal Qi) for current use. It is also responsible for the direction of the movement of Qi in the meridians (i.e. ascending or descending) and for the movement of Qi entering and leaving meridians.

The Triple Heater Official represents the outermost level of protection for the Heart. The Small Intestine Official is like the Emperor's personal servant and bodyguard; the Heart Protector Official is like the keeper of the castle gates; the Triple Heater Official is like the guard at the border of the kingdom.

At a physical level, this protection extends to keeping the body safe from external pathogens, a key part of the immune system. The acupoint TH 5 on the forearm, Outer Frontier Gate, succinctly describes this function. At the emotional level it is the Triple Heater which mediates our wider social interactions and determines appropriate levels of social intimacy.

Tongue

The tongue was considered by the ancient Chinese to be an offshoot of the Heart[19] and as such is the sense organ of Fire. The Heart opens to the tongue which is the vehicle of speech. Indeed, the tongue is so vital to the process of speech that it has become another word for language. People refer to their native language as the mother tongue and an eloquent speaker has a silver tongue. Malformation of the tongue can hinder speech. Without a tongue, we are literally speechless.

In Traditional Chinese Medicine, observation of the tongue is a pillar of diagnosis because it provides clearly visible clues to the patient's disharmony. Tongue diagnosis is remarkably reliable: whenever there are conflicting manifestations in a complicated condition, the tongue nearly always reflects the basic and underlying pattern.[20]

In this system of diagnosis, a practitioner assesses the colour, shape, coating and moisture of the tongue to determine patterns of disharmony. The state of the organs can be seen in different parts of the tongue. For example, the state of the Heart is reflected in the tip of the tongue, and a midline crack in the tongue indicates a weakness in the Heart itself, either physically or emotionally.

The tongue is also the main organ of taste. Its surface is covered with thousands of taste buds which are sensory receptors for saltiness, sourness, bitterness and sweetness. While the sense of taste is a resonance of the Earth Element (see Chapter 9), it is also dependent on the health of the Heart. 'Heart Qi communicates with the tongue. If the Heart is normal the tongue can distinguish the five tastes.'[21]

Blood Vessels

The blood vessels are the tissues of the Fire Element. The Heart governs both the Blood and the blood vessels; therefore, their health is a direct reflection of the health of the Heart. There is such a close relationship between the three that they can be viewed as part of a single system, the heart pumping Blood through the blood vessels. Indeed, Western medicine refers to it as the cardiovascular system.

There are several kinds of blood vessels: arteries, arterioles, capillaries, venules and veins. Arteries carry nutrient-rich oxygenated blood away from the heart. The arteries branch out to the small arterioles and further to the tiny capillaries. These microscopic blood vessels infuse all the cells of the body with blood and pick up the waste products of cell metabolism. The deoxygenated blood is then returned through the small venules to the veins and so back to the heart.

Diseases of the blood vessels or vascular system indicate an imbalance in the Fire Element and the Heart in particular. The most common of these are arteriosclerosis (hardening and narrowing of the arteries) and hypertension (high blood pressure). Vascular disease causes the build-up of plaque deposits on the walls of the arteries (atherosclerosis), increasing the risk of stroke. For all of these conditions, smoking is a significant risk factor.

Complexion

The external manifestation of Fire is the complexion.[22] The Heart and blood vessels distribute Blood throughout the body but it manifests most visibly in the complexion, particularly in the face. A healthy complexion is 'rosy and lustrous'[23] and indicates a healthy Heart. A complexion that is either dull white, pale, very red, dark or purplish indicates an imbalance of the Heart and therefore the Fire Element.

Diet and Lifestyle
Foods That Support Fire

Red is the colour that corresponds to Fire and so red foods are supportive of this Element. It is good news that most of the red vegetables and fruits are in season in the summer. Help yourself to plenty of red peppers, tomatoes, chillies, radishes, beets and red onions. Dive into strawberries, raspberries, cherries, watermelon, grapes, cranberries, pomegranates, plums, rhubarb, guava and red apples.

The red colour of foods such as tomatoes, red bell peppers, red carrots, watermelon and papaya comes from the presence of lycopene. This is a carotenoid (organic pigment) which is a powerful antioxidant and has been credited with reducing cardiovascular disease, cancer, diabetes, osteoporosis and, in men, infertility and prostate cancer.[24]

Beware the use of red food dye in processed foods. In the USA the food colouring Red 40 has been found to cause hyperactivity, aggressive behaviour, nervousness, difficulty concentrating or staying still. Moreover, it has been seen to exacerbate some conditions, such as attention deficit hyperactivity disorder and autism. Many of these signs and symptoms are typical of an excess of Fire.

Some suggestions to get more red food in your diet are as follows:[25]

- Drink fruit smoothies with strawberries and raspberries.

- Add sliced red peppers, radicchio, radishes and red onions to summer salads.

- Use red pepper sticks for dips instead of crackers or chips.

- Have a bowl of tomato soup for lunch.

- Roast cherry tomatoes, red peppers and red onions in olive oil and herbs.

- Choose red apple varieties over green.

- Add tomato puree to soups and stews.

- Get your face into a watermelon this summer!

The flavour of Fire is bitter, so bitter-tasting foods are also supportive of the Fire Element and its organs of heart and small intestine. This is especially so when Fire is in excess. Bitterness is a yin quality and therefore has properties of the Water Element, cooling Fire across the Control Cycle.[26]

Foods that are bitter include romaine lettuce, chicory, dandelion, bitter melon, citrus peel, unsweetened cocoa and quinine, which is used in tonic water.

While bitter foods are an important part of a healthy diet, problems can occur if there is overindulgence. 'Overindulgence in bitter foods will cause the skin to become shrivelled and dry and the body hair to fall out.'[27] This happens because the imbalance that is created in the Fire Element appears in the tissues and external manifestations of the Metal Element, namely the skin and body hair. Once again here, the principles of the Control Cycle are in operation.

Cardiovascular Health

CARDIOVASCULAR DISEASE

Cardiovascular disease is the leading health problem in the Western world and is the number-one cause of death in most of these countries. Cardiovascular disease is not an inevitable result of ageing. Many preventive measures can be taken to avoid heart disease.

STOPPING SMOKING

Despite vigorous campaigns by governments and health bodies, smoking continues to maintain an addictive hold over many people's lives. It impacts the cardiovascular system by accelerating arteriosclerosis, reducing the supply of oxygen to the cells, increasing blood pressure and reducing the supply of blood to the heart. The good news is that a smoker who does manage to quit for 15 years reduces his risk of heart disease to that of a person who has never smoked.

LOWERING BLOOD PRESSURE

Long-term hypertension damages the arteries and leads to arteriosclerosis, increasing the risk of heart disease and stroke. It also affects the brain and kidneys. Many people take medication for this condition, but these medications also have side effects. Lifestyle and dietary changes are important for those with this condition.

EXERCISING

We have all heard it countless times, and that is because it is true. Regular exercise is vital to a healthy heart, particularly aerobic exercise where the heart rate is increased for a sustained period. Examples of aerobic activities are walking, jogging, skipping, bicycling (stationary or outdoor), skating, rowing and low-impact aerobics or water aerobics. Exercising several times a week for 20–30 minutes is recommended.

LOWERING CHOLESTEROL

Low-density lipoprotein (LDL) cholesterol is called 'bad' cholesterol, because elevated levels of LDL cholesterol are associated with an increased risk of heart disease and arteriosclerosis. HDL (high-density lipoprotein) cholesterol is called the 'good cholesterol' because HDL cholesterol particles prevent atherosclerosis by extracting cholesterol from artery walls and disposing of them through liver metabolism. Lowering LDL and increasing HDL reduces the risks to the heart and arteries.[28] While medications can be successful in reducing LDL levels, there are also significant side effects, especially in the case of statins. Natural ways of improving cholesterol levels include reducing weight, reducing animal fats, eliminating trans fats, lowering alcohol intake, eating more whole grains and vegetables, and increasing consumption of omega-3 fatty acids.

IMPROVING DIET

A diet rich in whole grains and vegetables and low in processed foods will contribute greatly to a healthy heart. Fats should come mostly from unsaturated fats, so avoid large amounts of animal meat and dairy. The omega-3 fatty acids are very important to heart health. Main sources for this are oily fish such as salmon, mackerel and sardines. Krill oil contains high levels of omega-3. Of the plant sources, chia seed, flaxseed (also known as linseed) and flaxseed oil contain the highest levels. Other sources are walnuts, soybeans and canola oil.

LOSING WEIGHT

Being overweight is very taxing on the heart, so the more you approach an ideal weight, the happier your heart will be. A body-mass index (BMI) of 18.5–24.9 is a healthy range. You can find BMI calculators on the Internet and even as phone apps. One thing to note is that belly fat is particularly damaging to heart health. Men are more prone to put on weight around the abdomen. A waist measurement greater than 100 cm (40 in) makes for a high risk of heart disease.

REDUCING STRESS

High stress levels that come from working long hours, disharmonious relationships and from a type-A driven personality structure all contribute to stress upon the heart. Find ways to relax: meditation, yoga, walking in nature, listening to soothing music, getting a massage, taking a sauna. In short, do whatever works for you to slow down.

SUPPLEMENTS

Apart from the omega-3 fatty acids, top of the list of beneficial supplements for the heart is coenzyme Q10, which increases oxygenation of the heart tissue. Also important are calcium and magnesium to support the heart muscle, garlic to lower blood pressure and L-carnitine to reduce fat and triglyceride levels in the blood.[29] Also of note are vitamins B3, B6 and B12, psyllium, green tea, lecithin and artichoke leaf.

Warning: If you are taking prescription medications, consult your doctor about possible interactions with any of these supplements.

Small Intestine Health

Crohn's disease is an inflammatory disease of the digestive tract though it primarily affects the lower small intestine (ileum) and colon. It is a chronic inflammatory disorder in which the body's immune system attacks the gastrointestinal tract. It is believed to be caused by a combination of environmental factors and genetics.

Coeliac disease is also an inflammatory response and an autoimmune disease, though entirely genetic. It comes from a reaction to gluten, especially that found in wheat but also rye, barley and oats. It reduces the capacity of the small intestine to absorb nutrients. This is a debilitating condition. It is rare and affects about 1 in 5000 people.

Irritable Bowel Syndrome (IBS) is predominantly a colon condition, though there may be a link between IBS and small intestine bacterial overgrowth.

Gluten intolerance or sensitivity is becoming more common in Western countries where grains containing gluten have formed a substantial part of the diet over centuries. It is far more widespread than coeliac disease and often confused with it. Symptoms of gluten sensitivity include intestinal bloating, abdominal discomfort, pain or diarrhoea.

Summer in the Garden

Expansiveness

Everything about summer is expanding. The days are longer, the light is brighter, the temperatures are higher, and in the garden, foliage is rioting. The nature of Fire is to move outwards, filling space. Nature is certainly filling up the spaces in our gardens at this time. Melons, pumpkins and squash break out and snake across the lawns or into neighbouring beds. Vines that are untamed creep into every available opening. Tomatoes become unruly. Beans climb higher than their stakes. Fruit trees shoot through their netting. Beds are bursting with life and growth.

There is also an explosion of those plants we'd rather not have in the garden, also known as weeds. To bring some order to the chaos we need to prune, weed, stake, tie, cage and net. But it's a tall order and with so much happening, the gardener finds it hard to contain the proliferation. Much goes uncontrolled.

One of the qualities of Fire comes courtesy of the Small Intestine Official, also known as the Sorter. This is the capacity of discrimination. In the garden we choose what to weed and what to leave, what goes and what stays. Thinning the carrots, we need to choose which seedlings to keep and which to remove. Training the tomatoes, we choose which branches to trim in order to concentrate the plants' energy. The Small Intestine Official chooses that which can be let into the Heart and that which must be kept out. We must make wise choices in all areas of life; in the garden we get to practise in a way that produces the most bountiful results.

Community

One of the distinctive sounds of summer, especially on the weekends, is that of the lawnmower. Look outside and chances are you'll see people outside in shorts, singlets or bare-chested, sweating away trying to tame their patches. With so much heat, there is a need to stop frequently to take in fluids. This may coincide with opportunities to chat with neighbours over the fence.

Invite your friends and neighbours to visit your garden. Let them pluck ripe red tomatoes or luscious peaches still warm from the sun. Enjoy the delights of your produce with others. Share your love of nature with them.

Long summer days with their late sunsets and warm nights invite you to sit outside, enjoying the expanse of the garden, feeling the warmth on your skin, a comfortable fullness. Hang out with friends and a bottle of your favourite, cultivating your relationships in the realm of your husbandry.

Fun and Playfulness

The extended daylight hours of summer allow us lots of time outdoors, more than we need for actually tending the garden. So there is lots of time for simply enjoying it. Children can show us the way as they play, frolic and sport outdoors during their long summer holidays.

One of my favourite things to do in the garden in summer is to sit in the afternoon shade of a tree and survey my kingdom while listening to the cricket on the radio. After working hard in the heat, kick back and enjoy a good book, a cold drink, a snooze, a chat with friends. Or simply lie on your back in the grass and watch the clouds scud by. Enjoying all these activities in your garden puts you in touch at a deep level with the qualities of Fire.

Another way to explore your playful side is to make whimsical additions to your garden. Create sculptures from any natural materials to hand such as branches, pods, seeds and flowers. Make unusual planters out of recycled items. Place garden gnomes, fairies and animals in surprising places. Add windmills, flags, butterflies, colourful artwork, unusual rocks, painted palings. Make your garden a place that is fun, something that touches hearts. Fan your Fire and that of others.

Meridian Pathways

Of the six meridians of the arms, four are Fire meridians, reflecting the fact that the arms and hands are vehicles of contact and communication between our hearts and the world.

The pathway of the Heart meridian begins in the armpit and travels down the inside of the upper arm, the inside of the elbow and along the inside of the forearm to the little finger, ending at the inside corner of the little fingernail (see Figure 8.2).

Its partner meridian, the Small Intestine, begins at the outside corner of the little fingernail and travels along the side of the hand and forearm, through the point of the elbow, the back of the upper arm, and takes a detour through the shoulder blade before moving up the back of the neck and into the face, ending in front of the ear where the jaw hinges (see Figure 8.3).

The Heart Protector meridian follows the Heart meridian quite closely. It begins in the breast just outside the nipple and moves into the upper arm and through the biceps muscle. It continues down through the middle of the elbow crease, the middle of the forearm and into the palm of the hand, ending at the tip of the middle finger (see Figure 8.4).

Its partner meridian, the Triple Heater, follows the pathway of Small Intestine quite closely. It begins at the outside corner of the nail of the ring finger, passes up the back of the hand and the back of the forearm, the back of the upper arm and across the top of the shoulder blade, up the back of the neck and around the back of the ear before ending at the outside corner of the eyebrow (see Figure 8.5).

If you feel pain or discomfort in the arms, shoulders or neck, you can help to move the congested energy in these meridians by using your hand to stroke along each of these pathways in turn. As you do so, synchronise the strokes with your breath. Breathe out as you stroke down the inside of the arm to the hand; breathe in as you stroke up the back of the arm to the head. If you are able to visualise, imagine that a red-coloured light is flowing through the meridians, gently washing through any areas of congestion. If you have a particular area that feels stuck or painful, you can keep your hand there as you continue to move the energy along the meridians with your breath and your mind.

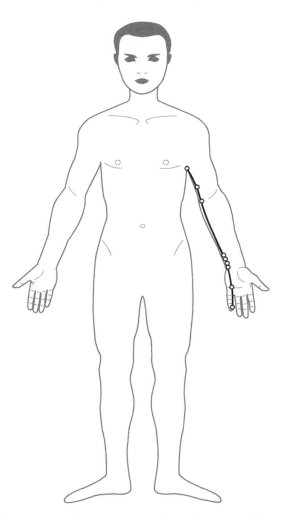

Figure 8.2 The pathway of the Heart meridian

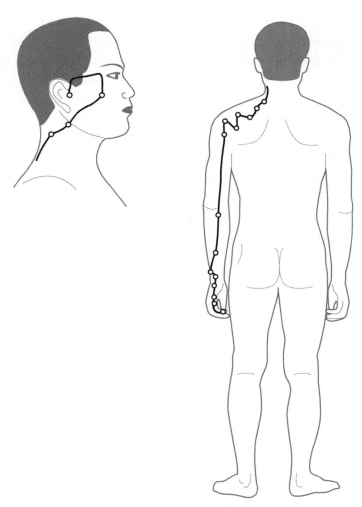

Figure 8.3 The pathway of the Small Intestine meridian

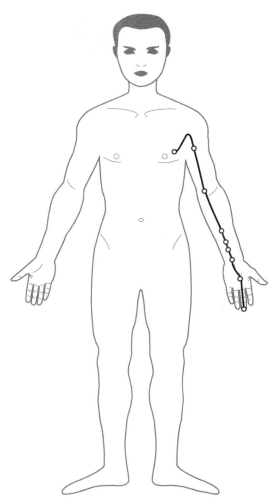

Figure 8.4 The pathway of the Heart Protector meridian

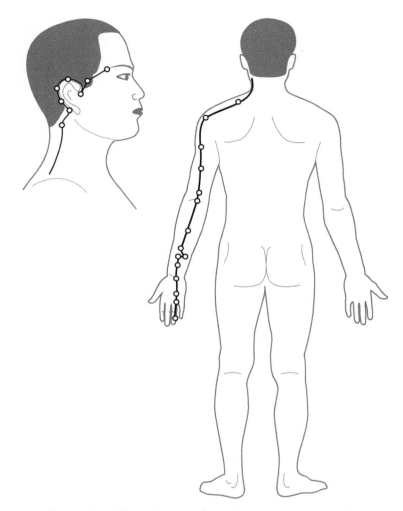

Figure 8.5 The pathway of the Triple Heater meridian

Organ Awareness

After doing the meridian visualisation practice, you can then do the organ awareness practice for the organs and functions of Fire. Place your right hand on the centre of your chest and place your left hand over the right. Tune into the organ of your heart, that steadily beating muscle whose health is vital to your life. Bring to mind the colour red. Perhaps remember a brilliant sunset or a bowl of raspberries. Allow the colour to infuse your heart. Acknowledge your heart for its steady, unfaltering work of circulating the blood that keeps you alive. Send love and gratitude to your heart. Notice how it responds to your attention and thanks. Notice how you feel as you do this.

When you are ready, move your hands onto your abdomen. The 6 m of your small intestine lies coiled throughout the abdomen, so you can place your hands anywhere that feels right. Once again, tune into this organ that is vital to the absorption of nutrition from the food you eat. Bring the red colour to mind and allow it to seep through the whole length of its tube and into the millions of cells that form the lining of the intestine. It is their tireless work that allows the absorption. Send your love and gratitude to your small intestine. Notice how the organ responds to your attention and thanks. Notice how you feel as you make contact.

Now bring your hands back to the centre of your chest. This time think of the pericardium that surrounds your heart. This fluid-filled sac protects your heart from shocks and jolts, both physically and emotionally. It is like a bodyguard that stands ever-vigilant to protect your heart. Again bring the colour red to suffuse this structure. Recognise all the work it does for you and send it your love and thanks. Notice how it responds. Notice how you feel.

Finally, we'll work with the Triple Heater. Imagine a structure of three interconnecting chambers that is responsible for keeping your body in just the right range of temperature. The lower chamber is below the navel, the middle chamber is above the navel and the upper chamber is in the chest. Since you only have two hands, you can take turns putting your hands over the chambers: first lower and middle, then lower and upper, then middle and upper. Each time bring to mind the colour red and acknowledge this amazing system for its work of keeping your body working harmoniously. Send it your love and gratitude. Notice its response and how it makes you feel.

Acupressure for Physical Health

After the meridian visualisation and organ awareness practices, you can focus specifically on the source points for each meridian. The source point heals the organ directly as well as balancing the meridian. They are powerful points while at the same time being very safe. They have the effect of tonifying the meridian if it is deficient, or sedating it if it is excess. It is the balancing point par excellence.

HE 7 *Shenmen* Spirit Gate

The Heart source point lies on the inner wrist crease towards the little finger side, about a fifth of the way across the wrist and between two tendons (see Figure 8.6).

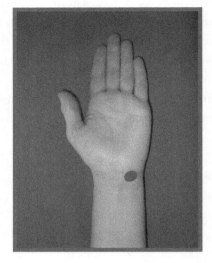

Figure 8.6 The Heart source point (HE 7 *Shenmen* Spirit Gate)

SI 4 *Wangu* Wrist Bone

The Small Intestine source point is found in a large hollow on the side of the hand between the wrist bone and the fifth metacarpal bone of the hand (see Figure 8.7).

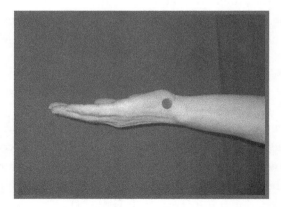

Figure 8.7 The Small Intestine source point (SI 4 *Wangu* Wrist Bone)

HP 7 *Daling* Great Mound

The Heart Protector source point is right in the middle of the inner wrist crease (see Figure 8.8).

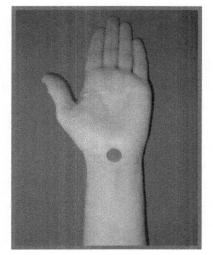

Figure 8.8 The Heart Protector source point (HP 7 *Daling* Great Mound)

TH 4 *Yangchi* Yang Pool

The Triple Heater source point is found on the back of the hand in a hollow below the wrist and between the heads of the fourth and fifth metacarpal bones. If you flex your wrist, a noticeable hollow appears (see Figure 8.9).

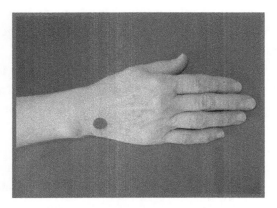

Figure 8.9 The Triple Heater source point (TH 4 *Yangchi* Yang Pool)

Press and hold each point for 2–3 minutes. Start with the left hand, then the right. Use a level of pressure that is comfortable for you. Don't press so much that it hurts. Tune into the point. Feel for the energetic pulse or wave. If you feel nothing, stay in tune and notice if things change.

After you have held each point singly, try holding Heart 7 and Small Intestine 4 together, first the left hand, then the right. Similarly hold Heart Protector 7 and Triple Heater 4 together. Points held in combination create a powerful synergistic healing effect.

Triple Heater Visualisation

Triple Heater Visualisation is helpful in balancing the three burners and supporting the Triple Heater Official in harmonising all of the organs and meridians. It can be done sitting in a chair or on a cushion, or lying down. Whichever position you are in, just be relaxed and comfortable.

Begin by placing your right hand over your lower abdomen at a place about two fingers' width below your navel. Then place your left hand over your right. Just tune into that centre, which we call the lower burner. Notice the sensations and energies, or lack of energy.

You are going to set up an imaginary windmill in your lower burner. This is an energetic wheel that turns around the point below your navel. The wheel can be any size and move at any speed that feels right for you. It turns in a clockwise direction, like a fan stirring the air. Notice if anything changes as the fan turns the energies in your lower burner.

Allow that wheel to continue to turn on its own as you bring your attention to the middle burner. Move your hands upwards to a place midway between your navel and your sternum, the solar plexus. Notice what is happening there. Are the energies moving or not? Now, imagine another wheel the same size and turning at the same speed as the wheel in the lower burner, like a fan gently turning the air. Notice what happens as that wheel turns.

Now there are two wheels in motion that continue to turn as you bring your attention to the upper burner. Move your hands to the centre of your chest. Notice what is happening there. Are the energies moving or not? Now imagine a third wheel, the same size and turning at the same speed as the other two. Like a fan turning the air, this wheel turns the energies in the upper burner.

Leave your right hand on the upper burner and move your left hand down to the lower burner. What do you notice as you hold the two spaces together? Is one more energised than the other? Does one have more heat? As you hold that combination, you may find that the two begin to equalise and resonate together.

Now move your left hand to the middle burner in the solar plexus. The right hand remains on the upper burner. Notice how these two burners feel in comparison. Are they similar or different in temperature and activity? Once again, as you hold this combination, you may find an equalisation taking place as the two burners resonate together.

Now move your left hand back to the lower burner and move your right hand to the middle burner. Notice how these two burners are in relationship with each other. Notice if anything changes as you continue to hold this combination.

Finally, bring your hands to rest in your lap and tune in to the three wheels turning together. Notice what has changed since you began, and what has remained the same. What has changed in each of the burning spaces and what has changed in the whole of you?

The Psycho-emotional Level of Fire

Having explored the ways in which Fire shapes us at the physical level, let's now look at the ways it shows up in our mental and emotional life. Thoughts and feelings are of a finer vibration than the body and so their energies are swifter and can change rapidly. But in another way, our emotional patterns, beliefs and attitudes can become fixed and entrenched. Here we will look at the ways in which the Fire Element can appear in us.

The Emotional Landscape of Fire

Joy

Many people, when they hear about the emotions of the Five Elements, want to be Fire types. They'd rather have joy than anger, fear or grief as their predominant emotion. It sounds like a much nicer life. But this arises out of a misunderstanding of the principles of Five Element diagnosis. For it is the emotion of the Constitutional Element that is the one most out of balance. So the Fire type is actually most out of balance when it comes to the emotion of joy.

When the classics tell us that joy injures the Heart, they are not referring to joy as a state of quiet contentment, but rather to a state of excessive excitement and agitation. Imagine the uncontrolled excitement on show at a children's party. When viewed like this, it is easy to see how overexcitement can have an unhealthy impact on the heart.

THE HEART OF THE MATTER

The Chinese ancients saw the body's organs as having functions far beyond their physiology. They saw the 12 organs as if they were 12 'officials' in a court, each with a ministerial role and a complex set of functions. They described the functions of the Officials much more in terms of mind and spirit than physiology.

From this perspective, the Heart Official is akin to an Emperor who sits on the throne and holds the kingdom together simply by being himself. When the Emperor is wise and moderate and all his ministers are taking care of business, then the kingdom functions harmoniously.

The Heart and its functioning are uniquely essential to life but are also very sensitive to disruption. Because of this, the other three Fire Officials (Small Intestine, Heart Protector and Triple Heater) act like an inner cabinet to the Emperor. They take on the job of protecting and supporting the Heart, which they do in their various ways, monitoring communications from the Heart to the world and from the world back to the Heart.

The particular job of the Small Intestine Official is to sort out what is good for the Heart and can be let in, and what is harmful and must be excluded. The Heart Protector Official negotiates close relationships, ensuring that there is a Heart connection and that the connection is safe for the Heart. The Triple Heater Official supports the Heart by ensuring balanced functioning in wider social relationships.

When the Heart is settled and protected, the spirit of the Heart, the *shen*, resides there quietly. But as we saw earlier, it is easily disturbed by shock and trauma. When the *shen* leaves the Heart, the connection with spirit is lost and the person tends to feel apathetic, depressed and separated from herself and the world. Others may see emptiness, vacancy and lifelessness in the eyes.

When the Officials cannot do their work properly, Fire becomes either excess or deficient, impacting not only the body but also the mind, thoughts, emotions and communication.

THE YANG RESPONSE: EXCESSIVE CONTROL, HYPERACTIVITY
Excess Fire produces a quickening at all levels. It creates a kind of feverish activity in the body, movement and speech. It appears as a rapid pulse and increased physiological activity, often producing heat in the body. At the psycho-emotional level, excess Fire can create a lack of boundaries in relationships, compulsive communication, and at its extreme, mania. Paradoxically, it can also create a need for control.

The need for control. When the Heart is in a state of balance, it does not need to do anything except to beat and to *be*. However, when the Heart energies become excessive, it is no longer possible simply to be and to flow with life. Instead, there is a desire to *do* and this doing directly opposes being. Doing becomes a way of controlling life and events, rather than simply allowing them to unfold.

When Fire is in excess, this control manifests particularly in relationships. When the protective Officials are no longer able to do their job effectively there is a need to protect the Heart from hurt. There is an attempt to achieve this by actively and compulsively controlling interactions with others. At its extreme, this behaviour can become domineering and even tyrannical.

Pushing boundaries. The uninhibited expansion of Fire energies causes the person literally to push the boundaries of what is appropriate in relationships. This can show up in close personal relationships as sexual innuendo or inappropriate intimacy and in the social context as exhibitionism.

Compulsive communication. The tongue, as used for speech rather than taste, is the sense organ of the Fire Element. Therefore, excess Fire tends to produce an excess of speaking, a chattering about every subject under the sun, often with linkages that are hard for the listener to follow. This flood of words is far greater than the content demands and repetition is common.

Mania. At its extreme, when a massive amount of energy sends Fire out of control, it produces behaviour that is characteristic of the manic phase of bipolar disorder. There is a lack of impulse control and a pushing against the boundaries of what is socially acceptable. There can be grandiosity, a sense of invincibility and an unrealistic view of capacities. This can all lead to reckless, dangerous and even criminal behaviour.

THE YIN RESPONSE: VULNERABILITY, DULLNESS, DEPRESSION
When the Fire Element is deficient, there is coldness, slowing and contracting at all levels. There is a feeling of flatness and joylessness, as if the spark has gone out of life. Because there is insufficient energy to maintain contact with others, relationships are particularly affected.

Vulnerability in relationships. The Heart Protector Official protects the Heart in relationships. When there is a deficiency of Fire in the Heart Protector, there is a diminished ability to protect the Heart. Such a person tends to become negatively merged with others, to fall in love easily and repeatedly, to form clinging attachments, to be easily exploited and vulnerable to abuse.

Dullness. When Fire is in excess, there is a tendency actively to exert control over the environment. In contrast, when Fire is deficient, the inclination is to look to the outside world for a set of rules which will allow for control with the least exertion. This can result in the personality of the uninspired bureaucrat: dull, boring, pedantic, lacking in spontaneity, unreceptive to change, mired in the past and looking to authority for approval.[30]

Yet, as we know, the tighter the control, the greater the resulting inner pressure. This repression produces an underlying sense of agitation and restlessness, of energy bottled up. This can sometimes lead to a kind of splitting where these energies are expressed in a hidden double life.

Depression. When the Fire energies are extremely deficient, depression is likely. In a Fire depression, the positive attributes and capacities of Fire are missing. There is a loss of pleasure in the usual activities, difficulties with thinking and concentrating, a loss of interest in sex and a decrease in communication. However, the fundamental nature of Fire is to expand, so these depressions tend to be self-limiting. This frequently results in a swing to the opposite polarity of mania. When episodes of mania and depression are extreme, the result can be bipolar disorder.

RETURNING TO BALANCE

For Fire Constitution types, Heart imbalances are accompanied by the belief that they are not loved and not loveable. Thus, their primary inner life work is not just with the energies of the Heart, but also with the issues of loving and being loved.

But as with all of the Elements, this wounding to the Heart is not the monopoly of Fire types. It is a core issue for all human beings. We are by nature gregarious, connected, social animals, yet we tend to see ourselves as separate individuals. One of the functions of the Fire energies is to navigate our real needs for both separateness and connectedness. When the Fire energies are in balance, we are able to meet both needs appropriately and harmoniously.

Modern psychology sees that the way we relate to others is learned very early in life. From birth, our mother becomes our primary model of what others are like and how best to relate to them. Our interactions with our father will also teach us about the nature of relationships. Later we learn to relate by observing how our parents interact. Later still, at about age five or six years, we are shaped by the way our opposite-gender parent meets our love in the Oedipal phase. All of these early imprints shape the way our Heart and its protectors operate, and how well the Officials of Small Intestine, Heart Protector and Triple Heater are able to support the Heart in its giving and receiving of love.

The more understanding we have of these early influences and how they determine our current behaviour, the more we can live from our hearts in the moment. We can bring the unconscious to consciousness by discovering what blocks the flow of love in and out of our heart. Is it fear, anger, hatred or something else? What is it that obscures the natural loving kindness that flows freely from an open heart?

It has been observed that everything we do in relationships derives from a desire to be connected. Even withdrawal is in the service of maintaining whatever contact of which we are capable. When we remember that our fundamental desire is to connect, however it is expressed, it allows us to find compassion for all humans, ourselves included. We are all doing the best that we can.

Fun

Years ago I made a new friend and early on in our friendship she asked me, 'What do you do for fun?' I had never been asked that question before and it actually took some thought to answer it. Lately, as I've been thinking and writing about the Fire Element, I have been asking others the same question and they, too, have to think about it for a while. First of all we have to think about what fun means. Something amusing, pleasurable and enjoyable. Something that is entertaining, diverting or comical. But above all something that is light-hearted and brings happiness. Then we think of the ways we seek to bring this sense of fun into our life.

In our fast-paced modern world, we can sometimes get very serious about taking care of the many strands of life and forget to have fun. The Heart needs to be tended and one of the ways to do that is to engage in activities that bring pleasure, amusement, laughter and light-heartedness.

Five Element acupuncturist Neil Gumenick offers this advice:

> Have fun on a regular basis, even if you have to work at it at first. Make it a priority – schedule your fun, if that's what it takes. Don't compromise. Consider fun as important to your well-being as work or anything else you do.[31]

Summer is a great time to work on your fun. For one thing there is just so much fun stuff happening in the summer, from parties and barbecues to fairs and festivals everywhere you look. Haven't you noticed how many events there are on the same weekend in summer? The energy of the Fire Element simply suffuses summer. It calls forth and supports anything that sustains and heals the heart.

Here's a suggestion: find one thing that you've always wanted to do for fun but never got around to and find time to do that this summer. Your heart will thank you.

Laughter and Humour

Laughter is the sound of joy bubbling out of the heart. What makes a person laugh? A good joke, a tickle under the arm, something unexpectedly delightful or just a moment of the sheer joy of being alive.

Children laugh much more than adults do. It is as if by becoming an adult, a cloak of seriousness descends upon us. Certainly the responsibilities and worries of work, money and modern living can dampen light-heartedness. If this is the case for you, behaving like a child can be a road back to laughter. Doing things just for fun, playing, having playtime, being playful, exploring things as if for the first time, having the wide-eyed wonder of children – all these things put us in touch with our hearts, and laughter is the spontaneous expression of the Heart.

Why is it important to laugh? At a physical level it provides a way of relieving tension and inducing relaxation. It has been discovered that laughter dilates the blood vessels and increases blood flow which makes it great therapy for the heart and the circulatory system.[32] Laughter is also a natural pain reliever. Norman Cousins discovered this for himself when watching Marx Brothers' films. 'I made the joyous discovery that ten minutes of genuine belly laughter had an anaesthetic effect and would give me at least two hours of pain-free sleep.'[33] Neurophysiology indicates that laughter is linked with the activation of the prefrontal cortex, the part of the brain that produces endorphins.[34] The old adage that laughter is the best medicine is being borne out by modern science.

Laughter also serves a valuable social function. In social settings it is used as a signal of acceptance and inclusion. We might laugh at something a friend says, not simply because it is funny, but as a way of signalling approval of them personally. Laughter conveys warmth to another person. It is well known that laughter in groups can be contagious, the laughter of one person provoking laughter in others. This principle underlies the use of laugh tracks in television sitcoms.

At an emotional level, laughter dispels gloom and raises the spirits, seemingly lightening the burdens of life. We have seen how it improves the condition of the cardiovascular system. It also benefits the emotional heart. It is no wonder that most of the movies made are comedies, and even in dramas the tension is often relieved by something funny. A good sense of humour is a great asset and support on the rocky road of life.

When it comes to humour, everyone is tickled by different things and by different things at different times. What causes uproarious laughter in one person may leave another quite unamused. Some people enjoy the slapstick style of humour of comedians like Charlie Chaplin and the Three Stooges – the whoopee cushion, the pie in the face, the banana-skin slide; others are more engaged by the clever, pithy one-liner style of stand-up comedians, like George Carlin's 'a dyslexic man walks into a bra'. Another favourite humour style is the pun, which suggests two or more meanings by exploiting multiple meanings of words, or of similar-sounding words. This is common in English humour because of the large number of homophones available in this language: 'I met a woman who said she'd met me at the vegetarian club but I've never seen herbivore.' Puns have been described as the lowest form of wit, but literary greats Shakespeare and Wilde were very clever punsters.

Deprecating humour is another way of raising a laugh. This is the art of the put-down. Groucho Marx was famous for this: 'I never forget a face, but in your case I'll be glad to make an exception.' Self-deprecating humour is common among comedians who want to get their audience on side. Woody Allen was famous for this: 'I have bad reflexes. I was once run over by a car being pushed by two guys.'

A more modern form is absurdist humour of which Monty Python is probably the most famous example. Devotees of this form are known to memorise whole passages of sketches to quote at one another.

Satire is a more complex form of humour that is less about raising a laugh than raising consciousness about an issue. It utilises strong irony and sarcasm. This originates in the work of the Greek playwright Aristophanes who made fun of individuals and institutions in ancient Athens.

But enough already of this introspection about humour. It is best enjoyed directly rather than by examination. As author E.B. White observed, 'Humour can be dissected as a frog can, but the thing dies in the process and the innards are discouraging to any but the pure scientific mind.'[35]

With that in mind, just have a good laugh and don't worry about why.

LAUGHTER YOGA

A few years ago when writing a newsletter on the Fire Element, I came across something called Laughter Yoga. I discovered that there is an international movement going on. There are hundreds of Laughter Yoga groups around the world. These groups meet and have a good laugh together, using particular exercises to stimulate and support laughter. One of these exercises is clapping the hands and fingers together. Since four of the six meridians of the arm and hand are Fire meridians, clapping stimulates important Fire points. Heart 8 and Heart Protector 8 on the palms of the hands are particularly stimulated and these points are the Fire points on the Fire meridians.

This is one sure-fire way to stir up the Fire in your life. Since laughter is the sound of Fire, it makes perfect sense that clapping the hands together will help get you in touch with your heart and get you giggling.

When I went searching the Web, I found a video on YouTube in which John Cleese goes to Mumbai to meet Dr Madan Kataria, founder of Laughter Yoga International. In this heart-tickling clip, you can see that some of the other exercises work directly on the heart. For example, sticking out the tongue is not only funny to look at but also stimulates the tongue as the sense organ of Fire. Another exercise has people pointing to the centre of the chest, CV 17, the alarm point of Heart Protector.

Kataria claims that laughing for 15–20 minutes a day, whether faked or real, relieves stress, boosts the immune system and reduces infections. So, get laughing, whether you like it or not!

Love

We have already looked at love as one of the Gifts of Fire. Let us now look more deeply into the part that love plays in the psychological and emotional framework.

What is love? I have been asking this question for decades and, still, a final answer eludes me. Many others are asking the same question. A quick look at iTunes shows there are currently nine songs and an album entitled *What Is Love?* In fact, if you were to listen to all the songs ever written, you'd find that most of them are about love of some kind. Love relationships also figure in most movie plots and works of fiction. Love is what people are most interested in. Love is the most common theme of human life. It is what people think and talk most about.

Countless philosophers, anthropologists, psychologists and other students of the human condition have addressed this subject and come up with many different ways of defining and analysing love in attempts to answer the age-old question, 'What is Love?' I have chosen just four of these ways as a sample of the different ways of looking at love.

THE ART OF LOVING

The psychologist Eric Fromm wrote a short book in 1956 called *The Art of Loving*. Some regard this as the original self-help manual of the modern age. Fromm argued that love is something that needs to be practised and mastered in the various arenas he identified: brotherly love, motherly love, erotic love, self-love and love of God. In order to practise this art, we need maturity, self-knowledge and courage. And we need to practise the art of loving in freedom, not out of controlling others as objects of love. Fromm also believed that 'Love is the only sane and satisfactory answer to the problem of human existence'.[36]

Love is not just a feeling, but a decision, a judgement and a promise. To love means to surrender and commit without guarantees. Love is an act of utter faith.

THE TRIANGULAR THEORY OF LOVE

Robert Sternberg developed a theory which he called the triangular theory of love.[37] Each of the different kinds of love involves varying degrees of three qualities: intimacy, commitment and passion (see Figure 8.10).

The ideal towards which most people strive, though few apparently achieve, is consummate love, a balance of intimacy, passion and commitment. At the three corners, love that involves only intimacy is liking, love that is only passion is infatuation, and love that only has commitment is empty love. Then there are three kinds of love that are missing one of the corners. Romantic love has passion and intimacy but no commitment, Companionate love has intimacy and commitment but no passion, and fatuous love has passion and commitment but no intimacy.

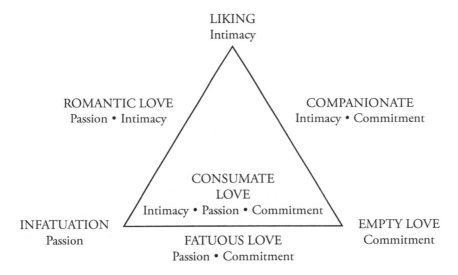

Figure 8.10 Sternberg's triangular theory of love[38]

By teasing out these seven kinds of love, Sternberg provides a useful framework for thinking about love and what it means to our lives.

THREE BRAIN SYSTEMS

Cultural anthropologist Dr Helen Fisher has developed another way of looking at love by dividing it into three brain systems that are driven by hormones: lust, romance and attachment.[39] These three systems can operate in any order and in any combination.

Lust is a craving for sexual gratification which can be felt for a whole range of people. Those caught up in romantic love focus all their attention on the object of their affection. Not only do they crave them but they also obsessively think about them and become sexually possessive. During this state the brain is driven by dopamine, a neurotransmitter central to the reward system.

Romantic love is more powerful even than the sex drive. It is a drive rather than an emotion and is very difficult to control, being one of the most powerful neural systems that has evolved.

Attachment is the sense of calm and security that you can feel for a long-term partner. It is associated with the hormones vasopressin and oxytocin, which are probably responsible for the sense of peacefulness and unity felt after having sex. Holding hands also drives up oxytocin levels, as does looking deeply into the loved one's eyes or simply sitting next to them.

LOVE AND FEAR

One perspective of love that has developed in recent years in the counter-consciousness movement is that there only two emotions that humans are capable of expressing, namely fear and love. All other emotions are subcategories of these two. On love's side there are things like joy, peacefulness, happiness and forgiveness. On the other hand, fear reflects things such as hate, depression, guilt, inadequacy, prejudice and anger. Moreover, love and fear cannot coexist but each displaces the other. In other words, love is an absence of fear, and fear is an absence of love.

Gerald Jampolsky's seminal work *Love Is Letting Go of Fear* has had a lot to do with the popularity of this perspective.[40] His short book was at least partly derived from *A Course in Miracles*.[41] These ideas have been presented by a number of people as diverse as John Lennon, Osho, Michael Leunig and channelled teachings by Kathryn Harwig.

FALLING IN LOVE

One of the greatest misunderstandings is that falling in love is actually a kind of love. In reality it is more like falling sick. It is a kind of illness that comes over a person and passes after a period of time. The myth that this illness is true love has been fostered by movies, television and novels, all of which exert a powerful influence on the psyche. Most romantic stories end with the getting together of the love-struck couple and assume a happily ever after continuation. They don't usually look several years ahead to see what happened to the relationship.

What happens when one falls in love? First of all there are powerful physiological effects. The heart beats faster when in the presence of the loved one. There may be sleep loss and appetite loss. Helen Fisher's work has shown there is a drop in the serotonin levels in the blood that is similar to cases of obsessive-compulsive disorder. Other hormones are affected, notably testosterone, dopamine and oxytocin. Testing 12 months later showed these hormonal levels reverting to normal even if the relationship continued.[42]

At a psychological level, what is happening when a person falls in love is that the love object is being seen through the eyes of the young-child part of us. This part is forever looking for the perfect parents to love us, take care of us, tell us how wonderful we are, see and mirror our gifts and skills. When we meet someone who closely matches our blueprint of 'perfect parents', there is the possibility of the falling-in-love process happening. When the other person feels the same, there is a feedback loop in which each person's idealisation amplifies that of the other. It is a compelling fantasy that one has indeed found the perfect person or soulmate. Even those who have psychological understanding can find themselves lost in this wonderful, blissful, merged state.

But all these projections of perfection onto the other eventually fade as we begin to see the person as they really are with all their flaws. It can be very distressing when these projections begin to disappear. For many, there is great disappointment and disillusion about love because the falling-in-love state has been confused with love. When there is a rush to marry based on this idealised projection, the consequences can be devastating. It is always a good idea to wait at least 12 months before making a lifetime commitment. Give the wild hormone swings time to settle. Travel through a cycle of seasons with your loved one. When you have recovered from your fall, you will have a much clearer idea of what is true.

I was never really insane except upon occasions when my heart was touched.

EDGAR ALLAN POE

SELF-LOVE

When I was at school, one of the sharpest schoolyard taunts was 'He loves himself.' Any hint of self-approval and self-acceptance was pounced upon and ridiculed as self-aggrandisement, grandiosity and narcissism. But self-love is none of these things. These schoolyard barbs confused self-care with self-centredness.

Self-love includes accepting, allowing, honouring and having compassion for all of the aspects of ourselves. This includes the critical, deficient and wounded parts. It also includes taking care of ourselves as much as we take care of others. It means not neglecting our needs. Self-neglect is an indication of a lack of self-love. If we love ourselves, we make healthy choices in diet and lifestyle, choosing not to consume foods that harm us, rejecting unhealthy habits such as drinking and smoking, taking up pursuits and forms of exercise that improve our physical health.

We demonstrate self-love when we engage in activities that improve us psychologically and spiritually, things that stretch us so that we can achieve more of our human potential. This might include study, philosophy, music and art, meditation and other spiritual practices.

More importantly still, we are self-loving when we choose relationships that support our growth. We do not count as friends those who denigrate, belittle, criticise and attack us. We choose an intimate partner who is supportive of our personal growth as much as he is dedicated to his own.

We choose a partner not because they can provide us with something we ourselves are lacking but rather as an equal in the journey of self-discovery. The seeking of love from the outside often comes from a lack of love for oneself. How can we truly love another if we do not love ourselves? We must include ourselves among the lovable.

Ultimately, self-love arises out of self-awareness which implies an attunement to our inner state. This means knowing what we are thinking, feeling and needing in each moment. Being here, being present to ourselves, is the deepest form of self-love.

At the beginning of the work of loving ourselves, we may need some modelling. Look at how others express their love for you and take that as a sign of your lovability. Try to receive compliments, recognition and acknowledgement with an open heart and an open mind. All of us are loved by someone. That is proof of our lovability. Being loved by others is fuel for the fire of self-love. We just have to let it in.

Here are some suggestions of ways to cultivate self-love:

- Keep a self-love journal. List all the compliments you get, all the things people appreciate about you. Write down the things that make you feel good about yourself. Note when someone tells you they love something about you.

- Stop comparing yourself to others. You are your own shining star, not dependent on reflected light. Celebrate your uniqueness.

- Keep a lookout for the unlovable self-critic. If your self-love work is hampered by this voice, see the activity 'Working with the Inner Critic' in Chapter 7.

- Take yourself out on dates. Go somewhere you love to go. Do something you love to do. Just do it in your own delightful company.

- Send a love letter to your adorable self. If you like, write an old-fashioned letter with pen and ink and mail it to yourself. Or send an email addressed to yourself from yourself. Think of all the love letters you have written to others. Smother yourself with the same loving, tender endearments you have lavished on others. Notice how you feel as you write, and again when you receive your letter.

- Check out Gala Darling's *Radical Self Love Project* including her *100 Ways You Can Start Self-loving Yourself Right Now*.[43]

You yourself, as much as anybody in the entire universe, deserve your love and affection.

BUDDHA

Acupressure for Psycho-emotional Health

The points I have chosen to support psycho-emotional health are known as the front mu points or alarm points of the yin Fire meridians.

CV 17 *Shanzhong* Within the Breast

The mu point of the Heart Protector meridian is located in a shallow depression in the centre of the sternum at the level of the space between the fourth and fifth ribs (see Figure 8.11). As such, it is very supportive of the emotional heart. The *Ling Shu* calls this place the palace of the Heart Governor, a protected place of power which enables communication of feelings, ideas, circulation, breath and speech from the Heart to the rest of the body, mind and spirit as well as outward to the rest of the world.[44] It activates the *shen* and allows the person to reconnect with Heaven. It is helpful when there is heartache from breakups or betrayal. This point can be held on its own or in combination with the source point, Heart Protector 7.

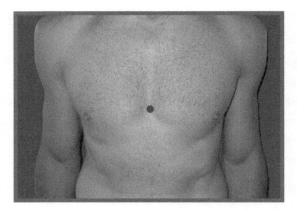

Figure 8.11 The mu point of the Heart Protector meridian
(CV 17 *Shanzhong* Within the Breast)

CV 14 *Juque* Great Deficiency

The mu point of the Heart meridian is located on the midline just below the tip of the xiphoid process which is the cartilage that attaches to the bottom of the sternum (see Figure 8.12). It provides even deeper access to the *shen* and is of great help when a person is low in spirit, lacks an inner sense of joy, is oversensitive to others' emotions or is lacking in confidence. It can be held alone or in combination with the source point, Heart 7.

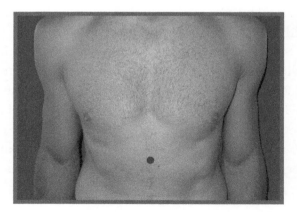

Figure 8.12 The mu point of the Heart meridian
(CV 14 *Juque* Great Deficiency)

The Spiritual Level of Fire

Our spiritual nature is not our body, thoughts, emotions or personality. If there is anything that remains of us when we die, it is the spirit. Here we examine how the Fire Element influences our spiritual life.

The Spirit of Fire: Shen

The character *shen* has two parts. The left part, *shih*, means influences from above, while the right part, *shen*, signifies a rope implying extension and expansion. 'Taken as a whole it suggests the sense of heaven extending its will towards earth and the consciousness of humankind.'[45]

In the classical literature, *shen* is used in two ways. In the first sense, it refers collectively to all five spirits (*wu shen*), five individual aspects of consciousness, each expressing the nature of its corresponding Element. In the second sense, *shen* refers particularly to the spirit of the Fire Element. This spirit is responsible for thoughts, feelings, emotions, perceptions and cognition. The Heart and the mind are so inextricably linked that the *shen* of the Heart is often translated as mind or heartmind.[46] The *shen* of Fire resides in the Heart during our lifetime; upon our death, the spirit returns to the Heavenly realm from whence it originated.

The *shen* is not directly visible, but it is reflected in a person's eyes as a sparkle, a point of contact, a 'thereness'. This inner radiance, called *shen ming*, is what gives each person his personal uniqueness. It is that which makes each of us like no other.

The *shen* is reflected also in a settled mind and clear thinking. When the *shen* is disturbed, has flown away, the eyes become dull and there is a sense that the person is not quite there. Shock, trauma and abuse are common reasons for the *shen* to fly. People who have experienced war, imprisonment or torture, or refugees who are fleeing persecution, are often likely to have *shen* disturbance and therefore Heart imbalance.

The Neijing says that the Heart houses the *shen*, the governing spirit;[47] therefore, anything that injures the Heart will also injure the *shen*. As it is the most yang of the spirits, the *shen* has the lightest, finest vibration with a delicacy that is easily disturbed.

The spirit of the Heart is also responsible for settled sleep, settled emotions and cognitive functions such as concentration, short-term memory and the ability to think clearly. *Shen* disturbance can therefore manifest as difficulty getting to sleep, dream disturbance, volatile emotions, anxiety, panic, depression and feelings of rejection. Since *shen* is the mind of the heart, any disturbance will result in disturbances of the mind. Indeed, all mental illness can be viewed as an imbalance in the *shen*.

A healthy and balanced Heart *shen* enables the capacity to form and maintain healthy and meaningful relationships. Heart boundaries are clear but also able to adapt appropriately to different relationships. Conversely, emotional problems that stem from relationships, such as abandonment and betrayal, weaken the Heart and hurt the *shen*.

What does *shen* look like when it is in perfect balance? Such a person is settled, calm and not easily distracted. She sleeps peacefully, undisturbed by dreams. She has an inner light that infuses her with a glow that can be seen in the eyes. She makes eye contact that shows her depth. Her speech is coherent, reflecting a balanced mind. The way she lives her life is congruent with who she is as a person. She gives and receives love with ease. In a way she lives a life of love. She may well be intuitive, her consciousness in open communication with universal consciousness.

The Virtue of Fire: Propriety

The classics teach that the virtue of Fire is *li*,[48] translated variously as propriety, ritual and ceremony. Propriety is therefore the quality which reflects and expresses the harmony of the Tao through the facet of the Fire Element.

We need to explore what is meant by propriety. This is a concept at the heart of Confucian thought, which was influential in the first century BCE when the virtues were assigned to the Elements. Central to that philosophy was adherence to a strict social order where everyone knew their place and was aware of their proper relationship with all others. Propriety is what allows for a well-ordered society with respect for others' and one's own place within it. It includes good manners and etiquette, courtesy and mindfulness of the rights of everyone.

This does not mean engaging in a mere show of politeness, of behaving in public in ways that are ritualistic and empty of meaning. Rather, propriety is about acting in ways that express real reverence for ourselves and others and the respective places we all have within society. It suggests mindfulness of our actions in the wider social context, of being present to ourselves and our situation, and recognising that cooperation with others is an indispensable part of living in the world.

'The virtue of propriety is evidenced by our capacity to be in the right place, at the right time, doing the right thing.'[49] This means living the life that is right for us, expressing our uniqueness in the way we live.

When we lose contact with our True Nature, the virtues of the Elements are also lost. They begin to degrade into the emotions of the Elements. In the case of Fire, propriety degrades to either excessive joy and overexcitement, on the one hand, or lack of joy and sorrow, on the other. When this happens, we no longer know what is the right life for us, the right place to be, the right way to be. The result is a move towards a need for either control or chaos.

As we grow spiritually and begin our return to our True Nature, we move away from needing to either control our surroundings or create chaos in our lives. As we come to know who we truly are, we also come to realise our true place in the universe and our connection to all.

The Spiritual Issue of Fire: Knowing the True Self
Who Am I?

There is much talk these days about people being themselves. Often it is a statement made in response to a criticism or a raised eyebrow about the way a person is behaving. 'I know that I'm loud and raucous at parties, but I'm just being myself.' Most of us have a sense of ourselves as a unique individual and of course we want to express that unique self in the world. Most of us want to be ourselves. But what is the self that is being referred to?

For most people, most of the time, this is the ego self. It is a constructed self, a collection of memories, impressions, ideas, beliefs, patterns and self-images that have been built over time into a fantastic edifice in our mind. It is the sum total of our history: the events in our lives, our relationships, the influences of parents, teachers, peers and culture. When we think we are being ourselves, it is more likely that we are actually being our mother, father, sibling, first-grade teacher, best friend, teen idol, political hero, spiritual guru and so on.

The big problem is not that we have an ego self but that we identify with that self and think that is who we really are. When we identify with that created self, we are suffering from a delusion. We are no more truly this ego self than we are the car we drive. Yet we cling so completely to the idea that we are this created self. Imagine if you were to walk around believing you are a 2010 Toyota Corolla. It sounds silly but, in effect, this is what we are doing when we identify entirely with the ego self.

This challenge of seeing beyond the false self to the true self represents the core spiritual issue of the Fire Element. This can be understood through the connection of Fire to Heaven. As the most yang Element, Fire is closest to Heaven and therefore closest to our Heavenly nature. *Shen*, the spirit of Fire, comes from the stars and resides in our heart during our lifetime. At our death, the *shen* rises up through the crown chakra and returns to the stars. Any distortion or imbalance in the Fire Element, and hence in the *shen*, will separate us from our Heavenly origin and from the knowledge that who we are is immeasurably greater than the collection of mental constructs that is the ego. While Fire constitutional types find this a particular theme in their lives, it is an issue for every human who begins to examine himself and his place in the cosmos.

For every human being, life's journey is one of the Fall and the Return. The first part of life is a fall from or moving away from Source, the second part a search for the way back. We are born as beings from the stars, pure and radiant. A newborn is at one with the starry realm from which she came but at the same time is unconscious of that fact. She is unable consciously to reflect upon her nature. Slowly she begins to develop a sense of a separate self, operating in relation to others, first to her mother, then to family and later to the wider world. By the age of five years or so, the ego self has been formed and the separation from Source is complete. Like the man who finally succumbed and drank the waters (see Chapter 6), the child has learned to fit into humanity but has forgotten her origins.

The Return to Source begins when we turn our attention inward. James Hollis refers to this as the 'second half of life',[50] which is not a point in chronological time but rather any moment when we inquire into ourselves and ask questions like 'What is the meaning of my life?', 'Why am I here?' and 'What is the point of my existence?' This turning inward can happen at any stage of life, but it most commonly happens in our forties or fifties when we are deep in the Fire stage of life, that of maturity. This quality of maturity of Fire offers the possibility of knowing the True Self. Having gained enough life experience upon which to reflect and having attained a certain level of ego maturity and strength, by this time we are equipped to make the inward turn and begin the Return journey.

How then do we find out who we really are if we are not who we have thought ourselves to be all these years? How do we return to our original nature? Of course, there are many paths back to the Source, many spiritual practices that help us to see through the veils of delusion, and each person needs to find the path that is right for her. But at the heart of all practices is seeing through the illusion of false self to True Self.

The Indian sage Sri Ramana Maharshi, a teacher in the Vedanta lineage, laid the greatest emphasis on the path of self-inquiry to discover the True Self. He taught that the first and foremost of all thoughts that arise in the mind is the primal 'I' thought. It is only after the rise or origin of the 'I' thought that innumerable other thoughts arise. If we go inward in quest of the 'I', the 'I' topples down revealing the 'I, I' that is the one perfect existence.[51]

So, who *are* you?

JOURNALING INQUIRY: WHO AM I?

'Who am I?' is a simple question of three words, but one with profound ramifications. A question for a lifetime. For now, you might devote a section of your journal to this question and keep coming back to it. Write down all the things you think you are as you go in quest of the Essential Self.

Another way of working with this question is with a partner in a repeating-question exercise. Set aside, say, ten minutes for each person. One asks the other, 'Who are you?' She replies with whatever spontaneous answer arises. The first person repeats the same question and the second responds. There is no commentary or conversation about the answers. When the time is up, change roles. The longer you set the time, the more you will exhaust the easy answers and begin to plumb the depths of the question. This exercise can be repeated as many times as you wish.

The Diamond Approach

Joy

From the Five Element perspective a balanced Fire Element will allow a joy that is neither overexcited nor depressed, a kind of quiet contentment of the heart. Almaas observes that true joy manifests when there is fulfilment and there are no remaining unconscious desires or wishes. Since there can be no lasting fulfilment as long as there is any aspect of Being that is not realised, true joy is one of the more difficult essential aspects to experience as a permanent station.[52]

Joy is usually associated with pleasure and pleasurable experiences. However, if we are only open to pleasure and closed to painful experiences, we close ourselves off from joy. True joy arises when we are open to all of our experience. It is therefore not about experiencing only pleasure.

> When there is no prejudice about what should happen, there is joy. Joy is openness to experience. There is no striving. Joy is not the result of anything. If you are yourself, there is joy. If you are accepting and are open to your experience, if you're being yourself, you are naturally joyful because you are the source of the joy.[53]

Essential Love

The usual view of love is that it is an action that has a subject and an object, frequently expressed by the phrase 'I love you'. However, when we examine who is the I, who is the you and what is the doing, the sentence falls apart – for the I is the ego and the ego is not capable of real love, only constructed love. Moreover, who is it who is being loved, if not another constructed self?

> When you say, 'I love you', it is always a lie, because the person who says, 'I' cannot love, and doesn't know what love is. The personality does not know how to love. The personality is the product of the lack of love, so how can it know love? The personality is what you usually think is you, what you call 'I', 'myself'. When you say 'I', it is a lie. 'I' doesn't love. 'I' doesn't know how to love. 'I' is there because you don't know how to love. 'I' is there from the beginning because of the loss of love. The very existence of an 'I' is the absence of love, the blockage and distortion of love. The 'I' knows how to need; the 'I' does not know how to love. It is not possible. What we call 'I', our separate identity, is our self-image. Even if the self-image knows what love is, it does not have the love and cannot be a source of love. In fact, when there is love, love tends to melt away the 'I'. The 'I' relaxes and gets out of the way.[54]

Love is not an emotion. Since the ego is incapable of love and emotions come from ego, love therefore cannot be an emotion. Neither is love an activity or a reaction. It is not a thought. If love is none of these things, what is it?

Love is an existence.

> It is as substantial, as real as Essence is, because it is Essence. You cannot have love as you are love. Whenever you feel you have love, there is a contradiction… When you experience love as a movement, a reaction, an emotion, a fantasy, an action, an idea it is not love. Love can bring these things about, but love is more basic and more profound than any reaction. Your nature is not your identity tag. It is you, who you are. When love is there, then who you are is love.[55]

Aspects of Love

Love manifests as more than one aspect of Essence. When essential love is first discovered, it is often experienced as a sweetness that feels like a light, fluffy, pink presence. This is one of the simplest and easiest aspects of love to experience. Love is often experienced this way at the beginning. When someone says, 'I love you,' it is usually this pink love they are experiencing. But it is the ego which takes this feeling and attaches it to certain people and certain conditions. Essential love is not conditional.

Another aspect of love is merging love, which has a melting quality.

> It has to do with the loss of boundaries between you and your environment; you experience merging with your environment. Your boundaries melt away, and you have no shields around you. You experience yourself as a delicateness, an exquisiteness that does not feel itself separate from anything else. This experience brings about a sense of contentment, and a deeper letting go, a deeper satisfaction. It feels like you are your own nourishment, and actually that you and the nourishment are the same. This is the kind of love people want when they desire closeness or oneness with someone else.[56]

There is a third kind of love that is passionate, powerful, consuming and ecstatic.

> You feel you've been taken by storm. Your mind is gone. You feel power and lustiness, passion and zest. You feel your whole being is burning like a flame and that flame is full, and that fullness is the love. You feel ecstasy, passion and no difference between desire, wanting, giving, receiving. It is all one consuming thing. I call it ecstatic, passionate love. This love is not only directed toward a person. It is again your beingness. You are the passion.[57]

So far we have looked at ways that love expresses through the heart, manifesting in qualities such as joy, fulfilment, contentment, gratitude and satisfaction. Not only are the qualities of the heart aspects of love, all essential aspects include love. There is no part of Essence that is not loving. The action of any aspect of Essence is always loving or in the service of love. Strength is loving. Will is loving. Intelligence is loving. Love is a quality of all Essence, though it is not always experienced as sweet.

> In short, everything in the universe is made out of love. The body, the walls, the air, the space, the atoms, all seem to made out of the same continuum of cosmic consciousness. All physical forms arise out of an infinite and boundless ocean of loving presence.[58]

> For one human being to love another, that is perhaps the most difficult of all our tasks, the ultimate, the last test and proof, the work for which all other work is but preparation.
>
> RILKE

Acupressure for Spiritual Health

Here we look at the outer shu points of the Heart and Heart Protector meridians. These points are located on the back of the body along the outer line of the Bladder meridian. They are particularly effective in healing at the level of mind and spirit. Their effectiveness can be increased by using them in combination with the source points and the mu points learned earlier.

BL 43 *Gaohuangshu* Rich for the Vitals

BL 43 *Gaohuangshu* Rich for the Vitals is located four fingers' width out from the spine against the border of the scapula and at the level of the space between the fourth and fifth vertebrae (see Figure 8.13). It exerts a strong influence over the Official of the Heart Protector, especially at emotional and psychological levels. However, the point name itself refers to the *Gaohuang*, a region in the chest, whose influence is much wider and deeper than that of the Heart Protector alone.

The *Gaohuang* or Vital Region is an area in the chest about four body inches in diameter, lying between the centre and base of the sternum, and extending laterally to the edges of the sternum. When there is illness that is caused by deep heartbreak, betrayal, abuse, shame, or isolation, this vital region is deeply impacted and the effects go deep. Jarrett sees this as a place where deep karmic issues and conflicts reside, and where dark family secrets live.[59] Chronic or incurable disease is said to lodge there.

Classical texts observe that BL 43 *Gaohuangshu* deeply nourishes and calms the Heart as well as Kidney and Spleen. The action of this point was considered so great that it was said to strengthen the original Qi, and treat every kind of deficiency. Sun Si-miao went so far as to say that there is no disorder it cannot treat.

BL 43 *Gaohuangshu* is a great tonic point for the physical body, treating exhaustion and general deficiency, increasing stamina and supporting all the organs. It brings warmth and strength and increases blood circulation.

At the emotional level, the point brings warmth when a person is emotionally cold and shut down. It helps to dispel depression and mental negativity. When someone has little capacity for intimacy and humour because they are too depleted or vulnerable, this point lifts the spirit.

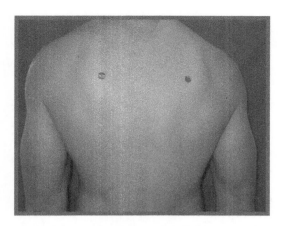

Figure 8.13 The outer shu point of the Heart Protector
(BL 43 *Gaohuangshu* Rich for the Vitals)

BL 44 *Shentang* Spirit Hall

BL 44 *Shentang* Spirit Hall is located four fingers' width out from the spine against the border of the scapula and at the level of the space between the fifth and sixth vertebrae (see Figure 8.14). It is the outer shu point of the Heart and as such exerts a powerful influence over the Heart Official and the *shen*. BL 44 *Shentang* addresses the spiritual nature of the *shen* as it radiates to direct affairs within both the heart and the mind. With this one point, heart and mind can be united in purpose as the *shen* is brought back to centre in all realms of being.[60]

This point makes direct contact with the spirit of the Heart. In health, the *shen* is seen as the sparkle in our eyes. It informs our intelligence and our responses to life. When the *shen* is disturbed and there is anxiety, depression or heartbreak, or when we are resigned, in a state of shock or without the capacity to act, then this point can restore the spirit and encourage participation once more in the richness of life.

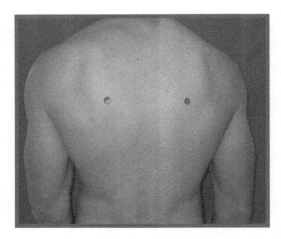

Figure 8.14 The outer shu point of the Heart (BL 44 *Shentang* Spirit Hall)

Meditation: The Heart

The Heart meditation can be done alone. In a group it can be vey powerful as the group field amplifies the energies of the heart.[61]

Find a comfortable position for yourself, relaxed and upright. Feel your pelvic bones in the chair or on the cushion. Feel your feet or legs on the ground. Let your hands rest lightly on your thighs or in your lap.

Begin by bringing your attention to your heart centre, the place in the centre of your chest. Notice what is there. Notice the sensation or lack of sensation. Notice any emotions or feelings that are there. And if there is nothing there, notice that. Allow your breath to be long, slow and rhythmic.

Now, whatever is in your chest, your heart centre, allow that to expand downwards. Your heart centre is becoming elongated, down through your body, down into the floor, down deep into the earth – dropping the anchor of the heart.

If you are doing this practice with a group, the anchor of your heart will meet with all the other heart anchors of the people in your group. You are meeting in the group heart. Feel the depth of that group heart and your connection with it.

Without losing contact with that place of the grounded heart, bring your attention back to the heart centre. Now allow the heart to expand upwards – holding the ground as your heart expands up through your chest, your throat, through the top of your head and up to the heavens. You are connected to the earth, connected to the heavens through your heart.

Now, without losing contact with the ground and the heavens, allow your heart space to open from the back. Your heart is opening like a gate, allowing the love from Source to fill your heart. Your heart is filling from the Source of all that is. Feel that love from Source filling your heart centre.

I invite you to be greedy. Allow your heart to fill until it overflows. If you don't get to a point of overflowing, continue to allow the Source to fill your heart.

Now, without losing contact with the ground, the heavens and the love that is coming from Source, while continuing to hold all of that, and only when your heart is full to overflowing, allow your heart to open at the front. Allow all that overflowing love to come out through the front of your heart and to flow into the room, filling the whole space of the room and all those in it. If the bubbling continues to flow, allow it to move out into the local neighbourhood, to the suburb, the city, out into your state, your country, spreading throughout the earth, and beyond the earth to the solar system, the galaxy, to the infinite reaches of the universe…all the while, connected to Earth, to Heaven, to Source, and now to all that exists.

When you're ready, you can open your eyes. Without losing contact with all of those things, come back into the room, to the here, to the now.

Transition from Fire to Earth

There comes a day when summer feels as though it has finally burnt itself out. It is reminiscent of a boisterous party which has talked and laughed and danced away the night but which finally runs out of energy and needs to take a rest. Nature's riotous summer foliage has reached its peak and now begins to droop. The sun's angle begins to drop and its heat is no longer intense. The light is softer, more golden. The shorter days become more noticeable. Overall there is a sense of lessening and decreasing. The summer holiday and party season is over. School goes back.

For some this is a time of sadness that the great summer party is over for another year. For those who love the summer heat, the end of the warmest season can engender a longing for it to continue. Some even fear the coming cold. There may be a feeling of poignancy at its ending. For those who find the high temperatures unbearable, there is a relief that the intense heat is finally over.

Because the season of late summer is itself a transition, the transitions from summer to late summer and from late summer to autumn happen quickly over the space of a few weeks. As with all transitions, there can be a going back and forth between the seasons. In some climates the hottest days are at this time of year, as if the summer is having one last dance at the party, one last drink for the road.

Whatever your feelings about heat and summer, whether you love it and don't want it to end, or you hate it and can't wait for it to leave, or you are somewhere in between, take time to be as fully present as you can with the changes that are happening both around you and within you. This transition will come again in other years, but never again in quite the way it is this year. This is a unique moment in your life and in the life of the planet. Just be. Right here. Now.

Chapter 9 ———————————————————————

Earth

The Nature of Earth

The importance of Earth is reflected in the many meanings of the word. Earth is one of the Five Elements. It is also the name of the planet, our home in space. It describes the soil which grows the food that sustains us. And it is the supportive ground upon which we stand and move.

All of the other Elements have a direction of movement. Wood is upwards, Fire is outwards, Metal is downwards and Water is inwards. Earth is unique in that, rather than having a direction of movement, it acts as an axis, fulcrum or centre around which all the other Elements move.

Earth energy is therefore neutral and is not classified as either yin or yang. It is the place of balance. It is like the hub of a wheel from which spokes radiate, the central point of reference to which other things are oriented.

This characteristic of centrality is central to the nature of the Earth Element. We will see this expressed again and again at all levels of its manifestation. At the physical level the organs of Stomach and Spleen are central to digestion and lie in the middle of the body. Emotionally, Earth wants to mediate and to connect others together. At a cosmic level it provides the pivotal point of balance between the heavens and the mundane world.

Earth energy is also seen in the principle of gravity. Gravity is the force which attracts a body to the centre of the Earth. Whatever is thrown into the air returns to Earth, comes back to centre. It is Earth's gravity which gives us weight and keeps us grounded.

Earth also creates shape, form and holding. It provides the banks that give shape and form to rivers and lakes. It provides stable ground on which to build. It supports our every step.

The Chinese character for Earth is *tu* (see Figure 9.1). The top horizontal line represents the surface of the soil while the bottom line represents the subsoil or bedrock. The vertical line represents all that is produced by the earth. The character therefore conveys two significant qualities of Earth, those of nourishment and stability.[1]

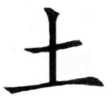

Figure 9.1 The Chinese character for Earth

The Resonances of Earth

The Season: Late Summer and Transitions

The Earth Element has its own special season of late summer and is also the facilitator of transitions between the seasons. The *Neijing* says that Earth energy is at its height in late summer.[2] But it also states that Earth's season is the last 18 days of each season and that it does not have a distinct season of its own.[3] From this we understand that Earth energy is evident four times a year at the changing of the four seasons, but most particularly at the end of the summer.

The late summer is the harvest time, Keats' season of 'mellow fruitfulness'[4] when nature takes a well-earned rest from producing and lies about in the warm fields, lazily listening to the humming of bees. The last fruit hangs heavy and round on the trees, oozing and dripping ripeness.

Many annual plants are looking droopy, drying out and going to seed. While the temperatures are still warm, the sting has gone out of the sun whose angle in the sky begins to dip. Days shorten noticeably and early sunsets allow for cooler evenings.

When does late summer begin? This will vary widely depending on your location. Jarrett places this season between the middle of August until the first frost,[5] which describes his experience in New England. Warmer climates may feel the change later, in September or March depending on your hemisphere. The *Neijing* definition would put the late summer at the beginning of August or February. Overall there is a sense of a decrease in nature, a lowering of intensity, a softening and rounding. You may feel these qualities within yourself.

The concept of the Earth Element acting as a transition between seasons means that the shortness of the season of late summer is compensated by the fact that there is also a late autumn, a late winter and a late spring, at which times the Earth energy reappears to mediate between the differing qualities of the four seasons.

The Chinese word *doyo* describes this time of transition. In the same way that 'twilight' and 'dusk' refer to the transition between day and night, so the word *doyo* denotes each of the four seasonal transitions. These periods are about 2–3 weeks in length.

This offers an explanation of the times between seasons when it is neither one nor the other. This is most evident in the transition between winter and spring when one day you are sure spring has begun, only to find you are plunged back into winter the next.

Why is it then that Earth is most specifically awarded the place between Fire and Metal? The qualities of nurturance, abundance, fullness and ripeness align it naturally to the time of harvest, that time of year when the energy is neither rising (Fire) nor falling (Metal), a period of balance and harmony. Earth finds its natural place in the season of nature's maturing.

The ease with which you are able to flow with the transitions between seasons will offer insights into the health and stability of the Earth Element within you. When you start wondering whether a new season has started, it already has!

The Sense: Taste
One of the newborn baby's first experiences is of the taste of mother's milk. At a very early stage in life, taste becomes associated with mother's comfort, support and love. In later life this sense can become strongly linked to deriving comfort from food.

The sense of taste is closely related to the stomach because it is the taste buds that identify foods that are good for us to eat. The mouth, lips, oesophagus and stomach are all part of the system that identifies, chooses and ingests food. The same receptors identify things that are not good for us; for example, many poisonous foods are bitter in flavour.

The sensation of taste, or gustation, originates in the taste buds, but also includes the sense of smell in rounding out the experience of flavour. The taste buds are taste receptor cells which identify the various flavours from food dissolved in saliva. There are five flavours which correspond to the five Elements: salty (Water), sour (Wood), bitter (Fire), sweet (Earth) and pungent or savoury (Metal).

Craving for or aversion to a particular flavour can indicate an imbalance in the corresponding Element. It is important to have a balance of flavours in our diet so that no one flavour is either absent or dominant. We will look more at the use of flavours in cooking in the section 'Diet and Lifestyle'.

The Colour: Yellow

In China, where the Five Element system originated, the colour yellow was associated with the colour of soil, ploughed earth and the famous Yellow River. This waterway is famous for silting up, its high soil content producing the yellow colour.

The golden-brownish yellow of a field of ripening grain is emblematic of both the colour and ripe fullness of the Earth Element. Other examples of yellow in nature include the bright yellow of lemons, bananas and egg yolks; the orange yellow of turmeric, peaches, pumpkins and squash; the golden yellow of leaves turning in early autumn; and the amber colour of honey. It is the most common colour of flowers, attracting the bees (also yellow) to pollenate them. It is the colour of gold, the ancient treasure.

In clothing, yellow is less common and yellow garments are rarely fashionable in Western countries. Perhaps this colour does not suit people with pale skin. Yellow clothing is more common in Asian and African countries where the bright colour goes well with darker skin tones. The saffron robes of Buddhist monks abound in Asia. In Hinduism it is the colour worn by *sanyasis* who have abandoned materialism and family in their wandering quest for ultimate truth.

What is your feeling about yellow? Do you have any yellow in your wardrobe? When might you choose to wear yellow clothes? How much yellow is in your home? It is good to have some yellow in your surroundings. According to feng shui principles, while the other four Elements relate to the four walls of a room, the Earth Element rules the middle of the room. Some yellow cushions, yellow flowers on a table or some yellow in a tablecloth can bring Earth energy into a room. The kitchen is more closely related to Earth than are the other rooms of the house, since it is the place where nourishing food is prepared. Bringing yellow-coloured and earth-toned objects into the kitchen is very beneficial to the energy of the home.

In Five Element diagnosis, a yellow colour in the face can indicate an imbalance in the Spleen and Stomach, the organs of Earth. The presence of dampness in the Spleen can often be observed as yellow around the mouth or cheeks.[6] (A yellow colour throughout the face can be caused by liver diseases such as hepatitis or jaundice.) People of an Earth constitution exhibit a yellow colour at the sides of the eyes. This colour can range from the bright yellow of a canary to a muddy, brown colour and sometimes appears as the colour of cream where the yellow is almost white.

The Sound: Singing

The sound of the Earth voice is one that has the widest variation. While the Wood and Fire voices are predominantly up and the Metal and Water voices are predominantly down, the Earth voice goes both up and down, often in the same sentence. I once was able to recognise a client as an Earth constitution because when I heard the person speaking in the hallway, I thought there were two people, so varied was the pitch of the voice.

The sound of someone's voice is diagnostic of their Constitutional Element and those of an Earth constitution will reveal this singing voice. The sound of singing carries the emotion of sympathy. Imagine a mother expressing sympathy to her child who has just fallen over. 'Oh, you poor baby. There, there, we'll make that better.' Such a tone would be caring, soothing, rounded in shape, not harsh. Think also of a rider soothing a frightened horse and how that voice would be modulated and soft.

People who are of an Earth constitution demonstrate this singing quality in their normal speaking voice. Even if they are talking about something sad or something that made them angry or afraid, the sing-song quality shows through the emotion being discussed.

There are some cultures in which people naturally speak in this way. The Welsh accent is a prime example of the singing voice, and Irish to some extent also. Scandinavians who speak English often sound as if their voice is going up and down in rapid alternation. In such cases, we must compare the person's voice to the norm within their culture. Not all people from Wales are Earth types!

The Odour: Fragrant

A person's subtle body odour is the third of the diagnostic tools that help to identify a person's Constitutional Element. Those of an Earth constitution will emanate an odour that is described as fragrant. Before you decide that you want to be an Earth type because this sounds like the most flattering of the odours, I must point out that this description is quite misleading. It is not the smell of fresh cut roses or honeysuckle in spring. While a healthy Earth person will have an odour that is somewhat sweet, it tends towards an excessive sweetness that can be cloying or sickly. When the person is out of balance, the odour becomes even stronger and can resemble that of fermenting grain or even the partly digested breast milk in a baby's vomit.

The odour arises from the organs of the Constitutional Element not doing their job optimally. In this case it is the Stomach that is not functioning well enough to digest properly, producing an odour of partially digested food.

The Emotion: Sympathy and Worry
Traditional Chinese Medicine regards worry as the emotion of Earth. Sometimes
it is described as pensiveness or overthinking. Like the planet Earth, the activity
of worry goes round and round in ceaseless repetition. This overactive mental
activity injures the Spleen.[7] It also keeps too much energy in the head, leaving the
worrier top-heavy and ungrounded, out of contact with the belly, legs and feet.

In the Five Element tradition, the emotion assigned to Earth is sympathy. To
discover the origin of this divergence, we need to look at the period of the 1960s
when acupuncture was first practised in England. The only English translation of
the *Neijing* available at that time was Ilza Veith's 1949 edition, which substitutes
sympathy for worry.[8] This was perpetuated by Felix Mann's 1962 book on
acupuncture,[9] which in turn influenced J.R. Worsley's understanding.[10]

In following this translation of the character as sympathy, Worsley discovered
that people of an Earth constitution tend to be out of balance in this emotion.
At one extreme they can be overly sympathetic towards other people. They focus
on the needs of others at the expense of their own needs and in ways that are
more concerned with their own need to give than the other's need to receive.
At the other extreme, the Earth person can be characteristically unsympathetic
to the needs and sufferings of other people, becoming self-focused, selfish and
narcissistic.

Some people argue that worry is not really an emotion at all but rather a
mental activity. Worry does not produce the intense movements of Qi as do the
emotions of fear, anger, joy and grief, and therefore sympathy more accurately
describes the core emotion of Earth.[11] Nonetheless, worry has a profound impact
on the Earth energies and cannot be ignored. We will explore both sympathy and
worry in the section 'The Pscycho-emotional Level of Earth'.

The Gifts of Earth
The Gifts of an Element are those qualities which are available when that Element
is in harmony and balance within us. When the Element is out of balance, these
qualities become less available or distorted. As you think about these Gifts of
Earth, consider to what extent they manifest in your life.

Stability
The ground upon which we stand provides stability and security. It is predictable
and reliable. It does not shift from moment to moment but provides a steady

platform for our feet. While there are some exceptions to this in the form of earthquakes and landslides, for the most part our experience is of the earth being solid. The planet's rotation and orbit of the sun is also reliably regular, giving us 24 hours in every day and 365 days every year.[12] While the seasons change four times a year, they also repeat with reliability.

These characteristics of stability, reliability and regularity are fundamental qualities of the Earth Element as it expresses itself in humans. When our Earth is in balance, we have regular sleeping patterns, keep regular mealtimes and make regular toilet visits. In addition, we are able to adapt to changing conditions in nature at the transition points between seasons, flowing easily from winter to spring to summer to autumn.

Earth needs the stability that can be provided by regularity and repetition. Developing steady routines and consistent patterns of action greatly support the cultivation of Earth energies. This is particularly important in the home. The place where we live provides a solid base from which to launch into the world and a haven of support to which we can return. When we can feel relaxed and at ease in our home, when home feels solid and supportive, then our Earth is nourished. It is no surprise that moving house is considered one of the biggest stresses in a person's life, for it challenges the Earth Element at a deep level. All of a sudden, the comfortable familiarity of the old home is gone. Everything changes, from where knives and forks are kept to how to get to the bathroom in the night. A whole new set of routines and patterns needs to be established before we once more feel at home.

Another way we can support our Earth is by being balanced and centred in the body. There is an acupuncture point beside the navel named Heavenly Pivot (Stomach 25). It is appropriate that this lies on an Earth meridian, for the Earth is the central pivot, in this case between the upper body and the lower body. When the Earth energies are balanced, there is a centring that occurs; our feet are firmly on the ground while at the same time we are connected to Heaven. This balance between Heaven and Earth was considered the natural human condition by the ancient Chinese. The character for a human being pictures a figure rooted like a tree in the earth with hands outstretched like branches towards the heavens, receiving support from above and below.[13]

How much stability and regularity do you experience in your life? What would it take for you to feel more stable?

Abundance

The season of Earth is that of the late summer or harvest time, when the year-long efforts of farmers and gardeners are rewarded with the bounty of the fruits of the earth. This harvest of the Earth Element is dependent on the full flourishing of the summer Fire which in turn is dependent on the rapid springtime growth of Wood. This in turn is founded on the restoration and rejuvenation of the Water in winter.

It is also true that the quality of the soil in which seeds are planted will determine the abundance of the harvest. Soil that is rich in organic matter, nutrients and moisture will repay the labour of cultivation far more than that which is poor, sterile and parched.

These principles of nature apply equally to human nature. The power of a person's Water Element, the growth of her Wood Element and the flourishing of her Fire Element will have a great impact on the way that her Earth Element manifests. But the Earth energy itself must be balanced for the abundance of life to be reaped and for there to be satisfaction and contentment. I am not referring to quantities of goods amassed, projects completed or accolades achieved, but rather to an inner state of satisfaction. Those who have much material wealth can be unhappy and dissatisfied, while those with little can be content.

Abundance is not a physical state but rather a condition of the mind and the spirit. When Earth energies are balanced, there is a natural recognition of the abundance that the universe offers us, from the bounty and the beauty of nature, to the love and connection with others, to the simple fact of being alive. Another acupuncture point on the Stomach meridian proclaims this gift of Earth. ST 40 on the leg is named Abundant Splendour for its capacity to connect us with the truth that we *are* already the cornucopia of life's abundance. When we understand that we are a living personification of abundance, there can be deep satisfaction from being alive and being present to life.

 What gets in the way of feeling satisfaction? Describe the ways you experience abundance.

Giving and Receiving

The soil of the earth provides us with abundance. It gives us the animal, vegetable and mineral of everything we need. We are the lucky recipients of the planet's generosity. However, this is not a one-way street. We must also give back to the earth in return. We must tend and nourish the soils, manage diversity, take only what we need and live sustainably. Failure to live in harmony with the ecology of the earth has historically resulted many times in the denuding of forests, depletion of soils and exhaustion of water supplies, situations which have resulted in the collapse of ecosystems and civilisations. Examples of this can be seen in the desertification of the once Fertile Crescent of Mesopotamia, the sudden end of the Maya civilisation in Central America and the disappearance of the culture of Easter Island.[14]

The lesson from nature is that for there to be a sustainable relationship, there needs to be a balance between giving and receiving. This has been described as the virtue of reciprocity and represents the expression of the Earth Element in any balanced relationship, whether it be in our relationship with the environment or in relationships between humans.[15] Reciprocity naturally arises out of an understanding that all things are interconnected. When we begin to recognise the interconnectedness and interdependence of all things, we realise that we are not separate. And if I am not separate from my neighbour, then giving and receiving amount to the same thing.

When Earth energy is balanced, both giving and receiving come easily and naturally. Giving happens when it is needed and appropriate. It arises from an attunement to what other people need and from a sense of generosity towards them. That which is given may be something material such as money, food or goods; or it may be through devoting time and effort to helping out on a project; or it may be the giving of attention, lending a sympathetic ear, providing reassurance or sharing wisdom. Healthy giving arises out of a recognition of another's needs and a willingness to meet those needs. At the same time healthy giving does not force the gift upon the other, nor does it give with strings attached. And it never gives out of a sense of obligation or responsibility.

Healthy receiving is that which has gratitude for the gift, is open and gracious. It receives without a feeling of entitlement to that which is given or a sense of guilt at receiving the gift. And it does not react by feeling a need to give something back in return.

Giving and receiving are two sides of the same thing, like the back of the hand and the front of the hand. Each is a part of the other. True giving cannot happen without true receiving, nor can there be receiving without giving.

How easy is it to give to others? What are the limits to your giving? How easy it is to receive? What are the limits to your receiving? Is there a balance between your giving and receiving?

Nourishment

Just as the whole world is nourished by the gifts of Mother Earth, every human begins life being nourished by his own mother.[16] One of the first experiences of the newborn infant is to nurse at his mother's breast. Connected intimately with his mother in the womb, after birth he reconnects with her by feeding from her milk. Nourishment, nurturing, support, satisfaction and comfort all become combined in a single rich experience, and all becomes associated with mother.

For the child, this first phase of life is one in which there is no experience of being a separate self. His whole world is a bubble that includes himself and mother. Sometimes called the dual-unity phase, it is a time in which the mother's experience and his own are not separate. And since mother is the source of supply for his needs of nourishment and nurturing, these early experiences profoundly influence the child's capacity to take nourishment and to be nourished, first from mother, later from others.

A positive experience of being nurtured and nourished by mother creates the foundation of a healthy Earth Element for the child. What follows is a healthy balance which allows the person to receive nourishment at all levels. At the physical level, a balanced Earth supports a healthy digestive system which extracts nutrition from food and drink. Emotionally, it enables the person to form connections with others that are rich and rewarding, to be nourished by contact with others, to receive love, affection, sympathy and caring. At the level of mind, the person can derive satisfaction and support from intellectual pursuits and abstract ideas. Spiritually, the person is nourished by art, music, nature and the connection to the divine.

At all of these levels, when one is nourished, there is a sense of being sated, richly satisfied, imbued with a round and pleasant fullness. As it was for Goldilocks in the bears' house, everything feels just right.

 What is it like to feel satisfied? What are the sensations and feelings? To what extent are you nourished by the different areas of your life?

Empathy

We have already learned that sympathy is the emotion of the Earth Element. Sympathy is the process of acknowledging another person's hardships and providing comfort and assurance. However, we might be sympathetic to someone's plight but have no real idea how it feels because we have not had our own experience of that condition. For example, we might feel sympathy for a friend whose husband has died, but if we ourselves have not had that experience or one like it, there is a way we do not quite comprehend how it is for them.

Empathy is deeper than sympathy because it includes an understanding of what others are feeling, because we have had a similar experience or at least we are able to really put ourselves in the other person's shoes. Empathy includes an understanding of the other's position, thoughtfulness for them and caring about them. The phrase 'I can relate' is perhaps a cliché, but it is appropriate in this circumstance. Empathy is the ability to relate to the needs of others.

Empathy has a specific affect or feeling. There is a deep sensitivity to the emotional vibrations of others, a capacity to tune into feelings, to understand people and know where they are coming from. There is a sense of deep engagement with the other, a focus on them and an attunement to their emotional state.

Empathy is a relatively new word in English, a psychological term coined in 1909. It has come to have a range of meanings from recognising and understanding another's feelings, to actually feeling those feelings as if they were one's own. Someone who directly feels another's feelings is sometimes called an empath. The word 'grok' has assumed widespread use since it was coined by Robert Heinlen in his science fiction novel *Stranger in a Strange Land* in 1961. In that work it is a Martian word meaning to understand another profoundly through intuition or empathy. This happens by a process of merging thoroughly with another person's world view.[17] Here is a Martian word whose meaning is replete with the qualities of Earth!

How do you experience empathy physically and emotionally? What gets in the way of truly empathising with another?

Connection

Humans are gregarious creatures. We naturally form into groups, tribes, communities and nations as a way of feeling connected to our fellows. Connection is just as much a human need as food, warmth and shelter. If children are isolated, they rarely survive, so important is their need for belonging. In tribal times people banded together for physical survival. Those who were ostracised from their communities, condemned to live 'beyond the pale', were effectively given a death sentence. In those times we needed connection with the tribe in order to survive. This need for connection is now embedded deeply into our human nature.

One of the ways our primitive ancestors bonded as a tribe was through telling stories. Before the advent of writing, storytelling was the way a tribe's history and identity were preserved. Having a common story meant that all members of the tribe had a common bond of connection. While the caves and fires are long gone, storytelling continues to have a significant place in our lives. Now, rather than sitting round the fire listening to the elders sing the exploits of legendary ancestors, we tell each other stories over dinner or immerse ourselves in others' stories in books, movies and television shows.

Across time and cultures, stories provide the medium that knits us together as humans, connecting us to our family, our community, our culture and our humanness. This connectivity is one of the Gifts of the Earth Element. It allows us to feel held, supported, nurtured and know that we belong.

Earth stands at the centre, connecting the other Elements to it and to one another. It weaves itself into the fabric of the whole, giving it unity and integrity. It is the energy of the Earth Element that establishes community, creates consensus, is friendly and welcoming to others. It likes to connect with others and to connect others together. Many Earth types naturally become a central point of mediation in groups and families. They often act as go-betweens.

This quality of connection is expressive of something even deeper. This gift of Earth is pointing to the reality of the interconnectedness of all things. One person, after a profound near-death experience, described her direct knowledge of this truth: 'I realised that I was at the centre of this universe, and knew that we all express from our perspective, as we're each at the centre of this great cosmic web.'[18]

 What are the ways you find connection with others? To what extent do you take the role of intermediary in your social network?

Altruism

Altruism is the highest form of giving. It is not simply giving to another in need but also includes a selfless concern for their well-being. It often involves some kind of sacrifice on the part of the giver, a sacrifice of energy, time or possessions, without any thought of receiving anything in return, either directly or indirectly. There is no expectation of recognition, gratitude or even a subtle desire to feel good about the giving.

Interestingly, when a person takes an altruistic action, it does feel good. Neurobiologists have found that when people placed the interests of others before their own, the generosity activated pleasure centres in a primitive part of the brain that also lights up in response to food or sex.[19] Even when the altruistic action is done with no expectation of reward, there is a pleasurable sensation.

Philanthropy is the concern for others which arises out of love for humanity and which has come to be associated with charitable giving. Altruism goes further in that it includes unselfishness. At its highest, there is actual selflessness, a lack of self. In this state, the giver has no sense of himself as a separate individual but rather as a part of the infinite web of manifestation. There is no sense of giving from one to another because there is no separation. No gift, no giver.

This brings to mind Lao Tzu's thoughts on the subject:

> *The Master stays behind;*
> *That is why she is ahead.*
> *She is detached from all things;*
> *That is why she is one with them.*
> *Because she has let go of herself*
> *She is perfectly fulfilled.*[20]

The ego is inherently selfish and self-serving. When there is no ego self, there is no selfishness. There is no self-centred action because there is no self there to act. Therefore, the way to true altruism is through disengagement from this false self and engagement with the True Self, which is not a separate individual but a manifestation of the Infinite. Then, fulfilment is not in the doing but in simply being.

What are your motives for giving? What is the most altruistic thing you have done?

And More…

Earth expresses itself in a cornucopia of Gifts. Here are some others to digest. Think or write about these qualities in yourself. How available are they to you?

Caring	Grounding	Reliability
Centring	Harvest	Satisfaction
Comfort	Home	Selflessness
Compassion	Integrity	Service
Contentment	Intention	Sharing
Devotion	Mother	Support
Fertility	Nurturing	Thoughtfulness
Generosity	Reciprocity	Understanding
Gratitude	Regularity	Welcoming

The Physical Level of Earth

Now that you have had a taste of the qualities of the Earth Element, it is now time to look at the ways these resonances manifest in the physical body. The ways in which you respond to the vibrations of the Earth Element will influence how it is revealed in its related organs and tissues.

Organs and Tissues

The Stomach

WESTERN MEDICAL PERSPECTIVE

The stomach is a J-shaped, muscular enlargement of the gastrointestinal tract that lies directly under the diaphragm in the upper left quadrant of the abdomen. Empty, it is the size of a long sausage. It comfortably holds about a litre of food but can expand to hold as much as three litres. Its upper portion is a continuation of the oesophagus, though separated from it by the oesophageal sphincter. The lower part of the stomach empties into the duodenum of the small intestine, separated from it by the pyloric sphincter. In between, the body of the stomach secretes gastric juice made up of hydrochloric acid and enzymes that break down food and begin the digestion of protein. At the same time peristaltic movements mix the food and the secreted enzymes into a liquid known as chyme that is passed to the small intestine for digestion.

Depending on the amount of food consumed, this process takes between 40 minutes and several hours. Emotions such as anger, fear and anxiety may slow down digestion in the stomach because they stimulate the sympathetic nervous system, which inhibits gastric activity.[21]

Stomach disorders are common and the cause of much suffering in humans. Factors which can affect the function of the stomach are bacterial infections, stress, overeating and medications such as non-steroidal anti-inflammatory drugs, which irritate the stomach lining. Ongoing stress is closely related to the development of peptic ulcers in the stomach, a condition which affects about 10% of the population.[22]

CHINESE MEDICINE PERSPECTIVE

The Earth organs hold a special importance because together they form a central axis in the body. The Stomach is the most important of the yang organs.[23] It is referred to as the Great Granary and is responsible for the nourishment of all the other organs. The Neijing says that 'the five yin organs and six yang organs derive their Qi and nutrition from the Stomach'.[24] The Stomach therefore has a wider significance and influence in Chinese medicine than from the Western perspective.

To begin with, it controls receiving. This function goes beyond merely being a repository for food taken in through the mouth. The Stomach is responsible for appetite which prompts the desire to take in food and also holds on to the food once it is ingested. Weak Stomach receiving may produce poor appetite, reflux and belching. This capacity of receiving also extends to the emotional level, as we will later explore.

It is said that the Stomach controls the rotting and ripening of food and drink, a process of transformation.[25] This can be compared to the Western view of the stomach organ's enzyme secretions and peristaltic action to produce chyme. Then the Stomach, together with the Spleen, controls the transport of the essences of food throughout the body. To have strong Stomach Qi is synonymous with robust health, while weak Stomach Qi will produce fatigue and ill health.

The Stomach also controls the descent of Qi. If the Qi does not properly descend, food will stagnate and produce bloating and belching. The Stomach is responsible not only for the downward movement of food to the Small Intestine, but also more generally for the movement of Qi down the body as well as the proper movement of Qi in the Three Burners. When the Stomach is not performing this task, there is a counter-flow of Qi which ascends rather than descends.

The Spleen/Pancreas
WESTERN MEDICAL PERSPECTIVE

The spleen is part of the lymphatic system which also includes the lymph nodes, tonsils and the thymus gland. The lymphatic system is closely allied to the circulatory system and is responsible for the collection and return of interstitial fluid to the bloodstream as well as creating the cells that assist in fighting infection. The spleen is the largest mass of lymphatic tissue in the body. Oval shaped and measuring 12 cm (5 in) in length, the spleen lies in the upper left abdomen. Its shape conforms to the organs around it: the stomach, left kidney, colon and diaphragm. It plays an important part in immune defence through phagocytosis (devouring) of bacteria, worn-out red blood cells and platelets. It creates lymphocytes, the cells that produce antibodies. It also stores blood for release during haemorrhage.

The pancreas is unrelated to the spleen in Western medicine. It has two separate functions that make it part of both the digestive and endocrine systems. It is a tube-shaped gland about 12 cm (5 in) in length and 2.5 cm (1 in) thick. It lies behind the stomach in the centre-right of the upper abdomen. Ninety-nine per cent of the cells of the pancreas secrete the enzymes which form pancreatic juice. This fluid is then carried into the duodenum of the small intestine to assist in digestion. The remaining 1% of the cells produce the hormones insulin and glucagon which together metabolise sugars and regulate blood sugar levels.

CHINESE MEDICINE PERSPECTIVE

Of all the organs, the Spleen is the most unlike its Western namesake. Some sources refer to the Spleen/Pancreas meridian because the functions of the Spleen do include some of the functions of the pancreas; however, purists eschew this practice, noting that the classics do not refer to the pancreas at all, except possibly in one place as 'the half pound of fatty tissue' surrounding the spleen.[26]

The main function of the Spleen is to assist the Stomach in the transformation of food essences and to transport these throughout the body. It is also responsible for the movements of Qi and fluids. In this sense it can be personified as the Minister for Transport. When the Spleen Qi is strong, there is good appetite, digestion and elimination. When it is weak, there may be poor digestion, bloating and loose stools. Spleen Qi deficiency is one of the most common patterns seen in clinical acupuncture practice in Western countries.

The second function of the Spleen is to control ascending Qi, partnering the Stomach's role of controlling descending Qi. One way this operates is that the Spleen sends food Qi upwards to the Lung to support its function of gathering Qi from the breath. It also sends food Qi upwards to the Heart to assist in forming Blood. In an overall way, the Spleen provides support and upward lift to the body.

One interpretation of the pathway of the Spleen meridian is that it is like a crutch under the armpit, supporting an upright stance (see Figure 9.3). When Spleen Qi is weak, there is often fatigue and sagging as if this upright support has been lost. The state of the Spleen is one of the most important factors in determining the amount of energy a person has.[27]

Mouth

The Spleen is said to open into the mouth, which is the sense organ or orifice of Earth. The mouth is used for tasting, the sense of Earth. When the Earth energies are balanced and healthy, the mouth is able to taste the five flavours. The mouth also produces saliva, which begins the process of digestion by breaking down the starches in food. The chewing of food is also a function of the Spleen. When the Earth energy is healthy, then tasting, salivating and chewing are normal and the appetite is good. If these capacities are impaired, or if there is a tendency to mouth sores, it indicates that the Spleen Qi is compromised.

Muscles

The muscles and flesh are the tissues of Earth. One of the functions of Spleen is to transport the food Qi to the muscles, especially those of the arms and legs. When Spleen Qi is weak, this function is impaired and there can be tiredness and heaviness in the limbs.

If there is a lack of smoothness and firmness to the muscles and flesh or if there are lumps and swellings under the skin, this can indicate an imbalance in Earth.

Another form of tissue that relates to Earth is the fascia. The myofascial sheath is perhaps even more resonant with Earth energies than the muscles themselves.[28] The fascia is a web of connective tissue that holds the body together and gives it integrity, shape and support. It includes the tough sheath of tissue that surrounds the muscles and muscle groups, yet also extends into the muscle cells, creating a completely integrated system within the body. It is a physical manifestation of Earth's Gift of connection.

Lips

The lips are considered to be the external manifestation of Earth and thus a reflection of the state of the Spleen. They are closely related to the mouth though not a part of it. The lips should be full, moist and red. If they are dull, pale and dry, or if there is a tendency to get lip sores, it is a sign of imbalance in Earth.

Hicks suggests that fat is the external manifestation or residue of Earth.[29] Excess fat on the body or lumps of fat under the skin are indicative of damp or phlegm, suggesting a weakness in the Earth.

Diet and Lifestyle

Foods That Support Earth

Yellow is the colour that corresponds to the Earth Element, so yellow-coloured foods are supportive of Earth. Orange is also included in the colour spectrum of Earth-related foods.

Yellow and orange fruits include banana, lemon, pineapple, orange, mandarin, apricot, cantaloupe, mango, nectarine, peach, papaya, satsuma and passionfruit.

Among the Earth-coloured vegetables are carrot, swede, sweet potato, butternut squash, pumpkin, yellow and orange pepper and sweet corn.

Other foods include the spices turmeric, saffron and mustard, as well as millet and sesame seed.

Most orange and yellow foods contain carotenes which are converted into vitamin A. This is well known to help with vision but is also important in maintaining a strong immune system and keeping the cells of the digestive tract healthy, both aspects of the Earth Element. Carotenes are better absorbed with the help of a little fat, so adding a little olive oil to your carrot, sweet corn and yellow pepper salad, or roasting your sweet potato and pumpkin in coconut oil, will aid in the absorption of these important carotenoids.

Here are some suggestions to get more yellow and orange food in your diet:

- Use mashed carrot, butternut squash and sweet potato as a substitute for mashed potatoes. Add this to cottage pie or serve as a side dish.

- Roast sweet potato and pumpkin to go with your Sunday roast.

- Make carrot or butternut pumpkin soup with leeks, nutmeg and ginger.

- Bake sweet potatoes instead of regular potatoes.

- Try Chinese sweet corn soup, with or without chicken.

- Use stewed apricots as a topping for porridge or cereal.

- Cool down with late summer fruit salads of mango, papaya, pineapple and cantaloupe.

The flavour of Earth is sweet; therefore, foods that are sweet are also supportive of the Element. Before you head off to the ice cream parlour or cake shop to support your Earth, we need to clarify what is meant by a sweet flavour. In the West most people associate the sweet flavour with that of sugar, and more usually refined sugar, which is increasingly being recognised as very damaging to health. The sweet flavour described in Chinese medicine is a more subtle one. It is the flavour of pumpkin, carrot, sweet corn and sesame, all of which also have the colour of Earth. Among the myriad of sweet foods are rice, potato, cabbage, tomatoes, beets, almonds, walnuts and chicken.

While small quantities of these foods will strengthen the Spleen and the Earth Element, overindulgence will weaken the Spleen and the muscles. Also, the Kidneys are impacted by too much sweetness, since the flavour of an Element has a negative impact on its grandson Element.

The Impact of Sugar on Health

It has been observed that Spleen Qi deficiency is the most common pattern, based on Traditional Chinese Medicine, encountered in Western acupuncture clinics. This begs the question, 'How much of this is due to the sweet-saturated Western diet?' We know that there is sugar in baked goods, desserts, jams and soft drinks, but there are large servings hidden in breakfast cereals, 'health food' snack bars, flavoured yoghurt, sports drinks, fruit juice, iced tea, pasta sauce and pizza. Almost all processed foods contain sugar, often used to mask the salt that is used as a preservative or simply to hook into the average person's sweet tooth.

If you look at the labels on packaged food, you will often see fructose listed as an ingredient. This might sound healthy, making us think of fruit, but the loading of high-fructose corn syrup into processed food is perhaps the leading cause of overweight and obesity. This in turn is responsible for much of the heart disease, diabetes and other chronic ailments in the population.[30] Fructose and other sugars are simple carbohydrates that contain lots of calories but few nutrients. They are broken down rapidly by the body and create the so-called sugar hit or sugar rush. These sudden spikes in blood sugar levels place great strain on the liver and the pancreas as they are suddenly called upon to process the glucose.

What is even more insidious is that sugar is highly addictive. Some people even argue that sugar is more addictive than opiates. Unlike fat or other foods, sugar interferes with the body's appetite, creating an insatiable desire to carry on eating. When we try to give up eating sugars, the body goes through a withdrawal, the symptoms of which are so unpleasant that we want to reach for something sweet to satisfy the craving.

Estimates of the average annual consumption of sugar in the USA vary between 36 kg (80 lbs) and 71 kg (156 lbs) per person. This amounts to between half and one cup of sugar per day. Similar figures apply to other Western countries. The American Heart Association recommends that women consume no more 6 teaspoons of sugar per day and men no more than 9 teaspoons. Some authorities are even moving to regulate or restrict the use of sugar in the food industry.[31]

As important as it is to reduce the total consumption of sugar, equally important is to replace refined sugars with unrefined alternatives.

If you want to reduce or eliminate bad sugars from your diet, here are some suggestions:

- Do not drink soft drinks. These are the biggest contributors to the high sugar intake.

- Read food labels and reject anything containing sugar, fructose or corn syrup.

- Prepare as much of your food as possible from fresh ingredients.

- Use honey instead of sugar. While honey is also a simple carbohydrate, it contains good nutrients. Get organic raw honey from local farmers' markets.

- Try stevia, a natural sweetener that is 300 times sweeter than sugar but does not raise blood sugar levels and has no calories.

- Agave syrup is lower on the glycaemic index (30) so it is processed by the body much more slowly than sugar (85), avoiding the blood sugar spike.

- Coconut sugar is also lower on the glycaemic index (35) and is packed with important minerals and vitamin C. Coconut palms are far more ecologically sustainable than sugar cane.

Stomach Health

Doctors are now finding that the main causes of stomach ulcers are bacteria and medications, not stress and spicy food as previously thought, though it is known that stress worsens the symptoms of ulcers. The main bacterial culprit is *Helicobacter pylori*, which causes inflammation of the lining of the stomach.[32] The regular use of pain relievers, including aspirin, ibuprofen and naproxen, especially among older people, can irritate and inflame the stomach lining. Alcohol can irritate and erode the mucous lining of your stomach. It also increases the amount of stomach acid that is produced.

Many digestive problems are associated with an imbalance in the level of hydrochloric acid (HCL) in the stomach. The correct pH level is required for the proper breakdown of proteins. Too much HCL (hyperchlorhydria) or too little HCL (achlorhydria) can both produce symptoms such as abdominal pain, heartburn, nausea, vomiting, gas and bloating, belching, flatulence and constipation. Because the symptoms of both conditions are so similar, many people who have low HCL are diagnosed as having high HCL and treated with antacids, which worsen the problem.[33] HCL production decreases steadily as we age, about 1% per year of life, so that a person age 70 years typically only has 30% of original HCL production in the stomach. Older people are therefore more likely to suffer from achlorhydria, a condition which is associated with impaired protein synthesis, bacterial overgrowth in the small intestine and decreased absorption of calcium, iron, vitamins B6 and B12 as well as folate.[34]

You can test whether you have too little HCL in your stomach by taking the Betaine HCL challenge test. This involves taking the Betaine HCL supplement with a protein meal and observing your body's reaction. If you have no reaction, this indicates that the stomach acid is low; if there is a warm sensation in the stomach, the HCL level is not low.[35] If you are experiencing stomach pain, another test is to take a tablespoon (15 ml) of apple cider vinegar. If it makes the pain go away, you likely have too little HCL; if it worsens, you probably have too much HCL.[36]

More generally, you can support the work of your stomach by developing good eating practices. Eat smaller meals more frequently. Chew food thoroughly. Avoid overeating. Only eat when relaxed and sitting. Do not eat while standing or walking.

Spleen Health

This section focuses on the Chinese medicine concept of the Spleen which, as we have already discussed, is quite different from and much broader than the Western one. It is an organ that is defined for its function, not for its anatomical location.

One of the most important ways to support the Spleen is to avoid cold food and drink. This means not drinking iced water, ice-cold beer and soft drinks, ice cream or indeed anything straight from the fridge or freezer. The Spleen is responsible for the transformation of food and the transportation of the energy derived from food. When food is cold, the Spleen has to work much harder to heat it up as part of the process of transformation. You can do your Spleen a favour by only taking warm food and drink into your body.

Foods that are challenging to the Spleen include refined sugars and flours, fried foods, cold raw foods, alcohol, coffee, milk, cheese and yoghurt. Foods that support the Spleen include warm foods, soups and the yellow/orange and sweet foods mentioned earlier. Being adequately hydrated is also important to support the Spleen's function of transporting fluids.

We have already seen that overthinking negatively affects the Spleen. This is especially true when eating, for the thinking process detracts from the process of digestion. You are probably familiar with the experience of eating a meal only to discover afterwards that your mind was somewhere else entirely. It is therefore important to eat with mindfulness. The more we can pay attention to the activity of eating, the more thorough will be the Spleen's digestion of the food. If eating can become a meditation, so much the better. Notice the placing of food in the mouth. Chew the food well, tasting the flavours and noticing how it becomes soft and mushy in the mouth. Swallow mindfully, noticing how the bolus of food is sent down to the stomach. Do all of these steps before putting the next forkful of food into your mouth.

One of the functions of Spleen is to digest information. We live in an increasingly information-driven society where we are bombarded with facts, ideas and images, as well as demands to respond. It is very helpful to take time out from this information overload, not just at mealtimes but at other times too. Finding times to turn off the TV, phone and computer, taking a break from email and Facebook, will make your Spleen happier. Finding time to meditate each day will also be very supportive.

Balancing the Five Flavours

When it comes to meal preparation, it can be fun to experiment with the five flavours. From the perspective of Chinese medicine, it is important to have a balance in our diet of salty, sour, bitter, sweet and pungent flavours. This does not mean that every dish or even every meal needs to contain all five, but over the course of a day, each should be making an appearance in our diet.

Different cultures tend to favour certain flavours, and individual preferences are strongly influenced by the foods we ate in childhood. For example, in China, the people of the northern province of Shanxi love vinegar with their food. They even have vinegar bars there. Meanwhile, in the southwestern province of Sichuan, people favour hot and spicy food. Sometimes these cultural preferences are based on conditions of climate or food availability that are no longer relevant today.

Notice which of the flavours you tend to favour and which you avoid. If there is a notable imbalance, try adding other flavours to your cooking.

One really useful tool in balancing flavours in cooking is to use the principles of the Control Cycle (see Chapter 2). From this we know that each Element controls its grandson, two Elements forward in the cycle. This applies also to flavours in the following way:

- Salty (Water) controls bitter (Fire).

- Bitter (Fire) controls pungent (Metal).

- Pungent (Metal) controls sour (Wood).

- Sour (Wood) controls sweet (Earth).

- Sweet (Earth) controls salty (Water).

If you have made a pot of soup and realise it is too salty, add something sweet to bring it under control. Eggplant, which is bitter, can be rubbed with salt before cooking to remove the bitterness. If you've been heavy-handed with the red hot chilli sauce, the pungent spice can be controlled with bitter herbs and greens such as parsley, dandelion, chicory, romaine lettuce and endive. If the pumpkin soup is just too sweet, add some cider vinegar or lemon juice. And if the vinegar in the borscht makes you pucker, add something spicy to calm it down.

Using these principles in the kitchen can be fun and satisfying, and will enable you to include all five flavours in your diet, even the ones you thought you didn't like.

The Way We Eat

An extraordinary amount of attention is placed on food and diet in our culture. On the one hand, the advertising of food tempts us everywhere we go and ubiquitous television cooking shows aim to make gourmands of us all. On the other hand, calls to lose weight shriek from television ads, Internet pop-ups and every magazine rack. Often these conflicting messages are sandwiched together.

Many of the dieting methods are contradictory, some advising to eat more protein and no carbs while others advocate a vegan diet as the only way to good health. There is the Atkins diet, the Zone diet, the Blood Type diet, the Mediterranean diet, the raw food diet, the Weight Watchers diet, the South Beach diet, the Paleo diet…and the list goes on.

All of these approaches focus on what we put in our mouths, which certainly is important. A plate of vegetables is almost always going to be better for you than a plate of ice cream. But there is rarely any focus on *how* we eat. Paying attention to the way we take the food into our bodies can make such a difference to the amount of food we consume that *what* we eat becomes less important.

Here are some suggestions of ways to cultivate healthy eating patterns:

- Eat only when you are hungry.

  Sometimes we eat because it is mealtime, not necessarily because we are hungry. Force-feeding is never a good path to healthy eating. Save the food for later, take it with you in a bag. You will enjoy it much more when your body calls for it.

- Eat slowly.

  Eating quickly is sometimes called inhaling your food. It can be like sucking up food with a vacuum cleaner. When we eat like this, the important predigestive processes of salivation and mastication are bypassed. This means that the stomach and intestines have a harder job extracting nutrition from the food.

- Chew thoroughly.

  I once met a person who tried to chew every mouthful 50 times before swallowing. She took a long time to eat her meals. While this may be a little extreme, it makes the point that completely pureeing food in the mouth along with saliva aids digestion greatly. Even drinks like juices can be chewed to add saliva before swallowing. A good maxim is 'Drink your food and eat your drink'.

- Stop eating while you are still hungry.

  It takes time for the hormones leptin (from the Greek word meaning thin) and ghrelin to register satiety. Especially if you are eating quickly, you can eat a whole lot more than you need to before the feeling of fullness arises. Try eating about three-quarters of what you would usually eat and wait 20–30 minutes. Then if you still feel hungry, go ahead and eat some more.

- Eat less, more often.

  Smaller, more frequent meals are less challenging to the digestive system than large intakes of food. Eating five or six small meals instead of two or three big ones has been shown to reduce conversion of food to fat, maintain steady blood sugar levels and reduce cholesterol.[37] Make sure the meals really are small and that your total daily caloric intake does not increase.

- Relax.

  Make sure that you are as relaxed as possible when eating. Do not eat while standing or walking, while sitting at the computer, in front of the TV or doing any other mental activity. If you are eating with others, avoid topics of conversation that are stressful. Arrange things so you can be as mindful as possible as you eat.

- Listen to your body.

  Your body knows what it needs. As you tune in to what it is telling you, you can discover which foods you need, which foods are not good and when you have eaten enough. The more relaxed and mindful you are, the easier it will be to hear your body's signals.

- Practise the one-bowl eating meditation.

  This practice suggests keeping a bowl from which to eat all your meals, to fill it once only for each meal, then eat mindfully until you are finished. You do not eat anything else until the next meal. This is a challenging practice and more difficult than it sounds. Even if you do this once a week or once a month, you may find it offers great support to your eating habits the rest of the time. And more generally it will support the cultivation of the Gifts of Earth such as stability, regularity and groundedness.[38]

- Fast.

  Fasting has long been used as part of religious and spiritual practice as a path to spiritual revelation. It has also been shown to deliver health benefits of weight loss, better insulin resistance and increased lifespan.[39] Intermittent fasting is the process of fasting for short periods regularly, say, one day a week or one day a month. A popular approach is the 5:2 method where you eat normally for five days a week, while on the other two days you eat 500 calories (women) or 600 calories (men).

As we all know, what and how we eat has much to do with our emotional and psychological state. No amount of good advice can help when we have parts of ourselves that use food for comfort, to suppress emotions or to fill a hole of pain. This is true for most people at least some of the time. We will look more into this issue later in the chapter, in the section 'The Psycho-emotional Level of Earth'.

Late Summer in the Garden
Harvest

Is there anything more delightful to a gardener than harvesting the fruits of his labours? Picking a plump ripe tomato from the vine and eating it still warm from the late summer sun, or plucking juicy, ripe strawberries and raspberries and popping them into the mouth one by one. This activity of savouring our harvest is one of the delights and Gifts of the Earth Element. The notion of harvest applies to all areas of life, not just our garden. But we can really practise the full enjoyment of savouring the harvest in our gardening activities. Notice how it feels in your body. Perhaps there is a feeling of fullness, roundness and juiciness within you – a feeling of deep satisfaction as if you have eaten a good meal or enjoyed a great wine. These are sensations and feelings of the Earth.

While the late summer may be the most abundant time in the garden, harvest comes in other seasons too. In my garden I harvest kale and collards in the winter and spring, potatoes, garlic and broad beans in the early summer, and lettuce all year round. But in every case the feeling is the same: the sense of fruition of all the love and labour that have gone into the project; of a job well done and rightly rewarded. Relish this. You are infusing yourself with the essential goodness of the Earth Element.

Sharing

If your garden is anything like mine, there is almost always more produce harvested than can be consumed fresh by one family. This gives rise to another Gift of the Earth Element, that of sharing. When we have more of something than we need, there is a natural tendency to want to share it with others who do not have it. My neighbour and I have different kinds of things growing in our gardens and it is a great satisfaction to me to pass over the fence the excess eggs from the chickens, the superfluity of leafy greens or the extra baskets of broad beans that inundate us in November each year. She, in turn, is happy to hand over her excess asparagus, cherries and figs that I do not grow. There is never any account kept, just a spontaneous sharing of surplus. And this, too, brings a sense of satisfaction similar to that of the harvesting.

After a while, I suspect my neighbours of hiding when they see me coming with yet more bags of zucchini. Then I take them down to the local goodwill store so they can be given away or sold cheaply to other people I do not know. This way I can share not only excess food but plants, seedlings and seeds. Though I have not tried it yet, I have an idea to set up a local street stall where all organic gardeners in the area can come and share their surplus.

Freezing and Preserving

It's almost impossible to avoid a glut. My little green apple tree produced 60 kg of apples last year, all within the space of a month. Even after giving away baskets of them, there were still hundreds of apples left. They kept well in the bottom of the fridge for the five months it took me to eat them, but there are many other things that will not keep and which need to be frozen or preserved.

These are some of the ways that I keep my surplus for a rainy day:

- Kale and collards

  Strip from stalks, chop roughly, immerse in boiling water for 2 minutes, drain and place in trays in the freezer, turning every 15 minutes to keep from clumping. When partly frozen, place in freezer bags. Keeps right through to next harvest.

- Green beans and carrots

  Similar to the kale, cut into pieces, blanch and partially freeze before bagging.

- Broad beans

  Popping the beans out of their shells, cook and mash them with butternut pumpkin and sautéed onion and spices to make a pâté which can then be frozen.

- Raspberries and strawberries

  Each day, pop the surplus into a jar in the freezer. When there are enough accumulated, time to make yummy jam, ice cream or sorbet.

- Peaches and nectarines

  No need to go to the trouble of bottling and canning; just cut the fruit into slices and place in freezer bags, being sure to squeeze out excess air from the bags.

- Zucchini

  There are never enough ways to use up these prolific vegetables. Try slicing them thinly and layering in a jar with garlic and salt. Press down firmly. When the jar is full, cover with olive oil. Preserves well for ages.

There are few fruits and veggies that cannot be preserved in some way (lettuce is a famous exception). Use your imagination or your search engine to find ways to save your surplus. Then you can have the Earthly satisfaction of your harvest all year round.

Meridian Pathways

The Stomach and Spleen meridians are the energy pathways of the Earth Element. The Stomach is the yang partner and its energy flows down the front of the body, helping us to ground to the earth. Usually the yang meridians pass along the back of the body, its yang aspect. The Stomach is unique in that its pathway is along the yin aspect, the front of the body. Its yin partner Spleen travels up the front of the body, bringing with it the supportive energy of Earth.

The Stomach meridian begins in the soft tissue immediately below the eye, directly under the pupil (see Figure 9.2). It travels down through the cheeks, does a loop around the mouth and goes into the jaw muscles. It has a side channel that goes up through the jaw hinge and into the temple. Meanwhile, the main pathway travels down the front of the throat to the collar bone. At this point it moves laterally and proceeds down through the nipple line (4 cun lateral to the midline) to the base of the ribs where it moves more medially (2 cun lateral to the midline) and down to the pubic bone. From here it moves onto the front of the thigh, down through the shin muscle of the lower leg and onto the top of the foot before ending at the lateral side of the second toe.

Its partner, the Spleen meridian, begins at the medial corner of the big toenail, travels through the arch of the foot and up the inside of the lower leg and thigh (see Figure 9.3). In the lower abdomen it runs 4 cun lateral to the midline, but when it reaches the base of the ribs, it becomes 6 cun lateral, on the edge of the ribcage. Just before it reaches the collarbone, it turns downward and ends on the side of the body at the level of the base of the sternum. In these latter stages, it resembles a crutch, an energetic support for our erect carriage.

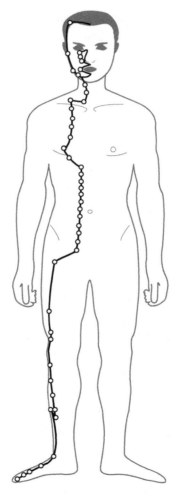

Figure 9.2 The pathway of the Stomach meridian

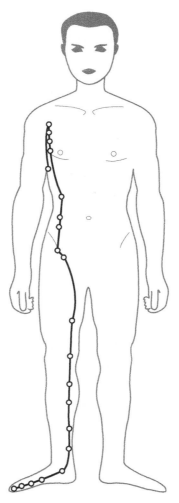

Figure 9.3 The pathway of the Spleen meridian

If you feel pain, discomfort, congestion or other symptoms along these pathways, or if you have issues that relate to these organs, you can help free the energy by doing a visualisation practice. Imagine a ball of yellow energy or light passing along the length of the meridians, freeing up any blocks in the energy flow. You can use your breath to support the practice by breathing out as you pass down the Stomach meridian and breathing in as you bring the energy up the Spleen meridian. You may also use your hands to stroke along the pathways. Do this several times. If you find a place where it is difficult to move the energy through, stay there and focus your mind, hand and breath to help free the block.

Organ Awareness

After doing the meridian visualisation practice, you can then bring your attention specifically to the organs themselves. Beginning with the stomach, place one hand over the area in the centre-left of your upper abdomen, then place your other hand over it. Tune in to this organ which has digested countless meals in your life. Bring to mind the colour yellow – maybe the golden yellow of a field of ripe wheat or the bright yellow of a sunflower. Allow this colour to permeate your stomach. Acknowledge your stomach for its lifetime of tireless work of receiving and breaking down your food so that you can be nourished by it. Send love and gratitude for its work. Notice how it responds to your attention and recognition. Notice how you feel as you do this.

When you are ready, move on to the Spleen. The Spleen in Chinese medicine is defined by its functions, not by its location. It is not the same as the organ of the spleen; therefore, the organ awareness practice needs to be modified. Imagine that the organs of spleen and pancreas in the middle of the body are the central railway station that is part of a whole body network of lines of distribution. Also, keep in mind the Spleen's function of maintaining the upward movement of Qi.

Move your hands slightly apart so that your left hand is over the left side of your upper abdomen (spleen) while your right hand is over the right side (pancreas). Bring to mind the colour yellow and allow this colour to infuse these organs with healing light. Allow this coloured light to spread outwards throughout the body like a rail network. Acknowledge your Spleen for its constant work in distributing the energy derived from your food, providing energy and support for all the functions of your body. Send it love and gratitude for its work. Notice how you feel as you do this.

Acupressure for Physical Health

After the meridian visualisation and organ awareness practices, you can focus specifically on the source points for each meridian. The source points heal the organs directly as well as balancing the meridians. They are powerful points while at the same time being very safe.

I have included an additional point here because it is just too important to be left out. This is Stomach 36, the Earth point of Stomach meridian. It is one of the most powerful tonic points of the body, tonifying Qi, treating any digestive disorder, supporting Spleen functions, combatting fatigue, helping with grounding and centring of the mind. As its name, Leg Three Miles, suggests, it provides the energy to go the extra distance.

It is worth noting here that the source points of the yin meridians are also the Earth points of those meridians. Kidney 3, Spleen 3, Liver 3, Lung 9, Heart 7 and Heart Protector 7 all influence the Earth as well as their respective organs and meridians, bringing their Officials back to centre.

SP 3 *Taibai* Supreme White
The Spleen source point is located on the inside of the foot, at the ball of the big toe and at the junction of the red and the white skin (see Figure 9.4).

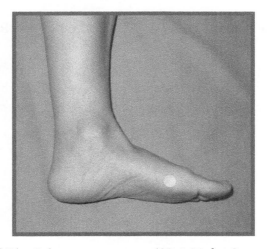

Figure 9.4 The Spleen source point (SP 3 *Taibai* Supreme White)

ST 42 *Chongyang* Rushing Yang

The Stomach source point is located in a shallow hollow on the middle of the top of the foot, 1.5 cun (two fingers' width) down from the 'crease' of the ankle (see Figure 9.5).

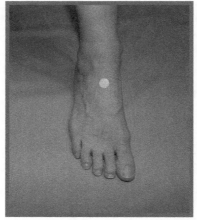

Figure 9.5 The Stomach source point (ST 42 *Chongyang* Rushing Yang)

ST 36 *Zusanli* Leg Three Miles

The Earth point of the Stomach meridian is located in the shin muscle, 3 cun (4 fingers' width) down from the base of the kneecap, and one finger's width lateral to the crest of the tibia bone (see Figure 9.6).

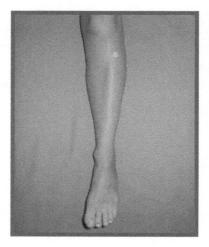

Figure 9.6 The Earth point of the Stomach meridian
(ST 36 *Zusanli* Leg Three Miles)

Journal Entry: 30 April 2012

This is not from my own journal but rather is a letter from a client who attended my Five Element workshops. Her experience shows the healing that is possible when we immerse ourselves deeply in all aspects of the Element of the season. I am grateful for her eloquent contribution.

About ten years ago I started having periods of extreme fatigue that became an underpinning of my days. For many years I'd looked after family members with serious illnesses while coping with stresses in my own life, and I had no energy reserves left to draw on. On a daily basis, and on every level, I pushed myself to do what needed to be done.

I ate a pretty healthy diet and was generally optimistic and coping, but when my energy levels dropped I would eat carbs or chocolate just to get by. On numerous occasions over the years I asked my GP [general practitioner] about my fatigue, menopausal symptoms, ongoing memory problems and mental fogginess, knee problems and early signs of oedema in my legs. She carried out numerous tests but suggested my fatigue and memory problems were probably a result of stress, menopause or just part of getting older – and recommended antidepressants (which I refused).

I didn't have much time to look after myself, but occasional treatments from Five Element acupuncture or acupressure practitioners seemed to make a significant difference.

Over the last two years the external stresses in my life lessened, but I was disappointed to find that the fatigue didn't disappear. Rather, it became a constant state which increasingly affected my life. I often had to go to bed for a whole day and, in addition to the other symptoms, I seemed to have lost a natural sense of when and what to eat, was putting on weight and had developed irritable bowel syndrome.

It was becoming increasingly hard for me to relax, meditate or be grounded in my body. I noticed changes in my personality – I seemed to have become less caring about others and to have developed a rolling anxiety about one thing after another that kept me feeling stressed and driven. All my energy seemed to be in my head, and in my thinking and efforts to solve problems – and my poor weary body was being dragged along behind it.

I noticed that the degree of fatigue had changed too. Something new and strange had happened: deep in my being, in addition to the feeling of 'running on empty', there was an almost audible dry 'grinding' sound – like dry gears in a large engine, or stone grinding on stone.

When I took part in a university research project I was diagnosed with pre-diabetes and became really concerned about what was happening to me on all levels. When John told me about his course, I was very excited and felt it was exactly what I needed.

The first session focused on the Earth Element and John guided us through a visualisation/meditation which left me feeling 'earthed' for the first time in a very long time. During the discussion that followed I was fascinated to hear that my diverse symptoms – physical, emotional, mental and spiritual – were indications of an imbalance in the Earth Element.

I was even more surprised when over the next two days all my physical, emotional and physical symptoms intensified. I seemed to go through a healing crisis and finally slept for 12 hours. When I woke on the third day, I was amazed to find myself feeling completely different.

I was still 'earthed' and my obsessive worrying had disappeared. The inner 'grinding' sound had gone completely and in its place was a sense of a 'smoothness', a 'bubbling spring' of energy – and the stirrings of some vitality where there had been none.

I practised the meditation a few more times, and also looked deeper into aspects of Earth energy and ways in which I could keep 'feeding' the healing that was happening. This included finding the Chinese symbol for Earth and having it in my house and my wallet.

The healing continued and after the second group session on Earth energy I looked to see if there were any more changes. I found an inner calm and contentment, and a quality of peace and happiness in the 'bubbling spring' that continues to this day.

Over the last two months I have had only two or three occasions when my energy has 'dropped' and I've become shaky – but these have been times when I hadn't eaten what I needed. It's apparent that my health isn't quite what it once was, but even the symptoms on those few occasions were not the same as the deep fatigue I experienced for so long. At other times my physical symptoms have almost disappeared and I have felt more energised, balanced, mentally calm, clear and happy to a degree that is hard to believe!

I may need to go for a 'tune-up' from time to time, but I feel my state of health has improved in a very fundamental way – and I'm so grateful for having the opportunity to continue to deepen my awareness and understanding through the course.

The Psycho-emotional Level of Earth

Having explored the ways in which Earth shapes us at the physical level, let's now look at the ways it shows up in our mental and emotional life. Thoughts and feelings are of a finer vibration than the body and so their energies are swifter and can change rapidly. But in another way, our emotional patterns, beliefs and attitudes can become fixed and entrenched. Here we will look at the ways in which the Earth Element can appear in us.

The Emotional Landscape of Earth

As we saw earlier, the Five Element tradition assigns sympathy as the emotion of the Earth Element, whereas other traditions describe it as worry, pensiveness or overthinking. One way we can see a connection between these two is in the way that sympathy can become an obsessive worrying about the needs of other people. I will begin by exploring the role that sympathy plays in our psychological framework. Later I will examine the effects of worry on the bodymind system.

Sympathy

The Earth Element occupies a unique place in the Five Element cycle. Not only does it have its place between Fire and Metal, it also manifests at the transition points between the other Elements and acts as the central point from which the other Elements spread out to the four directions. In this central position, Earth connects all the Elements and also acts as the bridge between the Elements as they cycle through the seasons.

From this we can infer several important qualities of Earth. It is a place of balance between the yin Elements and the yang Elements, it is the harmoniser of transitions between one state and another, and it is the central reference point to which everything is connected.

The function of sympathy is also to act as a bridge and connector, in this case between humans. It gives us the capacity to understand one another and to act in appropriately caring, sensitive ways. In this way, sympathy echoes Earth's role as a connector.

Nowhere are these functions of Earth and sympathy more clearly seen than in the role that our mother plays in our life. Our mother first provides her womb as the holding container for our physical development. Later, as she connects with us through sympathy, she is moved to provide for our needs, both physical and emotional. She gives us milk from her breast, and love and caring when we are helpless to take care of ourselves. As we grow older and make our way out into the world, she remains the central point of loving nurture to which we can return, allowing us to transition from dependence to independence in a smooth and healthy way.

Development of Earth Energies

Let us look more closely at the early years and the ways that the mother's parenting style influences the development of the Earth energies of her child.

THE BONDING PHASE

Earth energies are profoundly shaped by our time in the womb and in infancy. In particular, they are shaped by the extent to which our needs for nourishment and attachment are met. This means that our relationship with our mother is fundamental to the development of our Earth.

Mothers do an incredible job, sacrificing much to care for and nurture the development of their children. However, no mother is capable of providing absolutely everything all the time for her child. It simply is not physically possible. As a result, none of us gets all of our needs met. For example, a baby wakes from a nap in fright. Her mother takes a minute to arrive from the other room to comfort her. The mother is rushing as quickly as she can to soothe her child. But for the baby, it can feel like a whole world of abandonment in that minute.

There are many ways in which attachment, bonding and nurturance can be disrupted; many are simply unavoidable but can nevertheless affect a baby's Earth energies. If a mother is undernourished during pregnancy, the physical needs of her baby will not be fully met. She might suffer from anxiety or depression, or be ambivalent about having a baby, affecting the child's sense of holding and support. It might be necessary for the baby to be separated from mother immediately after birth and isolated in another part of the hospital. There could be insufficient breast milk to completely satisfy the newborn's needs. The baby might not get enough holding or attention. The mother may be sick and unavoidably absent for a period of time. The arrival of a younger sibling can make the child feel that the care and attention she was getting is suddenly cut off and given to the newborn.

THE SEPARATION PHASE

From about the age of 18 months, the child begins to separate gradually from the mother. The way in which this is handled will also shape the Earth energies. The child needs to be able to explore her world at greater and greater distances while still knowing that mother is there to return to. If this separation begins too early, the child feels pushed away and abandoned. On the other hand, if the mother does not initiate the separation, and the child remains too closely connected with her, then the normal process of individuation is not supported.

These two crucial phases of our childhood development determine the ways in which we give and receive, our capacity for sympathy and empathy, and our ability to bond with other humans in relationships.

Since it is impossible to get all of our needs met in these phases, it can be said that everyone carries issues in these areas. For people of the Earth constitution, these issues are particularly significant in their lives.

In a sense, we all had a deprived childhood, and the fundamental response to not having our needs met as children is to continue to try to meet them as adults. We go about this in two ways. One way is to try to directly meet our needs for caring by acting in ways that make us the centre of attention. I have called this the yin response. The other way is a reaction to, and a defence against, this yin response. If we are afraid that we will be judged or rejected for inhabiting the limelight, then we need a different strategy for meeting our needs. We hide them by giving excessively to others in the hope that the giving will be returned and our needs will be met that way. I have called this the yang response.

Unlike the other Elements, both the yin and yang responses are active and outwardly oriented. Thus, the labels yin and yang are not as suitable for Earth types as for the other four types, but I have continued to use them for the sake of consistency.

Most people move back and forth between the two polarities, but we all tend to have a preferred position in which we spend most of our time. Let us look in more detail at these two patterns.

THE YIN RESPONSE: LACK OF SYMPATHY, DEMANDING ATTENTION

A famous phrase that sums up the pattern of the yin response is 'Enough about me, what did *you* think of my performance?'

This imbalance in Earth is characterised by a focus on our own needs at the expense of others. We are all familiar with the person who dominates a conversation with talk about himself. He steers the conversation in such a way that the focus remains on him. He may ask questions of others but only so that it shifts the topic to something he wants to talk about. In short, it's all about him.

If a person has this orientation to the world, when sympathy is offered, the response is a pulling for more sympathy. To the sympathetic listener this can feel like being ensnared in a sticky web of attention-seeking need. Eventually, the behaviour of the attention seeker causes his listener to withdraw, reinforcing the feelings of abandonment.

Taken to the extreme, this becomes narcissism. Here, the person is grandiosely self-important, exaggerates his abilities, has a belief that he is special and has a sense of entitlement, but, most importantly, he lacks sympathy for others and is unwilling or unable to identify with their feelings.

This behaviour is almost always unconscious. The person is frantically trying to meet his own needs, which effectively blinds him to the needs of others. He is actually incapable of seeing their needs and responding to them. Like Narcissus of the Greek myth, he looks at the world and sees only a reflection of himself.

But before we start pointing fingers at others, we need to note that all of us are narcissistic to some degree. We all have an ego, and because the function of the ego is to ensure our own survival, we are all unavoidably focused on ourselves. The question is how much we balance that with our concern for others.

THE YANG RESPONSE: COMPULSIVE GIVING, REJECTING SYMPATHY
One of the primary characteristics of the yang response is an excessive focus on others. Such a person has an overly sympathetic response to others in a way that neglects her own needs. In addition, there is usually difficulty in receiving sympathy for herself and difficulty receiving from others in general. If there is one phrase that sums up this pattern, it is 'Oh, let me help you with that'.

Compulsive giving. One of the ways that an imbalance in Earth appears is in compulsive giving. While caring for others is a natural human tendency, when the giving occurs at a cost to the giver, things are clearly out of balance. We give our time, energy and resources without really recognising the cost to our own lives. It is only when we become exhausted that we are forced to stop and receive, often with great difficulty. This imbalance is common among Earth types.

When we look more closely at this pattern, we see that this kind of giving springs from the deep, unmet needs of the giver. We give to others what we crave for ourselves but cannot bring ourselves to request. Earth types often have trouble even recognising that they have needs, or that their giving springs from these unmet needs.

Many Earth types see themselves above all as generous, caring, helping people. This identity is deeply challenged by having needs and asking for help from others. To do so might lead others to think of them as selfish, inconsiderate and self-centred. So the giving continues, spurred by the longing that someone will eventually satisfy their needs without having to be asked.

Anger can also be a response when the gifts offered are not appreciated. Compulsive giving often results in inappropriate gifts that are actually not wanted by the hapless recipient. The giver has failed to see that the gift or the help offered is neither needed nor wanted.

Rejecting sympathy. The pattern of compulsive helping is often combined with a rejection of help or sympathy from others. This can be confusing, because we may sense that the Earth person is subtly pulling for help or attention, but when we offer what seems to be needed, she will often reject it with a response such as 'Oh no, I'll be fine, don't worry about me.'

It is difficult for her to simply open up to receiving the help, support or sympathy that is being offered. Sadly, she is unable to accept the thing that she actually longs for most.

Codependency. One of the ways that Earth out of balance can appear in the personality is in codependency. This is a relatively new term which surged to prominence with the publication of Melody Beattie's book *Codependent No More* in 1986.[40] It is used to describe a person who believes, often subconsciously, that their happiness is derived from other people, or from one person in particular whom they believe will make them happy. In this way they become dependent upon others to be happy and their behaviour then revolves around taking care of the desires of the other.

In particular, it leads to giving the other what they want rather than what they need. As a result many codependent people enter into relationships with addicts. The codependent person needs the other to need them, and so continues to maintain the other's addiction. While this behaviour may appear to come from a desire to help, it is in fact enabling the addict and really no help at all. It is a distortion of the true Gifts of the Earth Element.

Most of us are codependent to some degree. We get along with others so we can be supported by the feeling of connection that it brings. There are few people who do not have the need to be needed in some way. The challenge is to be able to avoid enmeshment without ceasing to care for others.

RETURNING TO BALANCE

How do we go about recovering from the early disruptions to our Earth energies that are still playing out in our adult lives? First of all, we must recognise that, as human beings, we do have needs.

In recent years, having legitimate needs has become confused with a judgement that we are being needy. We don't want to appear to be too needy or else we will be rejected. But the truth is that all humans have needs.

We have needs for food, for shelter and warmth, for satisfying work and, perhaps most of all, we have a need to feel loved and connected to others through friendship and family. These are essential needs that can only be satisfied from the outside.

Because of a fear of being labelled as needy, and for other reasons too, we often judge ourselves for the needs we have. This inner judgement is an impediment to recognising our true and legitimate needs. It is essential to set aside this judgement as best we can as we work with the issues that disrupt the balance of our Earth.

When we are inhabiting the narcissistic end of the polarity, it can be more difficult to recognise that we are being driven by our unmet needs. When we are the centre of attention, or getting ahead of others, there usually isn't a feeling that anything is wrong. But we might recognise our self-centredness if we find ourselves doing these kinds of things:

- exaggerating our problems, difficulties and/or successes

- dominating conversations

- taking more than our fair share

- getting ahead at the expense of others.

We need also to distinguish our ongoing needs as adults from the legitimate but unmet needs we had as children. These unmet needs from our infancy still remain within us and can never be met from the outside. It is these inner children who have been driving both our sense of need, and the yin and yang ways that we have responded to that drive.

However, it is possible for us to locate these inner children, recognise their pain, give them what they did not get and heal them with our own love and compassion. Many recent psychological therapies focus on healing the inner child.

Once the inner child heals and is no longer clamouring for our attention, our inner space becomes less cluttered. We are able to see ourselves with greater clarity, and see that our behaviours have been attempting to satisfy infant needs in an adult world. But most importantly, healing clears the space for us to see what it is we and others truly need for balanced well-being.

Ultimately, it is Being that resolves the issue of needs. As we spend more and more time in the present moment, we feel more and more whole, and need less and less. In this place of Presence, we feel emotionally and spiritually complete. Nothing is missing.

Am I taking too much?

It can be hard to see our own narcissism. You may need a good friend to give honest feedback about your behaviour. Consider how you behave in these situations:

- In conversations do you tend to speak much more than others, speak over others or talk in ways that do not leave space for others to enter the conversation? If so, consider why you do this. Try to become more of a listener and less of a speaker.

- Do you exaggerate, overplay or overdramatise? Do you make your problems look bigger than they are? Do you embellish stories about yourself by exaggerating the truth? If so, why do you do this? Observe yourself in conversations and try to represent yourself accurately.

- Do you complain a lot? If you are frequently complaining to others about how tired you are, or busy, broke, underpaid, undervalued and so on, you may be pulling for sympathy without realising it. Notice how often you complain and what is the subject of complaint. Simple recognition of such behaviour can lead to changes.

- What is the source of your dissatisfaction? Sometimes we have real needs that are not being met. But more often the need we have is not something that is satisfiable from the outside. Distinguish between these kinds of needs. There are some needs that can only be satisfied from the inside through self-love, self-acceptance and recognition of self-worth.

- Make a list of the things that you can do for yourself that bring you satisfaction, ways that you can nourish yourself without looking to others to provide it.

- Practise gratitude. Count all the things in your life for which you are grateful. Focus on the donut, not the *hole* in the donut.

- Be of service. Find ways to help others. Do some volunteer work at a local non-profit organisation. Donate your money, time or skills.

Am I giving too much?

Many people give to others in a way that ignores or denies their own needs. Since giving to others is considered a good and moral thing, this imbalance is often overlooked.[41] If you are the kind of person who gives more than is good for you, consider these questions:

- Why am I giving in this situation? How much am I doing this for the other person and how much am I doing it for myself?

- Is the giving really wanted? Is it a response to a request or am I deciding what the other person needs?

- Is the gift appropriate to the situation or the relationship?

- Can I really spare the time, effort and resources that this giving requires?

- Try saying no to a request for help. If you really cannot meet the other's needs without depleting yourself, it may be okay to say no. People who give a lot tend to be called on to keep giving. You have to decide when to say enough is enough. This can be challenging to your own identity as a giver.

- Put *yourself* in the line of people who need your help – and not at the *back* of the line. If you are used to putting yourself last, try putting yourself first, or at least in the middle of the line. This may not be an easy thing to do, so take slow steps in this process.

- Look in the mirror and say to yourself, 'I have needs.' What are your needs? Make a list. Speak them to others.

Below is an exercise on exploring needs. This is best done speaking with a partner but can be also be done as a written exercise.

Imagine that a very generous genie has granted you 100 wishes. For what would you wish? Try to let go of any judgements about what you want. Do this quickly without thinking too much. Say the first thing that comes into your mind. Spend 5–10 minutes. You may not get to use all 100 wishes.

When you have finished, choose one of the things that you wished for and consider whether this is reflecting some deeper need within you. Your partner may be able to help you with this. Is it so you will feel secure, happy, loved, appreciated or something else? Continue working through your list of wishes for 5–10 minutes. You may see a common theme to the things you want.

Then, if you are working with a partner, switch roles.

Worry

Worry is the emotion that is traditionally assigned to the Earth Element. What is meant by worry in this context? The Chinese character *si* depicts a brain above a heart, expressing the idea that thinking requires the heart to be engaged with the brain. 'When one is thinking, the vital fluid of the heart ascends to the brain.'[42] When this connection with the heart is lost, thoughts become scattered, unfocused and spin round in the head, unable to be anchored by the heart. This is what is meant by worry. Because this is a more nuanced emotion than, say, anger or fear, other English words have been used to describe it. Overthinking, cogitation, pensiveness, preoccupation, obsessive thought and rumination are some of the translations, all of which carry different shades of meaning.

Indeed, the Chinese themselves distinguished between worry and pensiveness, affording them separate billing in the list of emotions that cause disease. Worry is the pathological counterpart of the Spleen's mental activities of concentration and of generating ideas.[43] It is the act of constantly thinking about and brooding upon the events of life. It is frequently future-oriented. The worry is that a certain thing that is desired will not happen, or something will occur that is not wanted. It represents a disconnection from what is happening in the present moment.

The effect of worry is to knot the Qi, causing stagnation. This impairs the Spleen's function of transporting Qi throughout the body. The physical effects of this can be poor appetite, tiredness, epigastric discomfort, abdominal pain and distension. The expression 'worried sick' is apt.

Often the worry produces tension in the temples, tightening of the mouth and jaw, and clenching or grinding of the teeth. These locations lie along the pathway of the Stomach meridian whose Qi becomes knotted and stuck, unable to descend from the head and into the body. There is an imbalance of Qi in the upper body and the person can be ungrounded.

Distinct from worry is pensiveness, which involves constantly thinking but not necessarily worrying. The word 'rumination' is appropriate here, a chewing over of things that have happened in the past, a compulsive focus on the causes and consequences of one's distress rather than on taking action that would lead to solutions. In short, it is *thinking* intensely about life rather than living it. Pensiveness also includes excessive mental activity such as studying or doing a job that requires a lot of intense concentration.

The positive mental energy that corresponds to pensiveness is contemplation and meditation. This energy misguided leads to pensiveness.[44] Like worry, it knots the Qi and injures the Spleen, affecting digestion and causing bloating. At a spirit level, the spirit of Earth, the *yi* or intellect, is affected by the appropriation of a person's mental powers for negative ends.

One way that obsessive worry can manifest is in hypochondria. This is often seen in people of an Earth constitution or with a severe imbalance in their Earth. Here, the tendency to worry leads to an obsessive focus on their own health. They may become concerned at every twinge or slight problem that arises. This can lead to a lifelong quest for healing that results in visits to many practitioners either serially or simultaneously.

Here are some suggestions to reduce worry:

- *Don't worry, be happy.* This was a famous maxim of the Indian guru Meher Baba. It is easier said than done, but it is a reminder to reconnect with the heart so the brain does not spin off by itself. Try the heart meditation in Chapter 8.

- Overthinking results in too much energy in the head. Use your breath and visualisation to allow this energy to travel down the Stomach meridian from the head to the feet. Bring your awareness to your feet on the ground and feel them as keenly as you can.

- Walk barefoot and feel the ground under your feet. Try walking meditation.

- Hold the points learned earlier of ST 36, ST 42 and SP 3 to support your Earth.

- Take action. Worry is like spinning your wheels, a lot of energy going nowhere. Engage the gears and use your mental energy to focus on solutions. To do this, focus on one problem only. Get a friend to help you to prioritise and stay focused. Moving your body can often help break the cycle of mental spinning.

The Psychology of Eating

There is no doubt about it, this is a very big topic. It is the subject of countless books, articles, blog posts, conversations and jokes. The what, how and why of eating has assumed a very large space in our modern culture.

How are our Earth energies shaped by our relationship to food? How can we begin to change that relationship in ways that can support a healthy Earth?

When Earth energies are balanced and healthy, eating is pleasurable, satisfying and provides the optimum nutritional needs of the body. The food is enjoyable while it is being eaten, and when the body has satisfied its needs, we can easily stop eating until the next time we are hungry.

One of the ways that this balance is upset is by craving for food. Food cravings are sometimes biologically and nutritionally driven and arise out of the body's need for a particular essential component. For example, a craving for sugar may be a sign of vitamin B deficiency, a salt craving can indicate a need for a trace mineral and craving for fat may show a need for omega fatty acids. Cravings for chocolate have been linked to magnesium deficiency. However, most food cravings, especially those that drive people to overeat, have an emotional link. Emotional eating is (a) eating to supress feelings which are unbearable, unmanageable or overwhelming, and (b) eating to comfort parts of us that are in distress and which feel abandoned or unloved.

These behaviours are largely below the level of awareness. When we become aware that we are eating for emotional reasons, the behaviours begin to change. With full awareness, we no longer respond by eating to cover up or soothe difficult feelings but rather respond with love and care towards ourselves.

EATING TO SUPRESS FEELINGS

Most of us are not taught how to have feelings in a healthy way. Food is just one of the ways people try to manage their feelings. Other ways include drinking alcohol, taking drugs, watching TV or playing computer games. When we use food as an emotional manager, it has a significant effect on the Earth Element.

In our stressful modern world, anxiety is the most common feeling from which people try to escape. But also feelings of grief and loss, anger and frustration, hurt and betrayal can become too painful to bear. These feelings can arise suddenly and overwhelmingly or they can provide a constant background to our life. Sometimes it can feel as if we are going to die, so agonising are the feelings. It is an understandable response to want to make them go away.

The truth is that experiencing painful feelings is very rarely fatal. It might seem as if we are being swallowed up, buried, crushed, frozen, burned or generally tortured. But in the end we do survive. And the more we are able to fully feel our feelings, the sooner the pain passes.

Clinical psychologist Louise Adams observes:

We need to recognise that it's okay to have a strong feeling that makes you feel bad – yet we have this idea in our culture that a negative feeling must be banished straight away. Look how often we distract children with something like a biscuit if they're upset. We're not taught to ride out the feeling. Instead we learn to numb it with alcohol, eating or drugs. Yet if you learn to sit with the feeling, you realise that it's like a wave – it builds in intensity and then it passes. It's very empowering to realise you can handle it.[45]

It is important to try to avoid eating while feeling emotional. When we do this, we swallow the emotion along with the food. What is more, the emotion we are feeling will affect the internal organ associated with that emotion. Eating while feeling angry and frustrated will hurt the Liver; eating while feeling anxious and fearful will damage the Kidneys; eating while worrying will injure the Spleen; eating while experiencing betrayal and lack of love will wound the Heart; and eating while feeling grief and loss will harm the Lungs. Moreover, eating to supress any feelings undermines the Earth Element, affecting digestion, energy levels, vitality and overall balance. The Earth is the Element that connects all the others, so when it wobbles, so do all the Elements.

EATING FOR COMFORT

A comfort food is one that provides a nostalgic or sentimental feeling to the eater. It brings back good memories and comfortable feelings. Most comfort foods are ones that remind us of happy, safe, stable times in our lives, times we felt cared for. By eating these foods we are trying to rekindle these feelings. Most comfort foods take us back to childhood when food associations were first established. In a sense we are trying to replicate the very first comfort food: mother's milk.

Comfort foods vary widely between cultures and individuals. For an American it might be chicken soup and apple pie; for a German wurst and potatoes; for a Chinese person it may be dumplings. As someone with an English background, often when I have had a hard day, my mind turns to baked beans and chips, which was my childhood 'happy meal'.

But who is it that is being comforted? Almost all of us have parts of us that are still like young children who are in distress. It may be a part that feels unloved or unlovable, a part that is afraid of change, another part that feels lost and abandoned, another that has been abused.

If you find yourself eating for comfort, ask yourself, 'Who is eating this pie or cake or pizza or ice cream?' Consider which part of you needs comfort, and what does it need: love, nurturing, attention, acknowledgement or something else? The more you can discover what the comfort food represents, the more the need for it will dissolve.

 What are your comfort foods? Why do you choose these particular foods? What feelings are you trying to rekindle?

Try this mindful eating exercise,[46] doing it only when you feel hungry:

- Take a small amount of a single food.

- Look at it closely, observe its shape and colour. Feel its texture in your fingers.

- Smell the food. Notice the effects on your nose and what the smell reminds you of.

- Place the food on your tongue and notice the response of your mouth.

- Take a bite and be aware of the sounds and the textures in your mouth.

- Chew slowly until the food is mushy. Notice how it changes from solid to liquid.

- Enjoy the taste as the food makes its way to all parts of your mouth.

- Now swallow and follow the passage of the mouthful down your throat.

- Take a few breaths and sit with the totality of your mindful eating experience.

Try practising this mindful eating at least once during each meal.

Acupressure for Psycho-emotional Health

The points I have chosen to support the psycho-emotional health of Earth provide access to the rich source of nourishment that resides within.

ST 40 *Fenglong* Abundant Splendour

ST 40 *Fenglong* Abundant Splendour is located in the shin muscle midway between the base of the kneecap and the ankle crease and two fingers' width lateral to the crest of the tibia bone (see Figure 9.7). Stomach 40 brings balance between Stomach and Spleen, ensuring the proper transformation and distribution of all that we receive as nourishment. It is a grounding point, helping a person let go of worry and be more fully present in her body. When someone feels burdened by and unsatisfied by life or complains a lot about these burdens, Abundant Splendour provides access to a different perspective that all of life is a cornucopia from which we can derive nourishment, support and satisfaction.

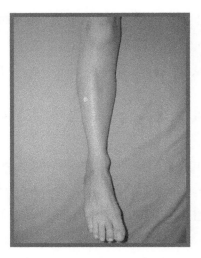

Figure 9.7 A grounding acupoint (ST 40 *Fenglong* Abundant Splendour)

SP 16 *Fuai* Abdomen Sorrow

SP 16 *Fuai* Abdomen Sorrow is located on the abdomen, 4 cun lateral to and 3 cun above the navel (see Figure 9.8). Spleen 16 is traditionally used to treat abdominal pain caused by indigestion and bloating. There is a deeper interpretation of this point, one which sees the Earth Element crying out from lack of nurturance and lack of fulfilment. For many people with an Earth imbalance, and particularly those of an Earth constitution, there may be a feeling that their plans, hopes and dreams seldom produce a satisfying outcome or bring them fulfilment. J.R. Worsley referred to this as 'lack of harvest'. Imagine the farmer who sows crops, tends them with care for months, only to see them ruined by drought, floods, pests or disease. What if this lack of harvest becomes a lifelong experience? Such a person can never enjoy the deep satisfaction of the fruition of her life. For the person who experiences life in this way, Abdomen Sorrow addresses the belief that her needs will never be satisfied. It can provide the support to find nurturance and satisfaction that can only come from within.

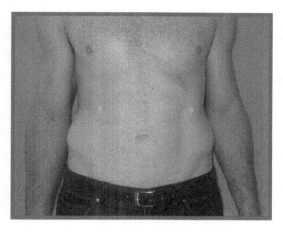

Figure 9.8 A nurturing acupoint (SP 16 *Fuai* Abdomen Sorrow)

The Spiritual Level of Earth

Our spiritual nature is that which lies beyond the body, the emotions and even what we think of as the mind. What role does the Earth Element play in our spiritual life?

The Spirit of Earth: Yi

The Chinese character *yi* has two parts. The upper part depicts an uttered sound, such as a word or a musical note. The lower part depicts the Heart. The character therefore portrays the intention of a man who speaks, manifested by the sounds he utters.[47] This intention emanates from the Heart, suggesting that the spoken words are founded on the sincerity and integrity of the speaker. As John D. Rockefeller put it, it is the sacredness of a promise, that a man's word should be as good as his bond.

Yi is most often translated as intention, thought or intellect, though another rendering is 'the consciousness of potentials'.[48] It is the spirit which supports the manifestation of new things to come into being. It unifies thought and action into a form of doing that, with applied purpose, produces desired ends.

One of the important qualities of intention is steadiness. The continued, sustained application of intention towards a goal is needed for the desired outcome to be achieved. It is the glue that sticks the writer to his chair in order to complete the manuscript; it is that which gets the athlete to training day in and day out; and it is what supports a mother to keep on being there for her children as she rears them to adulthood. It is the *yi* which sustains a practice of any kind, whether it is playing the violin, working on your backhand or perfecting your baking skills. It provides us with the support to keep on keeping on with the things to which we commit ourselves.

The classics say that the Spleen houses the *yi*;[49] therefore, anything that injures the Spleen will also injure the *yi*. Incessant worry is most injurious and undermines the steadiness of a balanced Earth. Going round and round in the head or chewing over something repeatedly will erode the *yi*. The resulting imbalance can cause a person to feel confusion, lethargy, boredom or indifference. Alternatively, she can show exaggerated sympathy, become sticky in her relationships and develop uncontrolled or even self-destructive generosity.[50]

Practice

On the spiritual path, we often encounter difficult places in ourselves, especially at the beginning. We are faced with the many old patterns and structures that a spiritual practice uncovers. Even after years of practice, the challenges and difficulties do not go away but become more subtle. It is the *yi* which supports our long-term practice through challenging times. Whatever your daily practice, whether it is meditation, chanting, prayer, movement, inquiry or something else, the ongoing repetition of practice becomes self-sustaining. Practice strengthens the *yi*, which in turn supports practice.[51]

One metaphor for working through our spiritual issues that seems appropriate to Earth is that of the two piles of dirt. At the beginning, there is one pile of dirt that is our unprocessed and undigested collection of beliefs, memories, ideas, habits, patterns and structures that make up the ego personality. As we sift through this morass and begin to see through the things that prevent us from recognising our True Nature, we gradually move the dirt to another pile that is our Essence, that which we truly are. Over time, the ego pile shrinks while the Essence pile grows, so that in time we are living less from ego and more from our essential nature. What gives us the support and steadiness to stay with this difficult task of sifting and metabolising our life is the spirit of *yi*.

At some point we begin to recognise that it is not really 'I' who is shovelling the dirt anyway. It is not 'I' who is practising anything, but that practice is simply happening in this location. What manifests through our actions does not belong to us. It is merely reality unfolding through a particular drop of the Tao. This is true practice.

The Virtue of Earth: Integrity

The classics teach that *xin* is the virtue of Earth.[52] The character depicts a man standing by his words and is variously translated as integrity, honesty, faithfulness, sincerity and devotion. These qualities are expressive of the Earth Element when it is in harmony at the level of spirit.

The word 'integrity' is a good one, for it combines the meanings of honesty and probity, which relate to a person's character, with the meaning of unity and wholeness, which echoes Earth's capacity to integrate.

The Confucian model upon which the virtues are based asserts that loss of contact with a virtue results in that virtue degrading into the emotion of its Element. Thus, when integrity is eroded, it transforms to a lack of sympathy.[53] In other words, when we lose our integrity, we become selfish and self-serving.

When a person is in alignment with his True Nature, he is completely balanced in his Earth Element and integrity is his natural condition. Such a person is aware of the needs of himself and others in equal measure. Altruistic actions naturally arise from this perspective of the world. Expecting nothing in return, he is able to care appropriately for himself and others without attachment to the results.[54]

As we lose contact with the virtue of integrity, we become less able to see the needs of ourselves and others objectively and either become selfish and self-serving or begin to care obsessively about the needs of others. This draws us to one or other of the polarities outlined in the psycho-emotional section above. Either we become focused on our own needs and are selfish and narcissistic, or we become focused on others' needs and become self-rejecting, ingratiating and codependent.

The way back to the virtue of integrity therefore lies in understanding that the Earth naturally supports and nourishes all beings equally, favouring no one above another, making no distinction between individuals. The sage therefore surrenders his personal intention, aligning himself with the intention of the Tao. His actions then proceed from a devotion to the service of all beings.

The Bodhisattva vow is perhaps the deepest example of selfless giving: the giving up or delaying the chance to achieve complete enlightenment in order to help others to do so.

The Spiritual Issue of Earth: Cultivating True Purpose

In Chapter 7 we saw that the spiritual issue of the Wood Element is finding our true path in the world. This means finding the direction our life will take and setting out boldly upon that road. The issue for the Earth Element is about finding the true purpose in our life that will manifest in ways that are satisfying and fulfilling for ourselves and be of genuine service to the world.

Discovering true purpose involves finding ground that will be fertile for you, where your efforts will bear fruit and your employment will be rewarded. People of an Earth constitution often do many different things in their lives, none of which is truly satisfying. They may be good at many things and develop skills in widely different areas throughout their life. And yet there is often a lack of deep satisfaction from any of them. There is a difference between what you are good at and what brings you satisfaction.

This pattern of chronic dissatisfaction that some people experience derives from not knowing what they need. Many Earth types do not know what they need. They need help in finding out what it is that they need. The perceived lack of nourishment in childhood patterns their behaviour in adulthood so that, at least in some areas of life, there is dissatisfaction that arises from an unsatisfiable hole.

J.R. Worsley observed that many people of an Earth constitution have a pervasive sense that their plans, hopes and dreams seldom produce a satisfying outcome or a sense of fulfilment. It is as if the whole span of their life is in some way deeply unsatisfying. He coined the term 'lack of harvest' to describe the Earth type who does not harvest the rewards of her endeavours in life.

How do we cultivate true purpose so that we can reap the harvest of our labours? The foundation for the harvest is the steady application of intention to that which we need. The first part of this prescription involves steadiness of purpose applied to whatever it is we are doing. This in turn requires practice. Practice involves repetition, devotion and commitment to whatever it is that we do. The second part of the prescription requires that we know what we need from our life. The more we can be clear about what it is that we ourselves need, and not what others need from us, the clearer it will be to us to what we need to devote our practice.

In our allotted years in this world of time and space, we spend our life doing things. We might ask ourselves, 'What am I *doing* here?' This is exactly the question for Earth. What am I going to do in my life that manifests my Essence as a mature human being? How is my particular drop of the Tao going to contribute to the unfolding of True Nature? What will be the colour and shape of my thread in the great tapestry of the universe?

The Diamond Approach

True Compassion

Some writers include compassion as a quality of the Fire Element, more aligned with love. I suggest that true compassion is the deepest form of caring for other beings and more related to the Earth Element. All emotions are distortions of an essential state (see Chapter 4). If sympathy is a distortion of a true or essential state, what is that state? I suggest that it is compassion.

Compassion is supportive and makes us feel supported. Compassion sits with the suffering of others or of ourselves in a way that is fully and openly present with the suffering without jumping in to help or fix. When we have sympathy, we want to fix, to make better, and we think we know how we can do that. This may lead to meddling with the other's experience in ways that are actually not helpful.

Compassion at its deepest level does not interfere. It recognises hurt but also understands that hurt is a portal to truth. If we move quickly to take away hurt, either our own or that of others, we may be denying the opportunity to understand something about ourselves, our life, of existence itself. If we can see through the distortion of sympathy to the deeper compassion that it imitates, we can begin to recognise Truth. True compassion is a kind of healing agent that helps us to tolerate the hurt of seeing the truth.

> In the beginning people take compassion to mean the feeling of wanting to alleviate the person's pain or take it away from them. That's usually what people think compassion is. A deeper level of compassion is, of course, taking action whether you feel inclined to or not. The third level of compassion could include hurting somebody else, or not taking their pain away when you see it. If you take their pain away they won't learn something. Sometimes they need the pain in order to learn something about themselves. They might not even learn about compassion, because the way to learn about compassion is to experience hurt. And if you take people's hurt away, they won't learn how to be compassionate themselves. The most objective compassion has to do with truth. The point is the truth; whether the person feels hurt or doesn't feel hurt is immaterial. The point is truth, the golden truth.[55]

Fulfilment

We have talked a lot so far about the qualities of satisfaction, contentment and harvest that Earth engenders. When the Earth Element is balanced, these qualities become available to us. However, as long as we are living from the ego, there can be no complete satisfaction and fulfilment in our life because the ego is never satisfied. It always wants more. More money, more goods, more recognition, more status, more love. It is dissatisfied with the way things are, whether it is our own appearance, our job, the way our partner or children behave, the condition of our house, the actions of the government. The list is endless. No matter how great our life is, the ego will always find something about which to complain.

The ego is a non-real structure – a collection of ideas, beliefs, memories and positions based on our personal history. The more we are identified with the ego, this sense of a separate self, the more we will feel the need to change ourselves and the world around us. Ultimate satisfaction and fulfilment come from being fully present to whatever is happening in our life and without any need for it to be different.

> This world we live in, the world of appearance and everything that is in it, has nothing wrong with it. In a sense, it is neutral in that the things are neither good nor bad. What makes it a place of suffering is that we are not present in it; what makes it a place of fulfilment is that we are present in it. For fulfillment is nothing but the fullness of our presence.[56]

> *A chickpea leaps almost over the rim of the pot where it is being boiled.*
> *'Why are you doing this to me?'*
> *The cook knocks him down with the ladle.*
> *'Don't you try to jump out. You think I'm torturing you. I'm giving you flavour so*
> *you can mix with spices and rice and be the lovely vitality of a human being.'*
>
> RUMI

Acupressure for Spiritual Health

Here we look at the outer shu point of the Spleen meridian, located on the back of the body along the outer line of the Bladder meridian. This point is particularly effective in healing at the level of mind and spirit. The effectiveness can be increased by using the point in combination with the Spleen points learned earlier.

BL 49 *Yishi* Thought Dwelling

BL 49 *Yishi* Thought Dwelling is located in the lower ribs and four fingers' width out from the spine. It is level with the space between the eleventh and twelfth thoracic vertebrae (see Figure 9.9). This point influences the spirit of Earth, *yi*, translated here as 'thought' but encompassing the quality of intention described earlier. What Kaptchuck describes as the consciousness of potentials, the highest form of thought, is nowhere more evident than in this point, the abode of the *yi*. 'Operationally, it is the spirit that is responsible for considering, deliberating and deciding on what is likely, possible or conceivable.'[57]

When these qualities of a healthy Earth Element become constrained and obscured by worry, repetitive thoughts and obsessions; when the mind is stuck in a rut and cannot get out of it; if there is stubbornness; if the mind is foggy and hazy and leaden, unable to process thoughts effectively; or if the person has lost their centre, swayed this way and that by all around them, then this point will help. It supports the Spleen to understand, grasp and work sequentially along a passage of thought. It helps us to digest our life experience in a way that is meaningful and will support fruitful action in the world. And it supports steadiness of intention that manifests a person's purpose.

The left-hand character of *yi* contains the heart radical at the bottom. It can be translated as meaning 'the process of establishing meaning in the world with words that come from the heart'.[58] *Yi* is not simply about thinking but includes the bringing of thought into manifestation through the vehicle of intention.

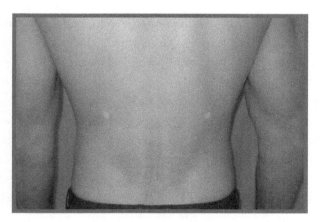

Figure 9.9 The outer shu point of the Spleen
meridian (BL 49 *Yishi* Thought Dwelling)

Meditation: Grounding and Centring

Imbalance in Earth can show up as too much energy in the upper body, especially the head, which needs to come down to earth, to be grounded. Alternatively, there can be too much energy in the lower body which does not rise upwards to support movement and action. This meditation exercise will help you to become more grounded, centred and balanced between your upper and lower halves.

Find a comfortable position, seated in a chair. Feel your feet on the ground, your pelvis firmly in the chair seat. Let your hands rest lightly on your thighs. Your back is relaxed and upright. Take a few breaths.

Bring your attention to the area of your navel. As you focus on this central point in your body, notice how much energy there is in your body above this point compared with how much energy there is below this point. How balanced are you between the upper and lower body? There is an acupoint to the sides of the navel named Heavenly Pivot. This really is a point of balance between the heaven and the earth within us, between the upper and lower body. How balanced are those parts of your body in relation to that pivot?

Now, allow your attention to drop down through the lower body, the pelvis and legs and to your feet. Feel your feet on the ground. There is a place in the centre of the pad of the foot that is like a portal that we are going to use to connect with the Earth energy. If you were to curl your toes, the hollow that is formed on the sole of the foot is the point to which I am referring.

Besides these two points in the feet, there is a third point of contact with the earth and that is through the energy that comes down through your tailbone. Imagine your spine has a long extension, like a monkey's tail, that is touching the ground. Feel those three points of contact with the earth, your feet and your tailbone, forming a tripod. Continue allowing your attention to travel downwards through your feet and tailbone into the earth. Imagine they are like three tree roots going down into the earth, through the floor, through the soil, through the subsoil, through the rock, anchoring you to the earth. Send those roots down as deeply as they will go into the earth. The deeper they go, the more anchored you will be to the earth and the more you will be supported by it. Imagine those roots going so far into the earth that they penetrate the core of the earth, go down through the other side and curl around the opposite side of the sphere. So you are absolutely grounded. Notice how this grounding feels to you.

Now, without losing contact with this feeling of grounding, imagine that the energy of the earth itself is rising back up through those roots, like sap rising, up through the roots and into your feet and tailbone, up through your legs, to your pelvis and abdomen. Rising up into your chest, filling the whole of your upper body, into your head, face, down through your arms to your fingers. Feel the supportive energy of the planet flowing completely throughout your body. At the same time feel the grounded connection with the earth.

Spend a few minutes experiencing that. Notice any differences here now compared with the beginning of the exercise. And when you get up out of the chair after this meditation, you can continue to take this feeling of being grounded and centred with you throughout the day.

Transition from Earth to Metal

You might say that the transition from Earth to Metal is a tautology (saying the same thing twice) since the Earth season is itself a transition between summer and autumn.

And yet the late summer does have its own unique qualities. Sometimes referred to as the Indian summer, it is a period of comforting warmth when the season seems to hang in the air for a time, when the bees think warm days will never cease, busily gathering the last of the pollens as if the summer will go on forever. Nature is infused with sweet warmth, roundness, plumpness. There is a feeling of lazy languor about the days where the sun's warmth is comforting without burning.

Eventually, there comes a day when the comfortable warmth vanishes and there are harbingers of the change to come. There is a crispness to the days, a nip in the air and a chill to the wind. In temperate areas, the first frost arrives to snap us out of our late summer haze. Leaves begin to leave their trees.

This transition from Earth to Metal marks the beginning of the yin half of the year's cycle, where nature's energy begins to descend and contract. Temperatures fall, leaves drop, days shorten. For many people this is the most challenging of the transitions. The falling energy of the year is a reminder that what goes up must come down. And the yin is sadly unappreciated in Western countries. Decline and decay are anathema to a culture which prizes only growth and fruition.

But for those who can appreciate and value the yin aspects of their nature – and this is fully half of who we are – this transition can seem like a welcome relief. The movement to autumn provides more space, more time to breathe. It invites reflection and contemplation, supports meditation.

The leaves that are falling from the trees outside your window inspire you to settle down into yourself.

Chapter 10 _____

Metal

The Nature of Metal

The movement of Metal is downwards.

After the uprising yang of Wood and Fire and the balanced axis of Earth, Metal represents the beginning of yin in the *sheng* cycle. Metal is representative of precious metals such as gold and silver, precious gems, crystals and minerals, all of which are stored underground, treasures awaiting discovery.

In the human body, Metal manifests as the minerals and trace minerals that are essential for biochemistry and the maintenance of health and life. We need minerals such as calcium, magnesium, copper, zinc, chromium and molybdenum. These minerals become available to us through plant and animal food sources, but all of them originate in the soil, hidden in the earth.

Metals can be fashioned into tools and weapons. The quintessential metal tool is the knife which is used for cutting away what is not needed from that which is required: peeling vegetables, scaling fish, cutting slices of pie, whittling wood. We even talk about budget cuts, tax cuts and spending cuts. Surgeons use the scalpel to cut away diseased tissue. All of these operations imply reduction, decrease, a dropping away of something in order to preserve what is essential to life.

At a metaphysical level, Metal represents the hidden treasure of our True Nature. There are countless tales of heroes and heroines defeating monsters and enduring terrible ordeals in search of precious treasures. The Golden Fleece, the Holy Grail, the dragon's hoard, rings of power and magical artefacts; these are all are metaphors for the priceless treasures of wisdom, self-knowledge and realisation which are obtained by cutting through the veils of ego and delusion.

The Chinese character for Metal is *jin* (see Figure 10.1). It represents nuggets of gold hidden within the earth. The symbol for the Earth Element is contained within the symbol for Metal, with an additional line suggesting greater depth and a sloping roof indicating concealment underground. Overall the suggestion is of something of value hidden within.

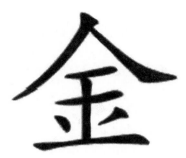

Figure 10.1 The Chinese character for Metal

The Resonances of Metal
The Season: Autumn or Fall
The Metal Element is most obvious in nature as the season of autumn or fall.

FALL
In North America autumn is referred to as fall, a word which succinctly describes the fundamental energy of Metal. In autumn everything is falling: the leaves, the temperature, the angle of the sun. Following the prolific expansion of summer and the warm fullness of harvest time, autumn begins the descent, the turning inwards. There is a sense of quieting. Autumn invites us to ponder the impermanence of all phenomena.

DECAY
The leaves and fruits of the trees drop to earth and begin to decay and rot. The nutrients and minerals of this material are returned to the earth to nourish future growth. Plants and trees drop the seeds that will ensure the continued survival of their species.

SPACE
Trees drop their leaves, leaving only bare branches. Fields which have given up their harvest lie fallow. Space is created. Space and spaciousness are qualities of Metal, which likes plenty of room to breathe.

LIGHT
As the angle of the sun drops closer to the horizon line, the light of the sun is gentler, no longer intense. Because of the low angle of the sun, it lights up the dust particles in the air, creating a sense of something ethereal. I call this 'cathedral light', resembling shafts of light filtering down from high windows in high-ceilinged churches. Indeed, autumn can have a quite spiritual feeling to it.

COOL

After the intense heat of summer, autumn heralds much cooler daytime temperatures, crisp mornings and cold nights. Sweaters and coats, hats and scarves are retrieved from the back of the closet. This is the beginning of movement from hot to cold, from yang to yin.

When does autumn begin? Depending on your latitude and climate, you can expect autumn to begin showing itself sometime in August in the northern hemisphere and February in the southern hemisphere. The cross-quarter day of Lammas (loaf mass) on 1 August is an ancient celebration of the end of summer and of the first fruits of the harvest. This Christian festival was based on a much earlier pagan celebration.

> No spring nor summer beauty hath such grace as I have seen in one autumnal face.
>
> JOHN DONNE

The Sense: Smell

Of all the senses, the sense of smell is the most instinctual, the closest to our animal nature. It is closely connected to survival. It tells us when we are in the presence of something dangerous or toxic like gas, harmful chemicals or smoke. Smell also helps us to ascertain whether food is good or bad for us, whether it is fresh or has gone off. And it informs us when something or someone is familiar and trusted.

The olfactory receptors in the nasal cavity detect molecules in the air that trigger a response. The information is transmitted to the limbic brain, which is one of the oldest systems in the human body, predating the thinking brain of the frontal cortex. While we may later interpret the smells in a cognitive way, the initial response is not at the level of thought but rather of emotion, since the limbic system is the part of the brain that deals with emotions. Smells also leave long-lasting impressions and are strongly linked to memories. Thus, we associate smells as good or bad depending on the memories they trigger.

There is a certain appropriateness to the fact that smell is a resonance of the Metal Element. The ancient Taoists regarded the spirit of Metal, the *po*, as the corporeal soul. This corporeal soul is the spirit that grounds us in the body. It is the only one of the five spirits that disappears at the time of death. It is the animal soul, the instinctual part of us. Smell is vital to the survival of wild animals; in humans, this sense is what connects us most directly to our animal nature

For many people, the sense of smell becomes more acute in the autumn. It is a good time to pay attention to this sense, which is often dulled by the proliferation of artificial scents in the environment. Watch how animals use their noses to give them information. Let your dog or cat teach you about getting more in touch with your animal self.

The Colour: White

The colour white has long been associated with purity. The Roman priestesses of Vesta wore white, which symbolised their purity, and the early Christian church adopted this symbolism of white as the colour of sacrifice and virtue. The association of this colour with spirituality is common, from the white of priestly garments to angels, heaven and healing white light.

While in the West people tend to wear black as a sign of mourning, in the East it is white that is used at times of grief. In China, when someone is gravely ill or has died, white clothes are worn, white candles are burned and white cloths are hung over doorways in the mourning household.

How do you feel when you wear white? Is it a colour you are particularly drawn to or is it one you tend to avoid? An extreme attitude to this colour may indicate an imbalance in your Metal. Is there much white in your home? Too much white can give a sense of coldness, but some white is good to invite the qualities of Metal into your living space. According to feng shui principles, it is good to have some white on the Metal wall of a room, the one on your right you as you enter.

In Five Element acupuncture diagnosis, the colour white at the sides of the eyes indicates a Metal constitution. This is a shiny, reflective kind of white, not to be confused with the grey, ashen colour that is the lack of red in a person of Fire constitution.

> The snow goose need not bathe to make itself white. Neither need you do anything but be yourself.
>
> LAO TZU

The Sound: Weeping

The energy of Metal is a downward movement, so it is natural that the sound of voice that relates to Metal should be one that goes down. Weeping or crying is one of the expressions of sadness, sorrow or grief. While people can also cry from joy or anger, it most usually arises from feelings of loss. It is a normal and natural response to emotional states and yet is commonly suppressed due to parental and cultural influences. Sayings like 'Big boys don't cry', 'Where's your happy face?'

or 'Stop or I'll really give you something to cry about' can lead to a lifetime of emotional suppression.

Cultures vary in the ways that sadness and crying are received and allowed. Men cry far less frequently than women, even though in childhood there is no difference between boys and girls. This suggests that men are expected to suppress their crying. The way people behave at funerals is also illustrative of cultural norms. Some cultures are very reserved in their expression of grief, while others are very demonstrative with loud wailing and sobbing being the norm.

Conscious or unconscious suppression of crying will inevitably affect the Metal Element in ways that can have harmful consequences for health, especially the lungs, as we will learn later.

The sound of a person's voice is diagnostic of their Constitutional Element. The weeping voice carries the emotion of grief. A person of Metal constitution has a weeping voice. What this means is that there is a sound in the voice as if the person were about to burst into tears, even when the topic of conversation is not sad. Many people of Metal constitution have difficulty expressing grief, so the weeping is suppressed in the chest and the sound comes out as a crack or a croak in the voice.

The Odour: Rotten

The resonance of odour is the third of the diagnostic tools in determining a person's Constitutional Element. People of a Metal constitution have a subtle odour emanating from their skin, which is described, rather unflatteringly, as rotten. When the person is in good health, this odour is faint and light, like the smell of leaves decomposing in autumn. When there is a serious imbalance in the person's health, the odour becomes stronger. The smell then becomes more like decaying meat.

The odour arises from the organs of the Element not functioning optimally. In this case when the large intestine is not eliminating waste in an efficient manner, the body gives off a smell of something rotting.

The Emotion: Grief

Since the movement of Metal is downwards, it follows that its emotion will have a falling energy. The overall feeling of the season of autumn is of descent, decay and loss. Loss of warmth, loss of light, loss of growth. This shedding and loss in nature confront the parts of us that have difficulty in letting go of the past. If we are unable to come to terms with the fact that something we cherished is no longer with us, there will be unresolved grief. This may be about a person, a pet, a house, a job, money, a favoured object or even an idea or dream. For many people, the ambient energy of autumn brings subtle reminders of past losses and can reawaken grief about them.

Grief is a normal and natural part of living a human life. In this world where everything that has a beginning also has an end, life becomes studded with many endings. When something we love ends, we are challenged to come to terms with its loss, to honour its place in our life, acknowledge its passing and move on with our life without its presence. The length of time it takes to make this adjustment to loss depends on the depth of its meaning to us. The loss of a parent, child or spouse is clearly going to take much longer to adjust to than the loss of money or possessions. But with all losses, the grief eases with the passage of time.

When there is difficulty in accepting loss, and grief and sadness continue unabated after a long period of time, this becomes damaging to health. So, too, the suppression of grief affects the health of body and mind. When these emotions are not fully dealt with and processed, they are stored in the lungs and the health of these organs suffers.

For a person of Metal constitution, these issues are primary. Either there is a suppression or denial of grief, or there is an ongoing keening sense of loss. The emotion of grief, feelings of sadness and issues of loss predominate in the Metal person's life.

We will look at these issues in more detail in the emotional landscape of Metal.

Tears are the silent language of grief.

VOLTAIRE

The Gifts of Metal

The Gifts of an Element are those qualities which are available when that Element is in harmony and balance within us. When the Element is out of balance, these qualities become less available or distorted. As you ponder these Gifts of Metal, consider to what extent you are letting them into your life.

Acceptance

In psychological terms, acceptance means assenting to the reality of a situation without attempting to change it, protest against it or run away from it. This does not mean that we like the situation or give whole-hearted support to it, but there is a simple recognition of the truth that this is the way things are in this moment.

It is a common view that we need to bring acceptance to the things we do not like, but really it applies to all the things of life. It can become an acceptance of everything that life has to offer. Acceptance is a posture that is full, alive, present to life and an active welcoming of whatever is happening. It is not resignation or submission or collapse. It is a breathing-in of life in all its manifestations. It is an active meeting of life in the moment, a simple recognition of that which is right here, right now.

This wider sense of the word is reminiscent of Rumi's poem 'The Guest House' in which the poet invites us to welcome and entertain all experiences, whether joyful or sorrowful, because all can be seen as guides for our growth:

> *This being human is a guest house.*
> *Every morning a new arrival.*
> *A joy, a depression, a meanness,*
> *some momentary awareness comes*
> *as an unexpected visitor.*
>
> *Welcome and entertain them all!*
> *Even if they're a crowd of sorrows,*
> *who violently sweep your house*
> *empty of its furniture,*
> *still, treat each guest honorably.*
> *He may be clearing you out*
> *for some new delight.*
>
> *The dark thought, the shame, the malice,*
> *meet them at the door laughing,*
> *and invite them in.*
>
> *Be grateful for whoever comes,*
> *because each has been sent*
> *as a guide from beyond.*[1]

 What are some of the things you are able to accept? What is difficult to accept? What lies in the way of accepting things as they are right now?

Non-attachment

Already we have seen that letting go is one of the key aspects of the Metal phase. In this realm of time and space that we inhabit, everything that has a beginning also has an end. This applies to everything we do, everything we own, everyone we know. And most of all, it applies to our own life. The more we are attached to the things of our life, the more we desire them.

Alobha is a word in Sanskrit that is defined as the absence of attachment or desire towards worldly things or worldly existence. This is a key tenet of Buddhism. Non-attachment is seen as a key to the enlightened state. The Dalai Lama has said, 'Attachment is the origin, the root of suffering; hence it is the cause of suffering.'[2] Therefore, non-attachment is key to escaping the cycle of suffering.

In the 1980s, I returned home from a long trip through India and Nepal where I had studied Tibetan Buddhism. I was filled with a spirit of non-attachment and decided to give away my whole vinyl record collection of hundreds of albums. My precious collection was divided and distributed among friends and relatives. But soon I began to miss my records and was filled with regret for my actions. Thus, I gained a salutary lesson that non-possession is not the same as non-attachment.

Desire and attachment are hard-wired into us through our survival as well as our sexual and social instincts; therefore, every human has some level of attachment. However, the degree to which we can let go tells us a lot about the state of the Metal Element in us.

We cannot will ourselves to be non-attached. It simply does not work. If we try, we are becoming attached to being non-attached. The solution is to become increasingly mindful of ourselves in every moment. The more we are present with the here and now, the less we are attached to what has happened in the past or to what we imagine will happen in the future.

Make a list of all the things to which you are attached. How does each of these attachments keep you from being present in the moment?

Acknowledgement

Acknowledgement implies recognition of a person, respect for their qualities and an appreciation for their being in the world.

The gesture of *Namaste* is a wonderful example of the acknowledgement that is meant here. The word literally means 'I bow to you', but it carries much more meaning than this. It recognises that there is a divine spark within us all and the bow to the other is both a recognition of the divine spark within the other person and to the divine within all. The word is accompanied by a slight bow with the palms pressed together at the level of the heart. The whole gesture is a succinct expression of this deeply respectful quality of Metal.

We all need acknowledgement from others and this is nowhere more necessary than in childhood when our sense of self is being formed. Therefore, the extent to which we were seen, recognised and acknowledged when we were children will have a profound influence on our sense of worth as adults. This is especially true of how we were acknowledged by our parents and whether we were recognised just for being ourselves or if we had to earn this recognition by achieving something or by being a particular way. The degree to which we were acknowledged for just being ourselves deeply affects the Metal Element in later life.

Acknowledgement and its related qualities flow two ways. We give acknowledgement to others and we receive it from others. A healthy Metal will allow us on the one hand to recognise qualities in others and to offer appreciation, while on the other hand being able to receive the acknowledgement of others in an open way that is neither rejecting nor grasping.

To what extent do you need recognition and acknowledgment from outside? How easy is it to acknowledge others?

Value

Metals such as platinum, gold and silver are valuable because of their relative rarity. Gems such as diamonds, rubies and emeralds are considered precious. These things become a store of value and wealth. Money also, whether it be paper money or a total in a bank account, is a store of value because of the purchasing power that it represents. A lot of energy has gone into accumulating these items of value and so you could say that the energy has been distilled down to its essence in the form of money, gems or minerals.

As people, we value the things that are precious to us, that have meaning for us, things we particularly appreciate and love. We ascribe value to people or things in our lives because of their usefulness, importance, worth or preciousness.

Value is often seen as relative. Things are given a value, then compared and ranked. Some things are seen as more valuable than others. This may be true in economic terms and from the acquisitive ego view. But from a wider perspective, one in which everything is seen as a manifestation of the Tao, everything has a value that is neither more nor less than the value in anything else.

When the Metal Element is balanced within us, we have a strong sense of our own value or self-worth. We feel confident in ourselves as a valuable human being and find little need to have our value recognised from the outside. The healthier our Metal Element is, the more we recognise our inherent value. Inherent value has nothing to do with how much we earn, what degrees we have or how useful we are to others. It is the value that is intrinsic to living a human life.

How do you respond when I tell you that you are you are infinitely valuable just the way you are right now?

Balance

The balance quality of Metal can be represented by a scale that is perfectly balanced between the two sides. This notion of balance in Metal is derived from the fact that some of the qualities of Metal relate to spirit and spiritual matters, while others relate to the body and mundane matters. The quality of balance is expressed in the notion that, as humans, we are beings of spirit inhabiting animal bodies.

For some people, there is an imbalance that is tilted towards spirit. This can produce ungroundedness and a lack of embodiment. Such people may appear spacey and ethereal, not quite in the world. For others, there may be an imbalance that is skewed towards the body. Such people are more aligned with the body, its desires and instincts, and may lose contact with the higher realms of human existence.

When Metal is perfectly balanced, these two aspects of our nature are in harmony. There is ease with both the spiritual and the corporeal sides of life. We can become lusty angels or angelic beasts, at home in both realms of human experience.

Are you balanced between body and spirit? If there is an imbalance, what prevents you from fully embracing both realms of your being?

Sacredness

Sacredness is the spiritual side of the balance scale. We are connected to spirit through the Lungs, which take in what the ancient Chinese referred to as the Breath of Heaven. This implies that we are continually being enlivened by the power of the source of all things. Other traditions also equate the breath with an ultimate source. The Bible states, 'And the Lord God formed man of the dust of the ground, and breathed into his nostrils the breath of life; and man became a living soul.'[3]

Our spiritual nature also resonates with the upper chakras, the fifth (throat), sixth (brow) and seventh (crown), those which lie above the heart and which, when open, connect us with the divine. There are a number of acupoints which contain the word heaven (*tian*), almost all of which are in the neck and head. Most of these points are called Windows of the Sky points and can be used to help us to realign with our Heavenly nature.

When we are in contact with our Heavenly origins, we are imbued with feelings such as awe and reverence. When we are moved by the presence of the sacred, we become awestruck and reverential. The mystical poet and artist William Blake turned his pen and brush to the task of expressing the sacred. His *Songs of Innocence* and *Songs of Experience* can be seen as a critique of his society's loss of contact with spirituality and the decay of purity in the corporeal world.[4] From the Five Element perspective, Blake was lamenting the imbalance of Metal in eighteenth-century English society.

Alignment with spirit gives us the capacity not only to contemplate our Heavenly origins and the sacredness of life, but also to respond to beauty, music, art, nature and to appreciate the refinements of life. Being touched by a painting, awed by a vista, inspired by a piece of music, enchanted by beauty: all are ways in which things of the world touch the spirit.

 To what extent are you connected to your spiritual nature? How does spirit influence the way you see the world?

Instinct

On the other side of the scale, we are endowed with a physical body that is very mundane and down to earth. It is a body that eats, digests, burps and farts, urinates and defecates, has sex and sleeps. A body that is able to perceive through its five senses. A body that gives us the animal power to respond instinctively.

These instincts are associated with the lower chakras, the ones below the heart. The first or base chakra in the lower pelvis provides us with the survival instinct which drives us to do whatever is necessary to stay alive as an individual. This propels us to do what we need to obtain food, shelter and safety. The second chakra at the level of the pubis provides us with the sexual instinct. This is the instinct that drives us to have sex and thereby procreate and ensure the survival of the species. The third chakra at the level of the navel provides us with the social instinct that drives us to seek relationships that will ensure our social survival. It propels us to find the safety of a mate, a family and a tribe to look out for us and provide the companionship that we need to live a satisfying life.

These three instinctual drives are extraordinarily powerful and mostly operate below the level of thought, if not of consciousness itself. These drives are intimately connected to the body, to the corporeal soul. They provide a balance with the more spiritual orientation of the upper chakras. Many traditions see the heart as the fulcrum of this balance between our animal and spiritual nature, the chakra that provides the place of connection between the upper and lower chakras, between the angel and the animal.

To what extent are you connected to your animal nature? How does your body influence the way you see the world?

Instinct is the nose of the mind.

DELPHINE DE GIRARDIN

And More…

The gifts we have examined here are a distillation of the many qualities in which Metal manifests. Here are some other expressions of the Element. Think or write about the ways these qualities appear in your own life.

Allowing	Perfection	Refinement
Appreciation	Preciousness	Respect
Awe	Precision	Reverence
Distillation	Purity	Sensitivity
Essence	Quality	Simplicity
Exactitude	Recognition	Spaciousness

Journal Entry: 23 April 2013

This morning as I sat down to edit the section on the Gifts of Metal, I noticed some fear arising. This persisted throughout the morning until I realised that the fear was related to my writing and to the book: Will I ever finish this book, will it ever get published, and if it does, will it sell? Looking more into this, I recognised that the fears were connected to the very qualities I was writing about, particularly the quality of value. My sense of my own value and self-worth were being challenged by my inner-critic voice.

Just as my issues of anger were brought up by writing the Wood chapter, and issues of love and relationship were front and centre while writing the Fire chapter, here now I see the issues of Metal rising to the surface. I realise that it is not only the issue of value that is arising, but also of letting go as the time draws near to leave this house and garden to which I have become so attached.

Once I notice that all of these things are related to the Element of the season I am writing about, I begin to relax and the fears recede. Once more I see that I am living in and living from the season. In short, I am living the book.

The Physical Level of Metal

Having looked at the resonances and gifts of the Metal Element, we turn our attention to the ways that these qualities manifest at the physical level in the human body. The ways in which we resonate with Metal qualities will shape the way the Element is structured in our physical form.

Organs and Tissues

Lungs

WESTERN MEDICAL PERSPECTIVE

The two lungs lie in the thoracic cavity on either side of the heart, extending from the diaphragm to a little above the collarbones. They are divided into sections called lobes, each of which receives a bronchus or tube through which air can pass. The bronchi divide into smaller bronchioles and further still into alveoli, which means 'bunch of grapes' in Italian. There are around 300 million of these alveoli in normal lungs. The whole system looks like an inverted tree. This creates a very large surface area for oxygen exchange to happen. If all the alveoli were laid out flat, they would cover an area the size of a doubles tennis court.

When we breathe, the principal muscle of respiration, the diaphragm, contracts and descends, expanding the lungs and drawing air through the nose and trachea into the lungs. This is an inhalation. When the diaphragm relaxes, the lungs expel the air in an exhalation. The whole purpose of this mechanism is to bring oxygen into the bloodstream. This takes place in the alveoli where oxygen from inhaled air diffuses into the blood and is transported to all the cells of the body. Carbon dioxide, a waste product of cellular metabolism, is extracted from the blood and expelled on the exhalation.

Because the lungs are exposed to the outside environment, there are a number of ways they are protected. First, hairs in the nose act as a filter so that large particles are kept out of the lungs. Second, a constant secretion of mucus in the breathing tubes traps smaller particles. The mucus is swept up towards the throat by tiny hairs called cilia that line the tubes. The mucus is then swallowed, a process that happens without us realising it. Third, if an irritant does enter the lungs, a cough can forcibly expel the irritant faster than the cilia can.

Because of the complexity of the respiratory system and its exposure to the outside air, lung diseases are among the most common medical conditions. Smoking, infections and genetics are the main causes. Conditions affecting the airways include asthma, allergies, bronchitis, chronic pulmonary obstructive disorder, emphysema and cystic fibrosis. Conditions affecting the alveoli include pneumonia, tuberculosis, lung cancer and pulmonary oedema.

CHINESE MEDICINE PERSPECTIVE

The organ of the Lung is considered to include the whole respiratory passage: the nose, nasal passages, trachea and lungs.

Governs Qi and respiration. As in the Western perspective, the lungs are responsible for inhaling air. However, from the Chinese medicine perspective, this also includes inhaling the Qi of the air, referred to as Heavenly Qi.[5] This is the most important function of the Lungs. This Qi is combined with the Qi extracted from food by the Spleen to form Gathering Qi (Zong Qi). This resulting Qi promotes lung and heart functions, circulation to the limbs and gives strength to the voice. It is said that 30% of our postnatal Qi comes from the air and the remaining 70% from food. If we do not breathe fully and deeply, we are not availing ourselves of the Qi available to us.

Regulates all physiological activity. The *Neijing* states, 'The Lung is the advisor [to the sovereign]. It helps the heart in regulating the body's *Qi*.'[6] This advisor is sometimes translated as Prime Minister – in other words, the senior minister of the emperor whose role is to oversee and regulate the activities of all other ministers. Since Qi is the vital substance that sustains life, and the Lung is responsible for its distribution to all parts of the body, the Lung governs all physiological activity. It controls all the channels through which Qi moves and, in conjunction with the Heart, controls the blood vessels. It also controls the ascending and descending as well as the entering and exiting of Qi.

In addition, the Lung serves the function of spreading the defensive or protective Qi throughout the body. This layer of protection lies just under the skin, which is the tissue that relates to Metal. Thus, a person with weak Lung Qi is less protected and therefore more susceptible to outside pernicious influences such as wind and cold, which can produce colds, flu and infections.

Houses the Po. The Lung is connected to Heaven through the breath and the inhaling of the Heavenly Qi. It is also home to the spirit of Metal, the *po* – the corporeal soul. We will look in detail at this aspect in the section 'The Spiritual Level of Metal'. For now it is enough to note that one of the functions of the Lung is to harmonise our spiritual nature with our animal nature, to resolve the conundrum of living as a spiritual being in the body of an animal. The health of our Metal will have much to do with how well we balance these two sides of our nature.

Large Intestine

WESTERN MEDICAL PERSPECTIVE

The large intestine is the final part of the digestive tract. It is a tube 1.5 m (5 ft) in length and averaging 6.5 cm (2.5 in) in diameter. It is divided into four regions: cecum, colon, rectum and anal canal. It connects to the small intestine at the ileocaecal valve. The colon is the largest part, forming an incomplete rectangle around the abdominal cavity. The rectum is the final 20 cm (8 in) of the digestive tract, which ends in the anus.[7]

The functions of the large intestine are to complete the absorption process begun in the small intestine, to manufacture certain vitamins and to form and expel faeces from the body. Bacteria in the colon contribute to a chemical process that breaks down amino acids to aid in the final absorption of nutrients. Absorption of water contributes to maintaining good water balance in the body and in producing faeces that are solid and suitable for expulsion.

The two most common problems of the large intestine are diarrhoea and constipation. Diarrhoea results from food passing too quickly through the digestive tract for the water to be absorbed. It can be caused by stress and microbial activity. Constipation is caused by insufficient intestinal motility where the food spends too long in the digestive tract and too much water is absorbed. It can be caused by insufficient fibre or water, lack of exercise and emotional upset. More serious disorders include diverticulosis, the formation of pouches in the wall of the colon which can then trap bacteria and become inflamed; and ulcerative colitis, an inflammation of the lining of the colon.

CHINESE MEDICINE PERSPECTIVE

At a physical level the functions of the Large Intestine are the same as in Western medicine, namely the conduction and passage of food and drink from the small intestine down the body, reabsorption of fluids and stool formation. The classical texts are brief on the functions of the Large Intestine because most of the pathologies which Western medicine attributes to it are seen in Chinese medicine as relating to Spleen and Liver patterns.[8]

Where there is a significant diversion from the Western view is in the Chinese perspective of the Large Intestine's relationship with the Lungs. Descending Lung Qi supports the Large Intestine's downward movement; in turn, the Large Intestine Qi helps descending Lung Qi. People with deficient Lung Qi often have problems with constipation.

At the mental level, the health of the Large Intestine is related to the ability to let go and not dwell upon the past. Hanging on to things that no longer serve, whether they be possessions, thoughts, beliefs or relationships, can be a reflection of Large Intestine imbalance.

Skin

The Neijing states that the Lung controls the skin and maintains its fullness and suppleness.[9] The skin is therefore the tissue of the Metal Element. The Lung is responsible for maintaining the defensive Qi of the body. It does this partly by maintaining the integrity of the skin as a defensive barrier, but also through controlling the space between the skin and the muscles. It therefore lubricates and nourishes the skin and allows for normal perspiration.

The skin is a direct reflection of the health of the Lung. Imbalance in the Lung can produce skin that is dry, rough, thin or easily broken. It can also manifest in excessive perspiration or lack of perspiration. Perspiration through the skin is one of the ways in which the body expels its toxins, so lack of perspiration can lead to a build-up of toxins in the body.

Body Hair

The body hair, as opposed to the hair of the head, is the external manifestation of Metal. The hair follicles of the body hair have their origins in the dermal layer, so body hair is seen as an extension of the skin. Moreover, the hair provides a certain level of protection, echoing the Lung's function of providing defensive Qi. The condition of the body hair, like that of the skin itself, will give an indication of the health of the Lung and the Metal Element.

Diet and Lifestyle

Foods That Support Metal

White is the colour that corresponds to the Metal Element; therefore, foods that are white are supportive of Metal. White foods are less plentiful than those of other colours. Fruits of this colour include white nectarines and white peaches. White vegetables include cauliflower, garlic, onions, leeks, parsnips, turnips, kohlrabi, mushrooms, white potatoes and Jerusalem artichokes.

The allium family of vegetables, which includes garlic, onions, leeks and shallots, is an excellent source of organic sulphur that binds to heavy metals in the body which are then excreted through the large intestine. In fact, the pungent odour of these vegetables derives from their sulphur content, so the more pungent they are, the more cleansing they are for the body.

A particularly important component of allium vegetables is quercetin, an anti-inflammatory antioxidant that may be helpful in treating inflammatory conditions such as arthritis.

Garlic is in a class of its own and regarded by many as the most beneficial vegetable there is. It is a natural antibiotic, aids in chelation and supports cardiovascular health. It contains the antioxidant allicin, which has been shown to have cancer-preventing properties.[10]

Here are some suggestions to get more white foods in your diet:

- Add sautéed onions and garlic to pastas, curries and rice dishes.

- Potato leek soup is a great warmer for the cooler autumn evenings.

- Try *aloo gobi*, an Indian dish of potatoes and cauliflower in a pungent sauce.

- If you're a garlic lover, roast whole heads of garlic drizzled with olive oil.

- If you are up for the intense flavour, use onions and garlic raw in salads.

- Make pear soup with cinnamon, ginger and honey as a delicious lung tonic.

The flavour of Metal is pungent; therefore, foods that have strong, intense or spicy flavours are supportive of the Element. Pungent foods include garlic and onions as well as many spices such as cloves, cinnamon, nutmeg, chilli, cayenne, ginger and black pepper. Pungent herbs include basil, rosemary, fennel, anise and dill. Pungence is a flavour that moves energy outwards, mimicking the nature of the Fire Element, the one that controls Metal; therefore, pungent foods act to counteract Metal's tendency to stagnate.[11] When there is an invasion of the Lung by external pathogens, pungent food can help to disperse the invasion. But if a person's Lung Qi is weak, pungent food should be avoided.

As with any flavour, the use of pungent foods must be moderate. Overconsumption can create imbalances in the Wood Element, the grandson of Metal. In particular, the liver may suffer. Those who pride themselves on eating fiery curries and red-hot chilli dishes may be in for more than just a burning bottom the next morning. Too much spicy food puts a strain on the functions of the liver.

Lung Health

The lungs are the only yin organs exposed to the exterior of the body and are therefore more vulnerable to invasion. Consequently, there is a wide variety of conditions that can affect the lungs and the respiratory tract, ranging from mild to serious. At the mild end of the spectrum are infections of the upper respiratory tract, which is most susceptible to viral infections. The most widespread of these infections is the common cold. Other infections include sinusitis, tonsillitis, laryngitis and some kinds of influenza. Symptoms include runny nose, sore throat, cough, nasal congestion, sneezing as well as facial and sinus pressure.

When infections penetrate below the throat and into the trachea, lungs and bronchioles, things can become more serious. These infections can be caused by viruses, bacteria or fungus. Bronchitis and pneumonia are the most common infections of the lower respiratory tract and can be life-threatening if untreated. Pernicious influenza that penetrates deep into the lungs is also a cause for concern. Symptoms include wheezing, shortness of breath, fatigue, fever, chills, muscle ache and excessive mucus.

The most common lung disease is asthma, affecting about 4% of the population. Hospitalisations from asthma attacks are rising. The underlying cause is inflammation and hypersensitivity of the bronchii, which go into spasm when exposed to certain stimuli. Individuals can have attacks when exposed to an allergen that is particular to themselves. Common allergens include chemicals, dust, cat or dog hair, feathers, food additives, mould and smoke. Increasing levels of environmental pollution are known to cause asthma epidemics. Emotion can also trigger an asthma attack and the attack can create fear, which worsens the attack. More serious lung diseases include emphysema or chronic obstructive pulmonary disease, mesothelioma and lung cancer.

The most common way to catch a cold or flu is to touch your eyes, nose or mouth after contacting the germs with your hands; therefore, when in the presence of people who are infected, keep your distance and avoid physical contact. Avoid touching your face and wash your hands often with soap and warm water for 30 seconds. Some people choose to wear surgical face masks when in the presence of people with lung infections because coughing can spread the airborne infection widely.

To avoid lung irritants such as excessive dust or chemical irritants like paint, glue or varnish, use a painter's mask. These masks are effective in keeping out the volatile organic compounds that not only irritate the lungs but also stress the immune system more generally. Make use of air filters in your home, especially in your bedroom where you spend a third of your life.

Cigarette smoke is now well known to injure the lungs, yet still a large minority of adults continue to smoke, harming themselves as well as others around them who are exposed to their second-hand smoke. If you are a smoker, use the season of autumn to tune in to your lungs and recognise their distress. This will help you to quit. Having been a smoker in my younger life, I know how difficult it is to stop. But now there are many ways to help, including nicotine patches, nicotine gum and electronic cigarettes. Ear acupuncture can support quitting by reducing addictions and addictive behaviour.

Foods to support lung health include those that are rich in antioxidants and which reduce inflammation in the body. Such foods include garlic, onions, green drinks and berries. Pears clear heat and moisten the lungs. Reduce or eliminate foods to which you are allergic. Common food allergens include dairy (especially from cow's milk), wheat and gluten.

The lungs also require protein. Deficient Lung Qi can point to an insufficiency of protein in the diet. While dairy foods can provide good protein support for the lungs, if there is an allergy to dairy, this is not recommended.

Herbs that help to cleanse the lungs and support their function include coltsfoot, comfrey, elecampane, fenugreek, ginger, ginseng, goldenseal, horehound, lobelia, lotus root, lungwort, mullein and osha root. These herbs can be used in cooking, drunk as teas or used as poultices.

Large Intestine Health

The large intestine, of which the colon is the largest segment, is the garbage disposal system of the body. When it is functioning well, it takes out the garbage smoothly and regularly. It disposes of the waste products of metabolism, indigestible matter and toxic materials including heavy metals.

When this system is not functioning well, it can lead to unpleasant conditions such as constipation or diarrhoea as well as more serious concerns such as diverticulitis, colon polyps and colorectal cancer.

Diarrhoea can be caused by hostile microorganisms in the digestive tract, food allergies such as lactose or gluten intolerance, stress or emotional upset. When the body is trying to eliminate an organism or food that is unwelcome, it tries to hurry the unwanted substance through the system as quickly as possible. The resulting diarrhoea is actually what the body needs. When you are undergoing stress in your life or experiencing emotions such as fear and anxiety, the autonomic nervous system is compromised. This part of the nervous system operates below conscious control and is what creates the contractions that push the waste along the large intestine. Emotions can interfere with this process, in this case speeding up the passage and expelling the waste before the water has been absorbed from it. This kind of diarrhoea is not helpful to the body and can prevent absorption of water and essential nutrients, leaving the body depleted.

The opposite of this is constipation, which results from a slowing down of the elimination process. Primary causes of constipation are certain medications, especially narcotics and antidepressants; not eating enough to stimulate peristalsis; insufficient water or fibre in the diet; insufficient mucous from the intestinal lining to smooth the flow; overriding the urge to defecate, which shuts down peristalsis; and emotional stress.

As with diarrhoea, emotion can interfere with the nervous system, this time slowing down elimination. Someone who is 'uptight' may have a tense colon which slows the passage of waste and reduces the frequency and ease of bowel movements. I once knew a receptionist who worked at an endoscopy clinic where people go for internal examinations of either colon or stomach. The receptionist was able to identify most of the patients who came for colonoscopies by the way they looked: tight, anxious and strained.

While constipation may seem just an unpleasant inconvenience, if it is chronic, its effects can become serious. Excess pressure on the walls of the colon can produce pouches which trap particles and produce an irritation known as diverticulitis. Other conditions include ulcerative colitis (ulcers in the colon), colonic polyps (excess tissue attached to the intestinal wall) and Irritable Bowel Syndrome, which causes abdominal cramping and bloating as well as affects the small intestine.

Most serious of all is colorectal cancer, the development of cancerous tumours on the intestinal wall. This is one of the more common forms of cancer but is treatable if detected early. Risk rises after the age of 50 years, which is why doctors recommend colonoscopies, especially for those with a family history of this condition.

WAYS TO SUPPORT YOUR LARGE INTESTINE
Health of the large intestine can be supported in the following ways:

- Eat a diet that is rich in fruits, vegetables and whole grains, thereby ensuring an adequate intake of fibre.

  Great sources of fibre are apples, pears, parsnips, broccoli, carrots, spinach, brown rice, quinoa, lentils, beans, flaxseed and chia seed.

- Drink water.

  While it is important to listen to your body and not drink so much water that it upsets your electrolyte balance, too little water puts stress on the colon. Are you thirsty or parched? Drink water. Some people confuse thirst with hunger. If you feel hungry between meals, perhaps you are thirsty. Drink some water and find out.

- Consume sufficient quantities of vitamin D.

  Vitamin D is necessary for the production of mucous in the colon and a deficiency can produce constipation. Optimal vitamin D levels help prevent all forms of cancer including colon cancer. Vitamin D is derived from sun exposure, so in sunless climates and in winter, you may need a supplement. Oily fish like salmon, mackerel and sardines are rich in vitamin D.

- Go to the toilet when you feel the urge.

  Don't hold on if you can help it. It is possible to override the urge to defecate, but doing so will leave toxic waste in the colon and the urge may not return for several hours.

- Engage in physical activity.

  Exercise increases blood circulation in the abdomen and abdominal exercise stimulates the colon. There are yoga poses that work the abdomen such as pawanmuktasana, the wind-relieving pose.

- Massage the abdomen.

  Massage it in a circular motion, following the pathway of the colon: up the right side, across under the ribs, down the left side and across the top of the pubic bone.

- Undergo enemas.

  Enemas or colon flushes can be effective in removing toxins, eliminating parasites and candida, and reducing fatigue. Coffee enemas are especially effective because the coffee stimulates the liver to produce glutathione, which is a powerful detoxifier. Consult with your health practitioner to ensure this is right for you.[12]

Skin Health

We have already seen that the skin is the tissue of the Metal Element and acts like an extra lung, 'breathing in' things on its surface and 'breathing out' sweat, oil and toxins. Among other functions, the skin acts as a protection against external pathogens, contains nerves that give us sensation and sweat glands which play a part in regulating body temperature.

One way the relationship between the skin and the lungs can be illustrated is in the connection between eczema and asthma. Naturopaths have long known that suppressing a skin condition by using steroids tends to drive the condition deeper into the body and especially into the lungs.

The skin is important to health because it manufactures 90% of the body's vitamin D as a result of exposure to sunlight. Vitamin D is vital to many systems of the body. It is essential for growth and development in childhood; it plays a part in the metabolism of calcium and phosphorus and is therefore important for bones and teeth; it keeps muscles strong and helps regulate heartbeat; and it supports the immune system and thyroid function. All this requires a healthy skin and adequate sunlight.

Thousands of skin disorders have been identified, ranging from dry skin, rashes, eczema and psoriasis, to serious skin cancers and melanomas. Many skin conditions reflect what is going on deeper in the body and the symptoms on the surface are a by-product of the body's detoxification.

WAYS TO SUPPORT YOUR SKIN
Healthy skin can be promoted in the following ways:

- Get some sun but not too much.

  The widespread use of sunscreen is preventing many people from getting enough sun to produce vitamin D. Strike a balance between too much and too little exposure.

- Eat fish and nuts.

  The omega-3 fatty acids found in these foods, especially in oily fish such as salmon, help maintain clear skin.

- Use pure water.

  Drink and bathe in non-chlorinated water. Get a shower filter that removes chlorine, which can irritate the skin. When you shower in chlorinated water, you take in the chlorine through your skin and lungs.

- Don't wash too often.

  While the Elizabethans went too far with their annual baths, washing too often denudes the skin of its natural oils. Some say that bathing too soon after sun exposure washes away the vitamin D in the oil on the skin.

- Sweat.

  Exercise regularly to make your sweat glands work. This clears the skin and expels toxins from the body. Wash afterwards to clear away these waste products.

- Eliminate allergens.

  Whether it is sugar, gluten and lactose on the inside, or laundry products, cleaning items and cosmetics on the outside, if something makes your skin itch, rash, pimple or boil, get it out of your life.

- Relax and let go.

  Stress is one of the big contributors to skin problems. Don't let things get under your skin. Do what you can to reduce stress in your life.

Autumn in the Garden

Tidying

'A place for everything and everything in its place.' This may remind you uncomfortably of a parental maxim. But at the heart of this saying are two qualities of metal: tidiness and neatness. When clutter is cleared away, the space that is created is echoed by a spaciousness inside us. We feel we have room to move and space to breathe.

In the garden, autumn is a time for tidying up after the excesses of summer. We can gather all the dead leaves and plants for the compost. We also need to prune trees, cutting back the prolific growth of summer to maintain their shape. There is the pulling up and putting away of the stakes, poles, frames, netting and shade cloth – each neatly stacked, folded and stored in the shed until needed next year. There is the neatening of garden beds and cutting back the edges of lawns. If you have a wood stove, there is the task of stripping branches into kindling, creating a neat stack to cure and season for next winter's fires.

As we perform these tasks, we can further explore the qualities of Metal within us by doing them with care, precision, exactitude and with mindfulness. Since there is little to do by way of tending the plants themselves, we are released from managing growth, given more space and time with the contracting of the year. As we work in the garden at this time of year, the dipping angle of the sun creates a different kind of light. The golden light of the late summer turns to the ethereal light of autumn evoking the qualities of reverence and respect.

Composting

There is perhaps no more Metal-like activity in the garden than making compost. While composting is a year-round activity for the gardener, autumn provides such a proliferation of leaves and leavings from the summer crops that the compost bins become full to bursting.

Every stage of the process evokes the qualities of Metal. By engaging in this alchemical activity, we put ourselves in touch with the vibration of the Metal Element in nature and in ourselves.

Like the alchemists who sought the process by which they could turn lead into gold, composting is alchemy in action in the garden. We are distilling what is rich and valuable from detritus and residue.

To many medieval alchemists, the search for the Philosopher's Stone that would turn base metals into noble ones was really a metaphor for spiritual transformation, a process of transmutation, purification and perfection of the soul. The art of composting is the gardener's alchemy. On the physical level, we are rewarded with a rich, dark, friable mixture that is ambrosia for plants, but on a deeper level, the composting process can put us in touch with Metal's spiritual qualities.

To begin with, it illustrates Metal's capacity to distil, finding the purity among the proliferation. It reminds us that all matter decays in time, including our own bodies, and that everything in our physical world is transitory. This in turn reminds us of our mortality and by extension draws our minds to the world of spirit, that which remains when the physical body dies.

In short, composting is a metaphor for the digestion of experience, the distillation of which transforms our base ego structures into their essential counterparts. Lead into gold. Ego into Essence.

Try this recipe for compost:

Veggie scraps from the kitchen

Tea leaves and coffee grounds

Egg shells

Poo and straw from the chicken pen

All the unused parts of plants from the veggie garden

Grass clippings

Leaves (brown and green) from deciduous trees (not eucalyptus leaves)

Algae and lilies from the fish pond

Weeds

Cow poo (dry and crumbled)

Pet fur

Hair and beard trimmings

Ash from the wood stove

A little compost from the previous batch

Any worms you can find who are willing to relocate

1. Water well.
2. Turn weekly.

Depending on the season and the frequency of turning, a cubic metre of these ingredients will produce a quarter of a cubic metre of rich, dark, crumbly compost in a month or two.

I've experimented with a number of compost bin structures over the years and I continue to search for the perfect method. Currently, I have a double bin, which allows me to easily turn the pile from one side to the other. The back wall of the bin is made of two bales of pea straw to allow the compost to breathe. The sides are made of wooden planks from an old pergola, kept in place by star droppers driven into the soil. The front removable 'gates' are made from the palings of old pallets. The pile is covered with an old cotton sheet folded.

Aeration is the key to generating the heat necessary to create the conditions which will accelerate the process; therefore, turning the pile as often as you can is important. Daily turning will be impractical for many of us (though strength-building), but weekly or even fortnightly turnings will suffice. Moisture is important too. Piles that are too dry will not begin to decompose, while those that are too wet will cool down and stagnate.

Remember, bring mindfulness to the process as you create your black gold.

The Breath

On average, we take 14 breaths per minute. That's about 20,000 breaths a day or around half a billion breaths in an average lifetime. Most of the time, breathing happens unconsciously as the diaphragm and other muscles of respiration expand the lungs to take in oxygen and then contract the lungs to expel carbon dioxide. And if you are still alive and reading this, the process must be working.

However, there are many things which can reduce the effectiveness of breathing. A tight diaphragm will limit the amount of air that can be taken in during inhalation. Other muscles in the ribs (intercostals) and in the neck (sternocleidomastoid and scalene muscles) contribute to respiration, especially when we take a deep breath. A tight neck can make it difficult to breathe deeply.

Emotions can also affect breathing, especially when they are suppressed. Unconsciously holding the breath for periods of time is usually an indication of emotional holding or distress. If you catch yourself holding your breath, take note of whether you are holding it in or out. Most people who hold their breath hold it in. If this describes you, when you discover you are holding your breath, you need first to breathe out. In fact, breathing out fully and forcefully is a great way to make room for a deeper breath. If you discover that you are holding your breath out, breathe in. In both cases, consider why you are holding you breath. Is it from fear, grief, a need for control or something else?

Posture is another way in which breathing can be restricted. Doing a job that requires constant stooping, sitting for long periods in a slumped posture and/or having rounded shoulders and a concave chest are all ways in which the posture of the body limits the ability to breathe deeply and easily. What is more, not breathing properly can lead to these physical traits.

Smoking seriously inhibits respiration besides being injurious to overall health. Tobacco smoke increases mucus production in the lungs and thickens the lining of the bronchioles, which in turn reduces lung capacity.

The ancient Chinese believed that we get 70% of our postnatal Qi from food and 30% from the air; therefore, the way we breathe determines how much of the Qi from air is available to us. This is why breathing practices are so critical to many martial arts, qi gong and meditation practices.

Ways to Breathe More Freely
You can promote better breathing in the following ways:

- Vigorous aerobic exercise activates and strengthens the muscles of respiration.

- Practise yoga. Breathing exercises (pranayama) are an essential component of yoga.

- Practices such as tai qi, qi gong and martial arts such as aikido, karate, kung fu and taekwondo all include breathing exercises as a fundamental part of their practice.

- Meditation practices that focus on the breath teach conscious breathing that can inculcate relaxed breathing in all of life, not just on the meditation cushion.

- Lie on the floor on a long bolster or rolled-up towel placed along the length of your spine. Place your arms out to the side. This allows the chest to open.

- Stand facing the corner of a room with you palms on the walls at shoulder height. Lean into the corner and hold this stretch for a minute. You should feel a deep stretch in the chest as well as a relaxation between the shoulder blades.

- If you find that your breathing is restricted, try this. First expel all the air from your lungs. Then take as deep a breath as you can and hold it for as long as you can. When you return to breathing normally, you will probably find that you are breathing more deeply. This practice works to lengthen and strengthen the muscles of respiration.

- Feel your emotions. Try to stay in contact with your emotions as much as you can. Feeling them as fully as possible while they are present is the best antidote to suppressing them. When emotions are not trapped in the body, you are more relaxed and breathing becomes easier.

A breath is not neutral or bland – it's cooked air; we live in a constant simmering. There is a furnace in our cells, and when we breathe we pass the world through our bodies, brew it lightly, and turn it loose again, gently altered for having known us.[13]

Quitting Smoking

I was impressed with an Australian Government billboard listing the practical benefits of stopping smoking:

Stop Smoking – Start Repairing

- In 8 hours excess carbon monoxide is out of your blood.

- Quit today, before getting pregnant, and the risk of premature birth reduces to that of a non-smoker.

- In 5 days most nicotine is out of your body.

- In 1 week your sense of taste and smell improves.

- In 1 month skin condition is likely to improve.

- In 3 months your lung function begins to improve.

- In 12 months your risk of heart disease has halved.

- In 1 year a pack-a-day smoker will save over $4000.

Every cigarette you DON'T smoke is doing you good.[14]

Meridian Pathways

The Lung and Large Intestine meridians are the energy pathways of the Metal Element, travelling along the arms from the chest out to the hands and returning to the face. Most acupuncture point location books begin with the first point of the Lung meridian as the first in the great cycle of all the points. This is because the ancients believed that when a newborn takes its first breath in life, the Heavenly Qi enters the body at this point. It represents the beginning of life.

The Lung meridian begins on the outside of the upper chest in the pectoralis major muscle, then rises up to the clavicle before crossing the shoulder joint and moving down the front face of the arm and forearm, through the place where the radial pulse is felt, and ending at the outside corner of the thumbnail (see Figure 10.2).

Its partner, the Large Intestine meridian, begins at the corner of the nail of the index finger, travels through the webbing of the thumb and forefinger and along the edge of the forearm, along the side of the upper arm, across the shoulder, up the side of the neck and around the mouth before finishing at the side of the nose on the opposite side of the body (see Figure 10.3).

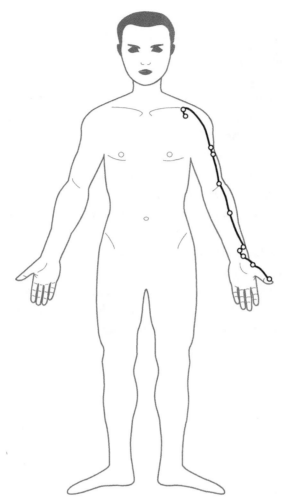

Figure 10.2 The pathway of the Lung meridian

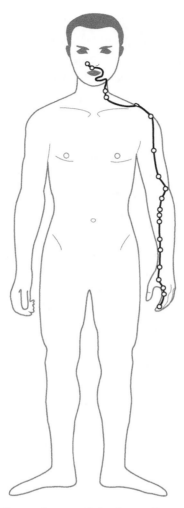

Figure 10.3 The pathway of the Large Intestine meridian

If you feel pain, discomfort, congestion or other symptoms along these pathways, or if you have issues that relate to these organs, you can help free the energy by doing a visualisation practice. Imagine a ball of white energy or light passing along the length of the meridians, freeing up any blocks in the energy flow. You can use your breath to support the practice by breathing out as you pass down the Lung meridian and breathing in as you bring the energy up the Large Intestine meridian. You may also use your hands to stroke along the pathways. Do this several times. If you find a place where it is difficult to move the energy through, stay there and focus your mind, hand and breath to help free the block.

Organ Awareness

After doing the meridian visualisation practice, you can bring your attention specifically to the organs themselves. Beginning with the lungs, place your right hand over the left side of your upper chest, then place your left hand over the right. Tune in to your left lung, which has drawn breath countless millions of times throughout your life, taking in not only life-giving oxygen but also the Heavenly Qi into your body. Bring to mind the colour white, maybe a field of snow or a swan's plumage. Allow this colour to infuse your lung. Acknowledge this organ for all its ceaseless work of respiration. Send love and gratitude to it. Notice how it responds to your recognition and appreciation. Notice how you feel as you do this. When you feel ready, turn your attention to your right lung and repeat this process.

Now move your awareness to your large intestine, which lies coiled around the perimeter of your abdomen like a sleeping snake. There are two ways you can work with this organ. Either put your hands at places along the length of the intestine, wherever it feels right, or you can slowly pass your hands along the length of the organ, starting in the lower right corner of the abdomen, moving up to the ribcage, across under the ribs, down the left side and across the lower edge of the abdomen. Again, bring the white colour to mind and allow white energy or light to infuse the organ, cleansing and healing it. Acknowledge your large intestine for its continuous work of extracting water and minerals and of eliminating the waste from your body. Send love and gratitude to it. Notice how it responds to your attention and acknowledgement. Notice how you feel as you do this.

Acupressure for Physical Health

After the meridian visualisation and organ awareness practices, you can focus specifically on the source points for each meridian. The source point heals the organ directly as well as balancing the meridian. It is a powerful point while at the same time being very safe. The source point has the effect of tonifying the meridian if it is deficient or sedating it if excess.

LU 9 *Taiyuan* Supreme Abyss

The Lung source point lies on the radial (thumb) side of the inside wrist crease, in a hollow between two tendons.

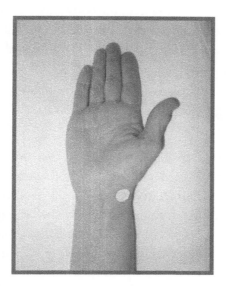

Figure 10.4 The Lung source point (LU 9 *Taiyuan* Supreme Abyss)

LI 4 *Hegu* Joining Valley

The Large Intestine source point lies in the webbing between the thumb and forefinger, halfway along the second metacarpal bone. Press towards the bone.

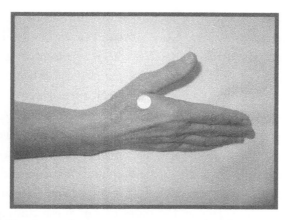

Figure 10.5 The Large Intestine source point (LI 4 *Hegu* Joining Valley)

The Psycho-emotional Level of Metal

Having explored the ways in which Metal shapes us at the physical level, let's now look at the ways it shows up in our mental and emotional life. Thoughts and feelings are of a finer vibration than the body and so their energies are swifter and can change rapidly. But in another way, our emotional patterns, beliefs and attitudes can become fixed and entrenched. Here we will look at the ways in which the Metal Element can appear in us.

The Emotional Landscape of Metal

What Is Grief?

The pioneering work of Elisabeth Kübler-Ross in the 1960s identified five stages of grief as denial, anger, bargaining, depression and acceptance.[15] While this was a useful model for grief counsellors at the time, it later became clear that the grieving process is anything but straightforward. Grief is a complex, multifaceted and highly individualised response to loss. People grieve in different ways and reactions to loss are very personal. It is therefore unhelpful to judge others regarding how well they are dealing with their loss. 'The severity of the loss is measured in how it is *felt*, not by some external metric, comparing situations with levels of grief.'[16]

A more recent model of the grieving process has been articulated by Susan Berger.[17] Rather than charting stages of grieving, she identified five different trajectories of grieving after conducting extensive interviews with people who had suffered various kinds of loss. These five different ways of processing grief she called 'identities'. These five identities she calls nomads, memorialisers, normalisers, activists and seekers. Nomads have not yet resolved their grief and may not understand how it affects their lives. Memorialisers preserve the memory of their loved ones by constructing concrete memorials to them. Normalisers try to recreate family structures that were in place before the loved one died. Activists help others who are dealing with similar losses through education. Seekers turn to philosophy, religion or spirituality to find meaning in their lives.

What is evident from both the stage theory and the trajectory theory is that grief is not a simple emotion in the way that, say, fear and anger are, but a complex mixture of feelings and states that vary from person to person and change from time to time. The final resolution of grief is a coming to terms with the loss – in other words, acceptance. 'Grief is the emotion that allows us to honor the memory of what we valued, release it, and move on with our lives.'[18]

Given the complexity of grief, it is perhaps more helpful here to focus on the feeling of sadness that arises from a sense of loss. Indeed, in translations of the classics, this emotion is most often referred to as sadness. It is the sadness which, if unexpressed or overly expressed, injures the Lungs.

We have all experienced loss many times. These losses may include possessions of varying degrees of value, important friendships or partnerships, a cherished dream that never comes to pass, an ideal that faded with the onset of reality, or the death of pets, dear friends, parents or children.

All humans experience loss; grief is the natural process of coming to terms with loss. It takes time to adjust to loss: hours or days in the case of objects, perhaps many years where loved ones are concerned. Grief is a process of letting go which, if healthy, leads eventually to a state of acceptance and surrender.

Father's Role in Letting Go of Attachment

In the Earth chapter (Chapter 9), we saw how our relationship with our mother is at the heart of the development of our Earth energies. The extent to which we were nurtured, nourished, supported and cared for by our mother, both in utero and in infancy, has a direct impact on our ability in later life to form healthy attachments and relationships, and to feel nourished and supported by the world.

On the other hand, our relationship with our father has much to do with the shaping of our Metal energies. While a mother's role is to support the creation of bonds and attachments and to make her child feel secure and supported, the father's role is to help his child in gradually letting go of these original attachments and creating attachments more widely.

The father takes his child out into the world, shows her how the world works and how to form attachments with others outside the family. Moreover the father's acknowledgement and appreciation for his child, just as she is, is instrumental in mirroring her intrinsic value. 'The father's role is appreciating the child for manifesting the potential he engendered.'[19]

There are many stages of letting go and reattaching. The first happens at birth when the child surrenders the attachment to the placenta and forms an attachment to the mother. Over time this single focus of attachment is widened as the child forms other attachments within the family. Later still, she forms attachments to teachers, school friends, peer groups and ultimately to love relationships. Each of these stages of letting go and reattaching is supported by the Metal energies as they were fostered by our father or father figure.

This process of letting come and letting go is closely associated with value. When Metal energies are healthy, we are able to recognise value and allow valued things into our life; conversely, when something is no longer of value to us, we can let it go.

These psycho-emotional processes are perfectly mirrored in the organs of the Metal Element, the Lung and Large Intestine. The Lung is responsible for taking in the Breath of Heaven, the air that is so valuable to life. At the same time, it acts as a barrier to harmful pathogens that are not of value. When the Lung is healthy, there is an effortless letting in of life.

The Large Intestine is responsible for discarding the waste products that are no longer of value to our bodies; indeed, it would be toxic for us if we did not let them go. At the same time, it extracts from the waste matter the fluid and minerals that are valuable to our body. When the Large Intestine is healthy, there is a smooth letting go on a daily basis.

As we saw in the Earth chapter (Chapter 9), the way our mother responds to our needs affects our Earth energies. These responses are inevitably limited. Similarly, even the most loving and attentive father is unable to provide perfect support for us as we move into the world. And this lack of support will impact our Metal energies.

Lack of support for moving into the world tends to polarise the ways we operate in the world, creating a yin response and a yang response to life events. While we each have both polarities within us, we tend to favour one over the other. Habitually taking either the yin position or the yang position determines our response to Metal's emotion of grief and issue of value.

THE YIN RESPONSE: CAN'T HOLD ON

The yin response is characterised by difficulty in recognising what is valuable. When we don't know what to value, or what is of value for us personally, we have difficulty letting things into our lives. And when we are able to let things in, we tend to have difficulty holding on to them. In other words, there is an imbalance in our ability to attach to the things of the world.

This can lead to difficulty in forming new relationships and holding on to those relationships. When we do form relationships, they may not be mutual because of our tendency to become dependent in the relationship and submit to the authority of the other. Sometimes this imbalance leads us to join groups, religious or otherwise, where there is a strong authority giving out directives that we can follow. This becomes a substitute for the mutual relationship that is so difficult to form. This inability to hold on can make us feel cut off and isolated from the world. When the Lung is not letting in, we tend to hold our breath, cutting ourselves off from life and whatever connects us to Heaven.

We may end up feeling a great deal of grief at our isolation. It may show up as a constant tone of sadness that is often close to the surface; or we may hold it inside and not express it, creating a sense of flatness or collapse. Our inability to hold on to things of value is reflected internally as a feeling of low self-worth. We feel that we are not worthy, that we have no intrinsic value. We find it difficult to see our own positive qualities. When others mirror our positive qualities, we tend to reject the acknowledgement. Even a compliment cannot hold.

THE YANG RESPONSE: CAN'T LET GO

The yang response is characterised by difficulty in letting go of attachments. In this position we have trouble letting go of things that are no longer of value to health and life and which may actually be harmful to our well-being.

One way we might manifest this is to focus on the accumulation of material possessions, be it money or objects. This can become compulsive and there is a drive to get just one more dollar, one more car, one more collectible. What is driving this obsession for accumulation is not fear about survival, but rather an attempt to fill the emptiness inside created by our sense of no value. We try to fill this void with material things.

This difficulty letting go is a kind of psychological constipation. It can extend to relationships, ideas and beliefs, and to the pursuit of reputation. In relationships, we tend to cling to others so strongly that we push away the very people to whom we are clinging. With ideas and beliefs we tend to become dogmatic, brooking no argument and tenaciously hanging on to, and defending, our beliefs against challenge. We elevate our qualifications and achievements as if they are a measure of and replacement for our missing value.

When the focus of our life is on acquisition, we tend to look constantly to the future and away from the here and now. This manifests as longing for what we imagine cannot be found in the present. Jarrett calls this longing 'grief directed towards the future'.[20]

When we are in the yang position, our general attitude tends to be critical, holding ourselves and others to a high standard of perfection. We are fixed and unyielding, tight and tightly held.

These behaviours create a protective barrier against our inner grief. If we never let go, then we never need to deal with the feelings of loss that might arise. Our grief is buried deep in our psyche and body where it tends to create mental and physical tensions and ultimately leads to physical imbalance and illness.

RETURNING TO BALANCE

We begin to return to balance as we start to appreciate that our value is not dependent on anything we do. It is not dependent on our looks, health, achievements, bank account or even our reputation. We are of value simply because we are emanations of True Nature, precious distillations of the Tao. We are Tao drops that are being created and recreated moment by moment without reference to past or future.

More than in any other Element, an imbalance in Metal is a removal from the present moment. Whether we are adrift and unable to attach, or we hold on tight to what we have, we are cut off from what is happening right here, right now. Paying attention to our every moment, being fully in the moment, allows us to unhook from the attachment to past or future. We can let in and let out, like an amoeba, permeable in an ocean of life-giving fluid.

Ultimately, we are beings of spirit living in physical bodies in a material world. The challenge of Metal is to be fully in contact with the Heaven that is our deepest nature, while fully inhabiting our bodies, which reflect our earthly selves. We are fully in the world, but we are not of it.

The Chinese ancients called the spirit of Metal *po*. It is our animal body, our animal soul. It is the only one of the five spirits that dies when the body dies, returning to the earth, becoming fertiliser for the earth.

The key to full-on living is to embrace our body and life totally while being willing to let it go at any moment – in fact, letting it go moment by moment. Spiritual teachers have been telling us this for millennia. Be here now. Live in the moment. The moment is all we have.

From this place we accept that what is here is what is here, not with resignation but with a full breath. This essential acceptance is the greatest gift of Metal.

> Out beyond ideas of wrongdoing and rightdoing, there lies a field and I'll meet you there.
>
> RUMI

If you are the kind of person who has a hard time holding on:

- Do you have a strong sense of your own worth and value? If the answer is no, begin to reframe your view of yourself by focusing on your positive inner qualities, your talents, strengths and gifts.

- Are you doing what you want to be doing with your life? Do you feel fulfilled? What steps can you take to do what you want to be doing and bring more fulfilment to your life?

- Experience yourself as an anchor, not dependent on others. Trying to live up to others' expectations at the expense of your own path can degrade your sense of worth. What do you want for yourself?

- Spend time with people who love and believe in you rather than those who don't.

- Don't blame yourself and don't blame others for your problems. Forgive yourself. We are all really doing the best we can.

- Follow through on your plans and projects. Even small successes build a sense of self-worth (see 'Activity: Taking an Aim' in Chapter 7).

- Establish a belly-breathing practice (see 'Meditation' in Chapter 5). Bringing more Qi to the belly centre strengthens the sense of self.

- Reflect upon your relationship with your father as a child and throughout life. To what extent did you lack your father's guidance and appreciation? Understanding the ways our personality structure was shaped in childhood can begin to free us from its patterning.

If you are the kind of person who has a hard time letting go:

- Identify what it is you tend to hang on to: possessions, people, old relationships, money, ideas, beliefs. Do you identify worth with accumulation? Read the sections on value in this chapter.

- Make a list of all the things you are hanging on to. Consider what is superficial and what is truly of value in your life. Begin to let go of those things on your list that are least important to you.

- During the autumn, clear out your garage or any other area of your home where extraneous stuff has accumulated. Go to the dump and recycling centre, have a garage sale, give things away to friends. Read the later section on space.

- Obsessions (pervasive thoughts) and compulsions (repetitive behaviours) may be indicative of Metal imbalance. When these begin to interfere with day-to-day living, it can be called obsessive-compulsive disorder. Therapy can help to relabel, refocus, reattribute and revalue in ways that change brain chemistry and result in changes to behaviour.[21]

- Do you hold your breath? This can be a subtle way of holding on. Take up a mindful breathing practice. The breathing meditation below is a good place to begin.

- If you find yourself lamenting, regretting and holding on to the past, coming to acceptance is not an easy thing. Meditation helps to make space for change. As much as you can, bring yourself to the present moment. Be grateful for what you do have. Gratitude is one of the best paths to acceptance.

Reflection

In March 2011 a massive earthquake and tsunami off the eastern coast of Japan created enormous destruction and an extraordinary loss of life. Some villages in the north of Japan disappeared entirely. While the world looked on in shock and horror at the consequences of this disaster, many outsiders commented on the way that the Japanese people coped. They seemed to deal with a terrible situation in a way that was orderly, dignified and accepting. All of these are qualities of the Metal Element. Indeed, the Japanese culture has much to teach us about the Gifts of Metal, from the bare essentials of the Zen monastery, to the gracious precision of the tea ceremony, to the way that the spirit can rise above death and destruction.

Money

We have already seen that one of the associations of the Metal Element is precious metal such as gold and silver. Before the modern era these metals provided the materials for coins that became a means of exchange and formed the basis of a functioning economy. These days we are more likely to have money as paper or plastic notes, and as theoretical numbers in an account. What all these forms of money have in common is that they represent a store of energy and a store of value.

One of the qualities of Metal is distillation. Money can be viewed as a distillation of one's efforts over time, a representation of hours and days of effort stored into a convenient form. The fruits of this effort can then be retrieved at a later date and used in exchange for something we need.

Our attitudes to money can tell us a lot about the health of our Metal Element. How easy is it to have a balanced attitude to money, neither holding on tight to it nor letting it leak through our fingers? Think about the issues we explored earlier, whether you are the kind of person who has trouble holding on or someone who has difficulty letting go.

Expressions such tight-fisted, tight-assed, money-grubbing, penny-pinching and grasping all refer to the physical action as well as the mental attitude of holding on as it is expressed through money.

On the other hand, words like spendthrift, profligate, squandering, improvident, prodigal and the expressions 'to spend money like water' and 'money runs through his fingers' describe an attitude to money that makes it difficult to function in the world.

Money is a flow. In many ways it is like a pool that forms in a stream. Money comes into the pool from upstream and leaves the pool to continue its downstream flow. The pool is a store of money that is continually changing and refreshing. When we hold on tight to money and restrict its outflow, it can have toxic consequences for us. Our whole being tightens up around it, affecting us at physical, mental and spiritual levels. On the other hand, if the outflow is uncontrolled, there is a depletion of resources that doesn't allow for the appropriate support of our lives.

EXPLORING ATTITUDES REGARDING MONEY

Try this exercise: Take a piece of money. It doesn't matter its kind or denomination. Hold it in your hand. Sit with your eyes closed for a few minutes and notice what thoughts, feelings and attitudes arise. Just observe your mind as it responds to the money.

Afterwards you may wish to journal about the experience. What did it tell you about your unconscious ideas about money? Where do you find yourself on the continuum of holding on and letting go when it comes to money? Why do you think this is?

Journal Entry: 20 April 2013

Cutting Through That Which Is No Longer Needed

On a bright autumn day in April 2012 I was preparing a lettuce for lunch. I'd pulled the last of the red oak lettuce from the garden and sliced through the base with a heavy sharp knife, when out from the leaves walked the biggest earwig I'd ever seen. I picked him up from the counter with my left hand but he gave me a sharp pinch on my index finger. In a split-second reflex, I hit him with the only thing to hand, namely the super-sharp chopping knife.

Time stopped. I stared for ageless milliseconds at the mouth that appeared on my finger, at the bright white finger bone that shone briefly. Here was the moment that would forever mark my life into two parts: before the cut and after the cut; the moment that somehow I always knew would come. A thought arose in this endless second: here it is at last, the accident to change my life.

The bone disappeared in a gush of blood. A priceless finger ruined, all else receded. The earwig, the knife, the room all vanished. Pressing, staunching, rinsing, shock, disbelief, alone. Wrapping a towel around the clenched left hand, I picked up car keys and headed for the car, intending to drive to hospital until I realised that would not be a great idea. Finding help, I got to hospital and had emergency surgery to reconnect severed arteries, tendons and nerves. Home again the next day, splinted in a cast, looking at two months off work and intensive rehab. Plenty of time to reflect upon the split-second event that put me in this place.

It was not lost on me that the incident was redolent of the Metal Element. Using a sharp metal knife, and in the season of Metal, I cut through the Large Intestine channel of my left index finger. For those who are curious, the cut was on the phalangeal crease, midway between *Erjian* (LI 2) and *Sanjian* (LI 3), the Water and Wood points, respectively, of the Large Intestine channel. Since my constitutional Element is Wood and first within is Water, there seemed some great significance in this, as if I were unconsciously cutting through to some core relationship to the attributes of Metal.

It is well known that the function of the large intestine organ is to eliminate the waste products of digestion while retaining water and essential minerals. At the psycho-emotional level, the Large Intestine Official is charged with cutting away those things that are no longer of value to one's life, and which, if retained, may become toxic. I spent my convalescence pondering the particular significance for my life. What was I hanging on to that was not serving me? Taking this further, I wondered whether the Water and Wood points had something more specific to teach me.

Lonny Jarrett provides some useful insights about these two points. Of the Water point (LI 2) he writes:

> If the presence of water within is deficient, dryness can result in constipation. In the same way we can tend to cling to the people and things we value for fear of losing them, even after they have lost their worth to us.[22]

Water's emotion of fear impedes Metal's capacity to let go, producing fear of letting go. What Jarrett has to say about the Wood point (LI 3) is even more apposite:

> ...the wood element can help us manifest the metal element's virtues of inspiration and value through its own functions of planning and decision making. Empowering perspective within the metal can facilitate our ability to decisively let go of that which has lost its value.[23]

This 'accident' afforded me the opportunity of examining those parts of my life that were constipated and needed to be purged. It was a profound kick up the backside that got the Large Intestine moving again. As I look back on the past year, I am amazed at the many changes that have come about as a direct result of recognising these stuck places, understanding that changes were needed and taking decisive action to let go of all those things that were holding back the flow of my life.

And finally, if you are wondering what happened to the earwig which was the catalyst for the changes which followed, the evening I got home from hospital and was cleaning up the mess of the accident, I moved the cutting board and out scuttled the giant earwig, apparently unscathed by the incident. This time I made no attempt to capture him. I just let him go.

Space

In the season of autumn, nature appears to be clearing out, as if making space. Each year there is a de-cluttering as leaves drop and decompose, crops that are not harvested die back, fields that were once full of vegetation lie empty and bare.

In our lives, the capacity to make space is a gift and a teaching of the Metal Element. When we are healthy and our digestive system is functioning well, the colon empties out the waste products that are of no use to us, clearing us out for the coming day's food intake. We can take this somatic process into the rest of our lives. Making space in the home, garden, office, car and other areas we inhabit allows more of life to flow through it. Even making space in our calendar can allow things to flow more freely.

The Chinese art of feng shui pays a lot of attention to clear space in the home and warns against too much clutter, which is bad for one's health. One of its basic tenets is that nothing new flows into your life until you make room for it;[24] therefore, clearing clutter is crucial to allowing Qi to move through your living space and through your life in general. Clutter refers to anything that is unfinished, unused, unresolved or disorganised. Clutter in different areas of the home represents resistance to various aspects of life: relationships, emotions, self-care, change.

If you are a person who tends to live in a cluttered environment, then autumn is a good time to begin making space. Trying to organise the whole house at once is likely to be overwhelming and too challenging; therefore, work on one area at a time. Start with one room, one closet, one desk, even one drawer. And don't forget the shed, the attic and the garage. Wherever clutter accumulates is a place that Qi stagnates.

For people who are of a Metal constitution or whose Metal is strong within them, space becomes an issue of the life. For some people it appears as a significant need for things to be tidy, clean and spacious. Sometimes this can become an obsessive need for cleanliness and tidiness. Other Metal types struggle to maintain order and may appear disorganised, untidy and slovenly.

Some Metal people appear distant and stand-offish, maintaining space between themselves and others. This is not usually how they see themselves. One such person I met put it succinctly: 'I relate to people through space.' While others often experienced her as distant, she experienced herself in relationship as being in contact with others through space. This keen self-observation provides an insight into the world view of the Metal constitution.

Acupressure for Psycho-emotional Health

The points I have chosen to support psycho-emotional health are known as the front mu points or Alarm points of the Metal meridians.

LU 1 *Zhongfu* Middle Palace

The Lung alarm point is located on the outer edge of the upper chest (see Figure 10.6). Find the large hollow under the collarbone (deltopectoral triangle) and move down by a thumb width and slightly lateral. It is the first point of that meridian and lies on the outer part of the upper chest. LU 1 *Zhongfu* Middle Palace is a powerful point for opening the chest, allowing for deeper breathing and letting go of emotional holding. Emotions that are held inside tighten the chest and breathing. This point allows pent up emotions to rise for expression. The ancients believed that when a baby is born, the Breath of Heaven enters at Middle Palace, which represents the beginning of life. This point is therefore a connection to our spiritual nature as much as it is to the process of breathing. By opening the chest, we inspire and are inspired to open fully to life. The effect of this point can be increased by holding it in conjunction with the source point LU 9 learned earlier.

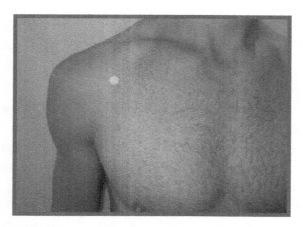

Figure 10.6 The Lung alarm point (LU 1 *Zhongfu* Middle Palace)

ST 25 *Tianshu* Heavenly Pivot

The Large Intestine alarm point is located two cun lateral to the navel. It lies on the Stomach Meridian. ST 25 *Tianshu* Heavenly Pivot reminds us of the fact that we are beings of spirit living in animal bodies. This point helps us to balance these two aspects of our nature so that we are neither too earthbound nor too heaven-centred. This point helps us to let go at the level of eliminating waste from the colon as well as at the psycho-emotional level, letting go of emotions, ideas and beliefs that no longer serve. This point can be further strengthened by holding it together with the source point LI 4 learned earlier. The two alarm points can also be held in combination to good effect, balancing both yin and yang of the Metal Element.

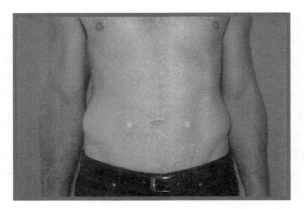

Figure 10.7 The Large Intestine alarm point (ST 25 *Tianshu* Heavenly Pivot)

The Spiritual Level of Metal

Our spiritual nature is not the body, the thoughts, the emotions or the personality. If there is anything that remains of us when we die, it is the spirit. Here we examine how the Metal Element influences spiritual life.

The Spirit of Metal: Po

The Chinese character *po* has two parts. The left part is the character for white, which is the colour of the Metal Element as well as the colour of bones that disintegrate upon death and return to the earth. The right part is the character for ghost or earthbound spirit. *Po* is therefore the spirit which is tied to the earth and the mundane.

The *po* is the corporeal soul (sometimes translated as animal soul) which enters the body at conception. In the first months after birth, the baby's whole life revolves around the corporeal soul as it forms the foundation of a healthy body for the life to come. Of the five spirits, it is the only one that disappears when we die. As soon as the lungs exhale for the last time and the body dies, the *po* exits through the anus and descends to mix with the earth from whence it came.

During life, the *po* is utterly tied to the physical body and to time and space. It is 'the unthinking and compelling passion that propels life.'[25] Like animal instinct, it is concerned with immediate reactions to what is happening in each moment. It is about the here and the now. This instinctual part of us lives on its senses, alert to all sights, sounds, smells, tastes and textures. It is our animal nature.

The *po* is paired with the *hun*, the ethereal soul which is the spirit of the Wood Element. While the *hun* roams the realm between the earth and the heavens, the *po* provides a counterpoint as the most physical and material part of the human soul. 'It could be said to be the somatic manifestation of the soul.'[26] It provides for clear and sharp sensations and movements; it is involved in all physiological processes. Of all these processes it is especially connected to breathing, which is its special province. In fact, the *po* is said to reside in the Lungs and is particularly affected by sadness and grief, which restrict its movement. Constricted breathing, holding of the breath and shallow breathing are all injurious to the Lung and to the *po*.

While the emotion of grief is the one most closely associated with the *po*, all emotions are ruled by it. It consists of the seven emotions (fear, anxiety, anger, joy, sorrow, worry and grief) which Jarrett neatly describes as 'the primal urges that facilitate the grasping of life.'[27]

Another function of the *po* is to perform a tricky balancing act of living life as a human being, anchoring the heavenly aspect within the density of the body. '*Po* is the embodiment of the spiritual father in the body, grounding the heavenly energy in flesh and blood.'[28]

Imbalance in the *po* produces a marked disparity between the Heavenly and earthly aspects of human life. On the one hand, there can be an obsessive attachment to material things and the accumulation of possessions, money and fame to the detriment of things spiritual. On the other hand, a person may have his head in the clouds and be unable or unwilling to navigate the ordinary world of human existence. There may even be a withdrawal from the world in order to focus on the spiritual search.

Other possible outcomes of *po* imbalance are ongoing physical pain with no identifiable cause, migrating pain, extreme sensitivity to outside psychic influences and chronic health problems associated with emotions that are stuck.

The Virtue of Metal: Righteousness

The Confucian virtues were first paired with the Five Elements in the *Bai Hu Dong* in 79 BCE. The virtue that relates to Metal is *yi*,[29] translated as righteousness or justice. The character *yi* is composed of two parts, the character for self placed below the character for king. It can be understood as the subjugation of the self to that which is above, namely the Will of Heaven.[30] Simply put, it is the moral disposition to do good. It represents the ability to recognise what is right and good and to intuit what is the right action to take in any given situation.

Many people throughout the ages have thought that they knew what was right and what was the right thing to do, and then proceeded to force their perspective onto others. This is amply illustrated by the actions of the medieval popes and Christian crusaders who believed they were doing God's work in killing Muslims. In our current era the situation is ironically reversed as Muslim fundamentalists carry out atrocities in the name of Allah. However, this outward-directed behaviour of rectifying and correcting the world is a distortion of the virtue and misunderstands the notion of righteousness. It is an inner state, a recognition of the rightness of all things as they are. 'The lesson, of course, is that justice arises through rectification of the self, not others, and that in fact there is nothing to rectify at all if one's true value is understood.'[31]

The ancients understood that as a human loses contact with his True Nature, the purity of the virtue of an Element is also lost. When this happens, the virtue begins to degrade into the emotion of that Element. When righteousness is eroded, it turns to grief. In other words, when we lose touch with the truth that everything that is happening in this moment is part of the perfect unfolding of True Nature, we descend into grasping and holding on, either to the past or to an imagined future.

This grasping manifests as an attempt to rectify the world in order to conform to a particular picture of what is right, good and perfect. This results in the setting of rules and limits, moralising, criticising and rebuking. Almost always these codes of honour and conduct are established for others to follow because the setter thinks he knows what is right for everyone.

Of course, this path is doomed to failure because the unfolding of True Nature is beyond the control of the ego. True righteousness comes from recognising the divine in all things and living in accord with divine law. This means honouring the natural cycles of the universe, in particular the cycle of life and death, letting go to the ultimate surrender of death.

The Spiritual Issue of Metal: Recognising the Preciousness of Now

In this world of time and space we inhabit, it is natural to think of time as a linear progression, the past stretching back and the future stretching forward. We normally see ourselves at a place on the time continuum, a place that we think of as the present and which we call now. But spiritual teachers from time immemorial have been telling us that this is an illusion. The only thing that is real is what is happening in this very moment. Whatever is happening in the now is all that there is. Everything else is either a memory of what has past or an imagination of what might be in the future. There is nothing but now.

Yet even as we contemplate the nature of this present moment, it has already gone and is no longer the present moment. It has passed into the past. The moments arise and fall away even as they are arising. There is nothing there that can be grasped. Spiritual teacher Adyashanti explains this in the context of endings:

> This moment, as soon as it comes into being, is ending. And since the arising and the disappearing are one event, there is nothing that can be grasped. That is the nature of all phenomena: it begins, it ends. And yet there is that which is neither beginning nor ending, that which notices the beginnings and the endings. And that is what it means to realise what is right now.[32]

Or as Eckhart Tolle puts it, 'Life is now. There was never a time when your life was not now, nor will there ever be.'[33]

Much of the time our minds are filled with thoughts that are nothing to do with the present moment. There are thoughts of the past, memories of pleasurable or unpleasant experiences, regrets over things we have done or said, reconstructions of what we might have done differently, self-attacks over our character or behaviour. There are projections into the future, anticipations of some long-awaited or dreaded event, plans and hopes and dreams, wanting to be somewhere else but now. And there are our emotional reactions, which are all based on patterns from the past.

These thoughts crowd and jostle in our mind for attention, constantly pulling us away from the present moment. This is the ceaseless activity of the ego, the false self which creates all this mental fabrication in order to preserve itself. The thought-chatter is the text of the ego's endless activity which is designed to keep the ego structure in place. Ego is not happy with stillness, with silence, with the space between thoughts. It needs to fill every single moment in order to protect its existence. For when there is cessation of thought, there is death for the ego.

To become more in touch with the now, we need to find the space between these thoughts, the space between the moments in order to find the now. Actually, we don't need to do anything, because to go looking for the now is just more ego activity. It is a conundrum: how to be fully present in the moment without trying to be present.

Why is this spiritual teaching of being in the moment of particular relevance to the Metal Element? Metal represents the process of stripping away the extraneous to discover what is truly of value. The precious gem inside each one of us is discovered by seeing through the clutter of the mind, recognising the false structure of the ego. When this begins to fall away, we experience the emptiness and stillness that is the True Nature of everything.

 What is happening right now? Find ways to express your direct experience of the present moment.

Impermanence

Shakyamuni Buddha observed that we live in a world where impermanence is the nature of all phenomena, that everything, without exception, is in a constant state of flux. Or as George Harrison more recently sang, 'All things must pass.'

How we deal with this truth tells us much about the state of our Metal Element. Metal gives us the capacity to confront loss, to let go of what we once possessed, to feel the pain of the loss and to move on. This describes the process of grief, letting go of attachment and coming to terms with loss.

This capacity derives from the Officials of Lung and Large Intestine. The Lung Official allows us to breathe in life in all of its fullness; the Large Intestine Official encourages us in letting go of attachment. Together they support us in being present in the moment, breathing in each moment of our existence, while simultaneously letting it go.

All endings, all losses, all deaths are but a training. They are training us for our own death. For ultimately we will all, at some point, be called upon to let go of our whole life and surrender to death. By contemplating our ability to let go of our attachments to possessions, people, ideas, beliefs, hopes and dreams, we gain insight into our greatest attachment of all: to life itself.

What is more, by anticipating this supreme loss, we get training in coming to terms with all the little losses. Death teaches us to let go day by day, moment by moment, and to live more and more fully in the present.

 The fact that the time of our death is unknown to us allows us to go to sleep to the fact that we will die. What if today were the last day of your life, and you knew it. How would you live?

Activity: Building an Altar

 One way to cultivate the Metal qualities of reverence, respect and ritual is to create an altar in your home or garden.

What is an altar? In the Western tradition an altar is a place in a church where religious rituals are performed. But in most religious and spiritual traditions it is common for people to have places in their home for private worship, devotion, prayer and meditation. An altar can become a place to honour the divine, express gratitude, give offerings and ask for blessings and protection. It is a focal point, a reminder of the spiritual realm. It implies recognition and honouring of those things in your life that represent the non-material part of your existence.

Here are some things to consider in creating an altar:

- Make a dedicated space.

  This will be a place for the activities of contemplation, meditation and prayer. Do not share it with other activities that will detract from the atmosphere.

- What is the purpose of your altar?

  Create personal meaning. Consider what will be the focal image of the altar as this will set its tone.

- Choose its location with care.

  One system of feng shui advises to locate the altar in the northwest corner of the house; another suggests having it on the Metal wall of the room (i.e. the wall to the right as you enter the door). But these suggestions are not essential. Intention is what is most important. Go with what feels right.

- Clean the area thoroughly and with mindfulness.

  Bring your intent to the whole process as this will express your commitment. You may wish to cleanse the area energetically with sage or crystals.

- Elevate the altar on a shelf or table.

  This will bring respect and lend special significance to your altar.

- Choose images, icons and artefacts that represent spirituality for you.

  This can be photographs of spiritual sages and teachers, paintings of deities, mandalas, statues, rocks and crystals, bells, bowls and other sacred items that you feel connected to. Some people like to make offerings of flowers, food and water. Candles, incense and oil infusers bring light and fragrance to the altar.

- The altar can be a place where you meditate, infusing that part of your home with spiritual intent. It then becomes a reminder and a support for spiritual practice.

- Establish a daily ritual.

  This may be to meditate, pray, make offerings or whatever it is that connects you to Spirit. Regularity of practice keeps the altar alive.

Your altar will be an organic thing, changing over time as you add to it and as your own spiritual unfolding continues. It becomes a reflection of your inner development. While the altar is an outward expression of your spirituality, ultimately it is honouring the divine within yourself, not as something external to you.

The Diamond Approach
Value

Many people define value in terms of what a thing is worth, its monetary exchange or its usefulness to us. From this ego perspective, people are also assigned a value according to what they contribute to the world. Even our own feeling of worth is often linked to our personal attributes, qualities and achievements.

As we take the spiritual journey, we begin to turn from valuing external things to valuing internal states. We value certain emotions, feelings or conditions. For example, we might value love, kindness and empathy but at the same time not value anger, fear and hatred. There is still a preference for this but not for that, a valuing of one thing over another.

From the view of Essence, value is nothing to do with these things, either internal or external. It is your *being* that has value. This is not to say that it is your existence that is valuable, but rather that your being *is* value. You don't *have* value, you *are* value.

> Value is truly nothing other than our heart's intimate contact with the immediacy of the moment, with each moment, with where we are precisely. In that contact, in that being with and knowing reality as it is, we recognize the unquestionable rightness and preciousness of where we are and what we are. Nothing touches us more deeply than the implicit value of our own beingness. It is value beyond mind, beyond concepts, beyond ideals and hopes and dreams. This preciousness of simply being here now with awareness and understanding fills our heart with contentment and satisfaction. We realize that where we are, which is what we are, is also the most real and precious nature of life itself.[34]

Change and Death

When we internalise the understanding that all forms in the universe are in constant change, we realise that holding on and not wanting things to change is a significant source of suffering. It is the ego which thinks that some changes are good while others are bad. Holding on to pleasure and pushing away pain, clinging to life and abhorring death: these are the choices of the ego. From the larger perspective, change is neither good nor bad; it is simply the nature of reality. This understanding radically changes our view of life and death.

> Personal death is simply Being manifesting at one moment with a particular person as part of the picture, and in the next moment without that person. From this perspective, all the issues about death change character. Death disappears into the continual flow of unfolding, self-arising change.[35]

> We cannot live if we don't live with death. There is no full, real living without dying. The wisdom we want to learn is the wisdom of life and death. Where we can see at some point that to live is to die and to die is to live. For we cannot separate the two. In many ways at many levels. To live fully is to die. To die correctly is to live fully. And that is relevant and true at each level of our awareness.[36]

Acupressure for Spiritual Health

Here we look at the outer shu point of the Lung meridian, located in the upper back on the outer line of the Bladder meridian. This point is particularly effective in healing at the level of mind and spirit. The effectiveness can be increased by using the point in combination with the source point and the mu point learned earlier.

BL 42 *Pohu* Door of the Corporeal Soul

BL 42 *Pohu* Door of the Corporeal Soul is located in the upper back at the level of the junction of the third and fourth thoracic vertebrae, and four fingers' width out from the spine. *Po* is the spirit of Metal, and *Pohu* offers a doorway to accessing this spirit. The Po is the most material aspect of the soul, sometimes referred to as our animal soul or animal instinct. Since it governs the instinctual parts of us, it is responsible for the automatic, rhythmic maintenance of life. Breathing, which happens without our conscious involvement, is an aspect of this. The *po* also guides our senses and our awareness of sensations in our body. Grief and sadness strongly affect the *po* and constrain its natural movement, constricting the inspiration of Qi through the breath, and so the revitalisation of the spirit.

It is no coincidence that our word 'inspire' means both to take a breath in and to instil a person with thought or feeling. Though our word derives from Latin, it reflects these two activities, which the Chinese ancients saw as emanating from the Metal Element.

It may seem something of a paradox that the *po*, which relates so much to our instinctual, animal side, is also paramount in connecting us to our spiritual nature. The *po* is concerned with balancing these aspects of our human nature, supporting us as beings of spirit who inhabit the bodies of animals.

Door of the Corporeal Soul is a point that helps with this balancing act. It can access the spirit of Metal at a very deep level and serve to reconnect a person with what she values in her life, with the preciousness of life itself and with her authentic being or Essence. Moreover, it supports us in valuing our essential spiritual nature.

All the longings that we feel are ultimately a desire to be reconnected with spirit, whether or not we are conscious of the underlying nature of our longing. *Pohu* supports reconnection with spirit and thus can treat all feelings of longing and desire for spirit.

These attributes of *Pohu* are particularly helpful in supporting people in their quest to find spiritual meaning in life on Earth. Where depression, long-term sadness, resignation or lack of inspiration derive from loss of contact with spirit, this soul door offers support.

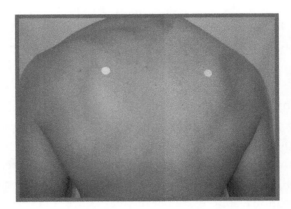

Figure 10.8 The outer shu point of the Lung meridian
(BL 42 *Pohu* Door of the Corporeal Soul)

Meditation: The Breath

Many meditation practices focus on the breath. Breathing is a natural and involuntary process and provides a useful focus for mindfulness practice. In this guided meditation you will be bringing your attention to the physiological processes involved in breathing as a way of tuning in to your body. Bringing awareness to the breathing process is an important step in developing a well-functioning respiratory system that is vital to your best health.

Find a comfortable sitting position. Let your hands rest in your lap or on your thighs. Sit in an upright yet relaxed posture.

Begin by bringing your attention to the tip of your nose, the place where the air enters your body as you breathe in and where it leaves the body as you breathe out. Notice the sensations at the tip of your nose. Notice the temperature, the feeling. Notice how you feel about the feeling.

Now bring your attention to your nasal passages where the air streams in. Notice how it feels at the back of your nose: the temperature, the sensations. How easy is it to breathe the air in and out? Whatever is going on, simply notice without trying to change anything.

Now bring your attention to your throat where the air moves down the larynx on its way to the lungs. There are muscles in the front of the neck that assist in respiration. Notice how these muscles feel. Are they loose or tight? What sensations are there in your neck and throat?

Now bring your attention to your upper chest. Notice the sensations of the air passing into the lungs. Is it comfortable? Is there discomfort? Is it neutral? Be aware of the rising and falling of your chest as the air comes in and goes out.

Now bring your attention to the deepest part of your lungs where a deep breath expands the lungs with air. In this area you will feel the diaphragm, which is the primary muscle of respiration. Notice what is happening in this area of your lower chest and upper abdomen as you breathe. Does it feel comfortable? Is there discomfort? Are there any constrictions? Try to simply notice without trying to change anything.

Now, finally, extend your attention to the whole process and pathway of the breath, from the tip of the nose, through the nasal passages, down the larynx, into the lungs, right down into the alveoli, at the end of the bronchial tree, and to the diaphragm and the chest muscles. Bring your attention to all aspects of breathing as you sit in meditation for a few minutes.

Transition from Metal to Water

In the Adelaide Hills where I live, the winter rains have come at last, plucking the final leaves from the deciduous trees. There are still warm days, but it is clear we are enjoying the last of them. Winter is waiting in the wings, ready to spread out across the landscape like spilled water.

For some people this can be a difficult transition if it brings with it a foreboding of the chilly days and long cold nights to come, and an unwillingness to let go of the bright days of autumn. For other people the transition to winter is welcome, a time to hunker down at home in front of a warm fire with a good book and an early bed, shutting out the world and retreating indoors.

During this transition between autumn and winter, the Metal and Water Elements dance with each other as cold days intersperse themselves in the last of the autumn warmth. We cannot ignore the sun as it dips lower and lower towards the horizon, heading for its rendezvous with the winter solstice. We reach for scarves, vests, extra layers and think of splitting wood for fires.

Before I began working with the Elements, I hated winter with a passion, dreaded the cold and the dark and the faint depression that descended. But gradually I began to see the rightness of the season, began to accept nature's invitation to go inside. The more we can rest and rejuvenate in this time, the more our internal batteries will be charged in readiness for the next round.

Take up nature's invitation and use this transition period to prepare for turning within. Secure the house against the cold winter winds; pare back your schedule to allow for early nights; stock up on books, movies, jigsaws, knitting or whatever keeps you comfortable indoors. Emulate the trees and drop the extraneous from your life. Prepare for the descent.

Into yourself.

Notes

Preface

1. The School of Philosophy and Healing in Action (SOPHIA) program was part of the TAI Institute, now the Maryland University of Integrative Health.
2. Almaas 2013.

Chapter 2

1. Throughout I have capitalised the word 'Element' to indicate a phase as distinct from lowercase 'element', which is a component.
2. Fung 1976, p.16.
3. Maoshing 1995, p.xii.
4. Maoshing 1995, p.1.
5. Eckman 1996, p.85.
6. Unschuld 1985, p.251.
7. Lawson-Wood 1959.
8. Mann 1962.
9. Austin 1972.
10. I have been unable to identify the date on which Worsley began to teach acupuncture. Even Eckman's (1996) brilliant detective work does not pin it down.
11. Reston 1971.
12. Mitchell 1992, p.1.
13. The four diagnostic tools of colour, sound, odour and emotion (CSOE) are the cornerstone of this method of diagnosis. While there can be a temptation to diagnose by behaviours, CSOE must always form the basis of finding the Constitutional Element.
14. Eckman 1996 (p.208) observed Worsley identifying the CF of a patient without any of the diagnostic factors, though Eckman declares this was a rare exception.

Chapter 3

1. The five notes of the Chinese pentatonic scale are assigned to the Five Elements: Water – La; Wood – Mi; Fire – So; Earth – Do; Metal – Re.
2. Maoshing 1995, p.34.

3. The use of the term 'Gifts' in this context originated, as far as I can tell, in the SOPHIA program described earlier.
4. Larre and Rochat de la Vallee 2003. The translations of the functions of the Officials are Larre's. I have used Worsley's order of the meridians, beginning with Heart rather than Lung, as occurs in most texts.

Chapter 4

1. Almaas 2002b, p.84.
2. Kaku 2007.
3. Al-Khalili 2010.
4. Al-Khalili 2010.
5. Hammer 2005, p.89.
6. Maciocia 2009, p.6. *Shen* meaning body and *shen* meaning mind are different characters but phonetically the same – what in English is called a homophone.
7. Maciocia 2009, p.6.
8. Brown 2013.
9. Reninger 2012.
10. McLellan 1998, p.229.
11. Morsella 2012.
12. Libet 1999.
13. Gyatso 1995.
14. Gurumaa 2013.
15. Maciocia 2005, p.69.
16. Maoshing 1995, p.34.
17. Maciocia 2005, p.69.
18. Maciocia 2005, p.70.
19. Solomon 2003, p.67.
20. Solomon 2003, p.2.
21. Solomon 2003, pp.271–283.
22. Scherer 2005.
23. Almaas 1987, p.25.
24. Almaas 1987, p.25.
25. Cleary 2003, p.57.
26. Maciocia 2009, p.8.
27. Almaas 1988, p.21.
28. Genesis 2:7.

29. For a detailed treatment of this subject see Dechar 2006.
30. Maciocia 2009, p.4.
31. Jarrett 1998.
32. Jarrett 1992, endnote 6.
33. Jarrett 1998, p.31.
34. Jarrett 1998, p.32.
35. Jarrett 1998, p.153.
36. Elijah 2009.
37. Almaas 2002b, p.249.
38. Almaas 1996, p.22.

Chapter 5

1. Kirkwood 2016 details the uses of 54 acupoints, arranged by Elements.
2. For beginners I recommend Jarmey and Bouratinos 2008, a book by two shiatsu practitioners.

Chapter 6

1. Wieger 1965, p.287.
2. Maciocia 2005, p.158.
3. Horowitz 2012.
4. Maoshing 1995 (p.43) translates the colour as black, while Maciocia 2005 (p.34) calls it 'dark purple, purplish, sometimes nearly black'.
5. Hicks, Hicks and Mole 2004, p.154.
6. Hicks, Hicks and Mole 2004, p.154.
7. Elijah 2013.
8. Bodymind is a term that refers to the interconnected levels of human experience (physical, mental, emotional and spiritual) as discussed in Chapter 4.
9. Suzuki 1970, p.21.
10. Mitchell 1992, p.71.
11. Fung 1983, p.41.
12. Jarrett 1998, pp.177–178; Moss 2010, pp.231–233.
13. Jarrett 1998, p.178.
14. Dechar 2006, p.276.
15. Dechar 2006, p.275.
16. Tortora and Anagnostakos 1990, p.846.
17. Maciocia 2005, p.205.
18. Tortora and Anagnostakos 1990, p.828.
19. Tortora and Anagnostakos 1990, p.520.
20. Hammer 1990, p.99.
21. Maciocia 2005, p.155.
22. Maciocia 2005, p.158.
23. Kellow 2013a.
24. Maoshing 1995, p.42.

25. Thompson 2006. There is debate about this, most refutations coming from creationists trying to debunk the theory of evolution. In fact, if saltwater is diluted with fresh water, the mineral constituents are very similar. Seawater has been used for blood transfusions in emergencies.
26. Batmanghelidj 2008.
27. Balch 1997, p.157.
28. Controlled use of fire was widespread 125,000 years ago, though there is strong evidence of its use 400,000 years ago.
29. Private teaching given by A.H. Almaas at Berkeley, California.
30. Merriam-Webster 2013.
31. American Psychiatric Association 2000, p.463.
32. Teeguarden 1996, pp.311–312.
33. Scaer 2005.
34. Scaer 2005, pp.214–251.
35. Levine 1997.
36. Levine 2005a.
37. Levine 2005b.
38. Cook et al. 1993.
39. American Psychiatric Association 2000, pp.463–464.
40. Brown 2007, p.173.
41. P.S. Maywald, interview with Internal Family Systems therapist, 7 July 2013.
42. Jarrett 1998, p.57.
43. Hicks, Hicks and Mole 2004, p.163.
44. Kaptchuk 2000, p.62.
45. Maoshing 1995, p.96.
46. Reninger 2013.
47. Fung 1983, p.41.
48. Kaptchuk 2000, p.63.
49. Keller 2006a.
50. Dechar 2006, p.321.
51. Shah 1967, p.21.
52. Jarrett 1998, p.176.
53. Maciocia 2005, p.154.
54. Willmont 1999.
55. Almaas 1988, p.303.
56. Almaas 1989, p.125.
57. Almaas 1989, p.126.
58. Almaas 1989, p.128.
59. Almaas 1989, p.127.
60. Almaas 1998, p.35.
61. Almaas 1999.
62. Raffel 2005, p.38.
63. Taylor 2008, p.139.

Chapter 7

1. Cohen 2001.
2. Maciocia 2005, p.117.
3. The capitalisation of 'Blood' distinguishes the Chinese notion of Blood from the Western notion. Blood is one of the five fundamental substances and is a dense form of Qi.
4. Maciocia 2005, p.200.
5. Zacks 2006.
6. Maciocia 2005, p.122.
7. Green Med TV 2013.
8. Many dentists advise not to drink lemon juice because of its effect on tooth enamel; however, rinsing the mouth with fresh water afterwards minimises the acidic effects on the teeth.
9. Simon 2012. One study of nursing home autopsies found over 50% with gallstones.
10. Hoffman 2013.
11. Balch 1997, p.286.
12. Waltz 2012.
13. Pears 2006, p.302.
14. Hizer 2012.
15. Harper 2012.
16. Hicks, Hicks and Mole 2004, p.57.
17. Greenfeld 1998.
18. Wetzler 1992, pp.14–15.
19. Benedict 1946.
20. Lewis 1971.
21. Freud 1960.
22. Miller 2011.
23. One of the Eight Strands of Brocade series of qigong exercises, of which there are many variations.
24. Brown 1999 is recommended for work with the inner critic.
25. Mahler, Pine and Bergman 2000, p.44.
26. Jarrett 1998, p.236.
27. Hicks, Hicks and Mole 2004, p.16.
28. Jarrett 1998, p.236.
29. Dechar 2006, p.199.
30. Wu 1993, p.40.
31. Dechar 2006, p.204.
32. Maciocia 2005, p.123.
33. Jarrett 2003, p.164.
34. Maciocia 2005, p.123.
35. *Bai Hu Dong* quoted in Jarrett 1998, p.239.
36. Gyatso 1990, p.135.
37. Almaas 2002b, p.271.
38. Almaas 1996, p.87.
39. Almaas 1988, p.42.
40. Almaas 1988, p.46.
41. This is one of the core practices I learned in the Diamond Approach. Hameed has recently brought this teaching into the public realm.

Chapter 8

1. Wieger 1965, p.290.
2. Hicks, Hicks and Mole 2004 (p.85) note that speech is the sense organ and the tongue is the orifice. I have taken some liberty here for simplicity.
3. The ancient Chinese regarded the Heart, rather than the brain, as the seat of the mind. See 'What Is Thought?' in Chapter 4.
4. Maciocia 2005, p.71.
5. Maitri 2000, p.263.
6. Franglen 2013, pp.204–208.
7. The Australian Institute of Health and Welfare 2010 reports that, in 2006, 17% of deaths were from heart attacks.
8. Hicks, Hicks and Mole 2004, p.88.
9. Maciocia 2005, p.107.
10. Larre and Rochat de la Vallee 1992, p.33.
11. Hicks, Hicks and Mole 2004, p.89.
12. Tortora and Anagnostakos 1990, p.759.
13. Maciocia 2005, p.191.
14. Campbell-McBride 2010.
15. Maciocia 2005, p.193.
16. Maoshing 1995, p.34.
17. Hicks, Hicks and Mole 2004, p.93.
18. Some authorities see the liver as more related to the lower burner despite its location in the middle burner.
19. Maciocia 2005, p.113.
20. Maciocia 2005, p.310.
21. Maciocia 2005, p.113.
22. Maoshing 1995, p.42. Hicks, Hicks and Mole 2004 identify head hair as the 'residue', but this is disputed and has no support elsewhere.
23. Maciocia 2005, p.109.
24. While not being dismissive, the US FDA and the Mayo Clinic have been cautious in allowing these claims.
25. Kellow 2012.
26. Reichstein 1998, p.75.
27. Maoshing 1995, p.42.
28. The standard medical view is challenged by a large body of medical opinion which now regards this linkage as a myth. In the ABC television program *Catalyst*, Demarsi 2013 interviewed physicians who pointed to a single flawed study as the foundation of this view.
29. Balch 1997, p.189.
30. Hammer 2005, p.166.
31. Gumenick 1997.
32. Miller *et al.* 2006.
33. Cousins 1983.
34. Gorman 2011.
35. White 2012.

36. Fromm 2006, p.123.
37. Sternberg 1988.
38. 'Triangular Theory of Love' licensed under public domain via Wikimedia Commons: https://commons.wikimedia.org/wiki/File:Triangular_Theory_of_Love.svg#/media/File:Triangular_Theory_of_Love.svg.
39. Stuart 2007.
40. Jampolsky 1979.
41. Foundation for Inner Peace 2008.
42. Gross 2012.
43. Darling 2013.
44. Hatton 2000.
45. Jarrett 1998, p.50.
46. Maciocia 2005, p.100.
47. Maoshing 1995, p.96.
48. Fung 1983, p.41.
49. Jarrett 1998, p.197.
50. Hollis 2006.
51. Maharshi 2008. 'I, I' is Ramana Maharshi's term for the True Self.
52. Almaas 1988, p.312.
53. Almaas 1990, p.86.
54. Almaas 1989, p.153.
55. Almaas 1989, p.157.
56. Almaas 1989, p.160.
57. Almaas 1989, p.162.
58. Almaas 1988, p.437.
59. Jarrett 2003, p.400.
60. Jarrett 2003, p.404.
61. Elijah 2013.

Chapter 9

1. Wieger 1965, p.209.
2. Maoshing 1995, p.90.
3. Maoshing 1995, p.116.
4. Barnard 1977, p.434. I find the first two stanzas of Keats' 'Ode to Autumn' to be one of the best transmissions of late summer.
5. Jarrett 1998, p.279.
6. Hicks, Hicks and Mole 2004, p.108.
7. Maoshing 1995, p.21.
8. Veith 1949, p.119.
9. Mann 1962, p.94.
10. Eckman 1996, p.206. I am grateful for Eckman's impeccable scholarship and detective work which has uncovered this origination.
11. Hicks, Hicks and Mole 2004, p.110.
12. While there are 366 days every fourth year, this too is reliable.
13. Beinfeld and Korngold 1991, p.29.
14. Diamond 2001 provides a detailed treatment of how failure to live in harmony with the earth can cause sudden catastrophe.
15. Jarrett 1998, p.282.
16. While some infants are removed from their mothers at birth, with profound consequences for the Earth energies, the experience of nourishment in the womb is one we all share.
17. Free Dictionary 2013.
18. Moorjani 2012, p.113.
19. Cherry 2013.
20. Mitchell 1992, p.7.
21. Tortora and Anagnostakos 1990, p.750.
22. Balch 1997, p.423.
23. Maciocia 2005, p.185.
24. Maoshing 1995, p.47.
25. Maciocia 2005, p.186.
26. Maciocia 2005, p.143.
27. Maciocia 2005, p.147.
28. These observations on fascia are from my own experience as a bodyworker and not from classical sources.
29. Hicks, Hicks and Mole 2004, p.114.
30. Mercola 2013.
31. Waterfield 2013.
32. Mayo Clinic 2013.
33. Lloyd 2013.
34. Brownie 2013.
35. Brownie 2013.
36. Balch 1997, p.423.
37. Titan *et al.* 2001.
38. Dechar 2006, p.228.
39. Mosley 2012.
40. Beattie 1986.
41. While the *Diagnostic and Statistical Manual of Mental Disorders* (published by the American Psychiatric Association) defines narcissism as a personality disorder, there is no such thing as compulsive giving disorder.
42. Wieger 1965, p.111.
43. Maciocia 2005, p.250.
44. Maciocia 2005, p.150.
45. Goodyer 2013.
46. Eating Disorders Foundation of Victoria 2013.
47. Wieger 1965, p.187.
48. Kaptchuk 2000, p.69.
49. Maoshing 1995, p.96.
50. Kaptchuck 2000, p.60.
51. Dechar 2012.
52. Fung 1983, pp.41–42.
53. Jarrett 1998, p.282.
54. Jarrett 1998, p.282.
55. Almaas 1987, p.92.

56. Almaas 2001, p.34.
57. Kaptchuck 2000, pp.59–60.
58. Hicks, Hicks and Mole 2004, p.118.

Chapter 10

1. Barks 2004, p.109.
2. Gyatso and Hopkins 1988, p.37.
3. Genesis 2:7
4. Vines 2005.
5. Maoshing 1995, p.17.
6. Maoshing 1995, p.34.
7. Tortora and Anagnostakos 1990, p.768.
8. Maciocia 2005, p.195.
9. Maoshing 1995, p.40.
10. Kellow 2013b.
11. Reichstein 1998, p.153.
12. Jarrett 1998 (p.275) observes that enemas can disempower the Large Intestine and that excessive use of enemas weakens the organ.
13. Ackerman 1991, p.6.
14. From OxyGen 2014 (website no longer online).
15. Kübler-Ross 1969.
16. Suttie 2012.
17. Berger 2009.
18. Gumenick 2013.
19. Jarrett 1998, p.265.
20. Jarrett 1998, p.262.
21. Schwartz 1997.
22. Jarrett 2003, p.591.
23. Jarrett 2003, p.592.
24. Olmstead 2014.
25. Kaptchuk 2000, p.65.
26. Maciocia 2005, p.138.
27. Jarrett 1998, p.260.
28. Moss 2010, p.204.
29. While it is spelled the same, this is a different word from *yi*, which is the spirit of the Earth Element.
30. Jarrett 1998, p.261.
31. Keller 2006b.
32. Adyashanti 2014.
33. Tolle 2004, p.49.
34. Almaas 2008, p.221.
35. Almaas 2002a, p.26.
36. Almaas 1999.

References

Ackerman, D. (1991) *A Natural History of the Senses.* New York, NY: Vintage.

Adyashanti (2014) *The Doorway to Now.* (Video). Available at www.adyashanti.org/index.php?file=watchvideo, accessed on 14 May 2014.

Al-Khalili, J. (2010) *The Observer Effect.* Video. Accessed on 9 January 2014; no longer available.

Almaas, A.H. (1987) *Diamond Heart Book 1.* Boston, MA: Shambala.

Almaas, A.H. (1988) *The Pearl Beyond Price.* Boston, MA: Shambala.

Almaas, A.H. (1989) *Diamond Heart Book 2.* Boston, MA: Shambala.

Almaas, A.H. (1990) *Diamond Heart Book 3.* Boston, MA: Shambala.

Almaas, A.H. (1996) *The Point of Existence.* Boston, MA: Shambala.

Almaas, A.H. (1998) *Facets of Unity.* Boston, MA: Shambala.

Almaas, A.H. (1999) *Wisdom of Life and Death.* (DVD). Berkeley, CA: Ridhwan Foundation.

Almaas, A.H. (2001) *Diamond Heart Book 4.* Boston, MA: Shambala.

Almaas, A.H. (2002a) *Facets of Unity.* Boston, MA: Shambala.

Almaas, A.H. (2002b) *Spacecruiser Inquiry.* Boston, MA: Shambala.

Almaas, A.H. (2008) *The Unfolding Now.* Boston, MA: Shambala.

Almaas, A.H. (2013) *The Diamond Approach.* Available at www.ahalmaas.com/articles/the-diamond-approach, accessed on 10 October 2013.

American Psychiatric Association (2000) *Diagnostic and Statistical Manual of Mental Disorders* (4th ed.). Arlington, VA: APA.

Austin, M. (1972) *Acupuncture Therapy.* New York, NY: ASI Publishers.

Australian Institute of Health and Welfare (2010) *Cardiovascular Disease Mortality.* Canberra, ACT, Australia: AIHW.

Balch P.A. (1997) *Prescription for Nutritional Healing* (2nd ed.). New York, NY: Avery.

Barks, C. (trans.) (2004) *The Essential Rumi.* New York, NY: Harper One.

Barnard, J. (ed.) (1977) *John Keats: The Complete Poems* (3rd ed.). London: Penguin.

Batmanghelidj, F. (2008) *Your Body's Many Cries for Water.* Rome, GA: Global Health Solutions.

Beattie, M. (1986) *Codependent No More.* Center City, MN: Hazelden.

Beinfeld, H. and Korngold, E. (1991) *Between Heaven and Earth.* New York, NY: Ballantine.

Benedict, R. (1946) *The Chrysanthemum and the Sword: Patterns of Japanese Culture.* Boston, MA: Houghton Mifflin.

Berger, S. (2009) *The Five Ways to Grieve.* Durban, South Africa: Trumpeter.

Brown, B. (1999) *Soul Without Shame.* Boston, MA: Shambala.

Brown, D. (2013) *Bioelectricity Qi and the Human Body.* Available at www.qigonginstitute.org/docsQiIsEnergy.pdf, accessed on 1 February 2016.

Brown, R.M. (2007) *All the Fishes Come Home to Roost.* London: Sceptre.

Brownie, S. (2013) 'Nutritional well-being for older people.' *Journal of the Australian Traditional Medicine Society 19*, 3, 141.

Campbell-McBride, N. (2010) *Gut and Psychology Syndrome: Natural Treatment for Autism, Dyspraxia, A.D.D., Dyslexia, A.D.H.D., Depression, Schizophrenia.* Medinform Publishing.

Cherry, K. (2013) *What is Altruism?* Available at http://psychology.about.com/od/aindex/g/what-is-altruism.htm, accessed on 10 October 2013.

Cleary, T. (trans.) (2003) *The Taoist Classics* (volume 1). Boston, MA: Shambala.

Cohen, P. (2001) 'Mental gymnastics increase bicep strength.' *New Scientist 24*, 17.

Cook, B., David, F. and Grant, A. (1993) *Sexual Violence in Australia*. Canberra, ACT, Australia: Australian Institute of Criminology.

Cousins, N. (1983) *The Healing Heart: Antidotes to Panic and Helplessness*. New York, NY: Norton.

Darling, G. (2013) *Adorn Yourself Adore Life*. Available at http://galadarling.com, accessed on 3 January 2013.

Dechar, L.E. (2006) *Five Spirits*. New York, NY: Lantern.

Dechar, L.E. (2012) *Yi: Intention, Practice and the Incubation of the Sage*. Previously available at www.fivespirits.com, accessed on 19 November 2013.

Demarsi, M. (2013) 'Heart of the Matter.' *Catalyst*, ABC television program, aired 31 October 2013.

Diamond, J. (2001) *Collapse*. New York, NY: Penguin.

Eating Disorders Foundation of Victoria (2013) *Mindful Eating*. Available at www.eatingdisorders.org.au/docman/fact-sheets/234-fact-sheet-mindful-eating, accessed on 22 October 2013.

Eckman, P. (1996) *In the Footsteps of the Yellow Emperor*. San Francisco, CA: Cypress.

Elijah, T. (2009) *5 Element Treatment Protocols*. Available at http://perennialmedicine.com/wp-content/uploads/2011/11/5%20Element%20Treatment%20Protocols.pdf, accessed on 2 December 2013.

Elijah, T. (2013) *The Perennial Medicine*. Available at http://perennialmedicine.com/wp-content/uploads/ThePerennialMedicine.pdf, accessed on 2 December 2013.

Foundation for Inner Peace (2008) *A Course in Miracles*. Mill Valley, CA: Foundation for Inner Peace.

Franglen, N. (2013) *Keepers of the Soul*. London: Singing Dragon.

Free Dictionary (2013) Available at www.thefreedictionary.com/grok, accessed on 10 October 2013.

Freud, S. (1960) *The Ego and the Id*. New York, NY: Norton.

Fromm, E. (2006) *The Art of Loving*. New York, NY: Harper Perennial.

Fung, Y.L. (1976) *A Short History of Chinese Philosophy*. New York, NY: Free Press. (Original work published 1949.)

Fung, Y.L. (1983) *A History of Chinese Philosophy* (volume 2). Princeton, NJ: Princeton University Press.

Goodyer, P. (2013) 'Fixing emotional eating.' *Sydney Morning Herald*, 25 March. Available at www.smh.com.au/lifestyle/diet-and-fitness/chew-on-this/fixing-emotional-eating-20130325-2gp0y, accessed on 12 October 2013.

Gorman, J. (2011) 'Scientists hint at why laughter feels so good.' *New York Times*, 13 September. Available at www.nytimes.com/2011/09/14/science/14laughter.html?_r=0, accessed on 3 December 2012.

Green Med TV (2013) *The #1 Anti Cancer Vegetable*. Available at http://tv.greenmedinfo.com/the-1-anti-cancer-vegetable, accessed on 6 September 2013.

Greenfeld, L.A. (1998) *Alcohol and Crime: An Analysis of National Data on the Prevalence of Alcohol Involvement in Crime*. Washington, DC: U.S. Department of Justice.

Gross, M. (2012) 'Cupids' chemistry.' *RSC*. Available at www.rsc.org/chemistryworld/Issues/2006/February/CupidChemistry.asp, accessed on 12 December 2012.

Gumenick, N.R. (1997) *Tending Our Fire*. Available at www.5elements.com/docs/elements/fire.html, accessed on 1 December 2012.

Gumenick, N.R. (2013) *The Metal Imbalanced Patient*. Available at www.5elements.com/articles/pract-px_metal_rapport.pdf, accessed on 29 January 2013.

Gurumaa, A. (2013) *What Is the Mind and Where Is It Located?* Available at www.gurumaa.com/library/what-is-mind-where-mind-located, accessed on 11 October 2013.

Gyatso, T. (1990) *Freedom in Exile*. New York, NY: Harper Collins.

Gyatso, T. (1995) 'What is the Mind?' *Mandala*, Nov–Dec. Available at http://fpmt.org/mandala/archives/older/mandala-issues-for-1995/november/what-is-the-mind, accessed on 7 January 2016.

Gyatso, T. and Hopkins, J. (1988) *The Dalai Lama at Harvard*. Boston, MA: Snow Lion.

Hammer, L. (2005) *Dragon Rises, Red Bird Flies (Revised ed.)*. Seattle, WA: Eastland.

Harper, D. (2012) *Online Etymology Dictionary*. Available at www.etymonline.com/index.php?term=anger&allowed_in_frame=0, accessed on 5 September 2012.

Hatton, C.L. (ed.) (2000) *Acupuncture Point Compendium*. Leamington Spa: College of Traditional Acupuncture.

Hicks, A., Hicks, J. and Mole, P. (2004) *Five Element Constitutional Acupuncture*. Edinburgh: Churchill Livingstone.

Hizer, C. (2012) *Yes You Can Practice Crop Rotation*. Available at www.vegetablegardener.com/item/2487/yes-you-can-practice-crop-rotation, accessed on 31 August 2012.

Hoffman, R. (2013) *Gall Bladder Disease*. Available at http://drhoffman.com/article/gallbladder-disease-2, accessed on 6 September 2013.

Hollis, J. (2006) *Finding Meaning in the Second Half of Life*. New York, NY: Gotham.

Horowitz, S. (2012) 'The Science of Art and Listening.' *New York Times*, 9 November, p.SR10.

Jampolsky, J.J. (1979) *Love is Letting Go of Fear*. Berkeley, CA: Celestial Arts.

Jarmey, C. and Bouratinos, I. (2008) *A Practical Guide to Acu-points*. Berkeley, CA: North Atlantic.

Jarrett, L.S. (1992) 'Myth and Meaning in Chinese medicine.' *Traditional Acupuncture Society Journal England* 11, 45–48.

Jarrett, L.S. (1998) *Nourishing Destiny*. Stockbridge, MA: Spirit Path Press.

Jarrett, L.S. (2003) *The Clinical Practice of Chinese Medicine*. Stockbridge, MA: Spirit Path Press.

Kaku, M. (2007) *Quantum Mechanics*. Available at www.youtube.com/watch?v=45KGS1Ro-sc, accessed on 11 October 2013.

Kaptchuk, T.J. (2000) *The Web That Has No Weaver*. Chicago, IL: Contemporary Books.

Keller, R. (2006a) *Wisdom: The Virtue of the Kidneys*. Available at www.robertkellerca.com/wisdom.htm, accessed on 19 August 2013.

Keller, R. (2006b) *Preciousness and Righteousness: The Virtues of the Lungs*. Available at www.robertkellerca.com/lungvirtues.htm, accessed on 12 May 2014.

Kellow, J. (2012) *Eat a Rainbow of Red Food*. Available at www.weightlossresources.co.uk/healthy_eating/eat-a-rainbow/lycopene-red-food.htm, accessed on 25 November 2012.

Kellow, J. (2013a) *Eat a Rainbow of Purple and Blue Food*. Available at www.weightlossresources.co.uk/healthy_eating/eat-a-rainbow/anthocyanins-blue-purple-food.htm, accessed on 30 August 2013.

Kellow, J. (2013b) *Eat a Rainbow of White Food*. Available at www.weightlossresources.co.uk/healthy_eating/eat-a-rainbow/quercetin-white-food.htm, accessed on 25 April 2013.

Kirkwood, J. (2016) *The Way of the Five Elements*. London: Singing Dragon.

Kübler-Ross, E. (1969) *On Death and Dying*. New York, NY: Macmillan.

Larre, C. and Rochat de la Vallee, E. (1992) *The Secret Treatise of the Spiritual Orchid*. Cambridge: Monkey Press.

Lawson-Wood, D. (1959) *Chinese System of Healing*. Hindhead: Health Sciences Press.

Levine, P.A. (1997) *Waking the Tiger*. Berkeley, CA: North Atlantic.

Levine, P.A. (2005a) *Healing Trauma*. Boulder, CO: Sounds True.

Levine, P.A. (2005b) *The Biological Process of Trauma*. (Audio CD). Boulder, CO: Sounds True.

Lewis, H.B. (1971) *Shame and Guilt in Neurosis*. Madison, CT: International Universities.

Libet, B. (1999) 'Do we have free will?' *Journal of Consciousness Studies 8–9*, 47–57.

Lloyd, I. (2013) *Hyperchlorhydria*. Available at www.ndhealthfacts.org/wiki/Hyperchlorhydria_%28High_Stomach_Acid%29, accessed on 30 September 2013.

Maciocia, G. (2005) *The Foundations of Chinese Medicine* (2nd ed.). Edinburgh: Churchill Livingstone.

Maciocia, G. (2009) *The Psyche in Chinese Medicine*. Edinburgh: Churchill Livingstone.

Mahler, M., Pine, F. and Bergman, A. (2000) *The Psychological Birth of the Human Infant*. New York, NY: Basic Books.

Maitri, S. (2000) *The Spiritual Dimension of the Enneagram*. New York, NY: Tarcher Putnam.

Maoshing, N. (trans.) (1995) *The Yellow Emperor's Classic of Medicine*. Boston, MA: Shambala.

Mann, F. (1962) *Acupuncture: The Ancient Chinese Art of Healing*. London: Heinemann.

Mayo Clinic (2013) *Peptic Ulcer*. Available at www.mayoclinic.org/diseases-conditions/peptic-ulcer/basics/definition/con-20028643, accessed on 30 September 2013.

McLellan, S. (1998) *Integrative Acupressure*. New York, NY: Perigree.

Mercola, D. (2013) *Fructose*. Available at http://articles.mercola.com/sites/articles/archive/2013/01/14/fructose-spurs-overeating.aspx, accessed on 27 September 2013.

Merriam-Webster (2013) Available at www.merriam-webster.com/dictionary/trauma, accessed on 27 July 2013.

Miller, M.C. (ed.) (2011) *Understanding Depression*. Available at www.health.harvard.edu/mind-and-mood/understanding-depression, accessed on 15 September 2012.

Miller, M., Mangano, C., Park, Y., Goel, R., Plotnick, G.D. and Vogel, R.A. (2006) 'Impact of cinematic viewing on endothelial function.' *National Institute of Health*. Available at www.ncbi.nlm.nih.gov/pmc/articles/PMC1860773, accessed on 1 December 2012.

Mitchell, S. (1992) *Tao Te Ching*. New York, NY: Harper Perennial.

Moorjani, A. (2012) *Dying To Be Me*. London: Hay House.

Morsella, E. (2012) 'What is a thought?' *Psychology Today 9*. Available at www.psychologytoday.com/blog/consciousness-and-the-brain/201202/what-is-thought, accessed on 7 January 2016.

Mosley, M. (2012) 'The power of intermittant fasting.' *BBC,* 5 August. Available at www.bbc.com/news/health-19112549, accessed on 3 October 2013.

Moss, C.A. (2010) *Power of the Five Elements,* Berkeley, CA: North Atlantic.

Olmstead, C. (2014) *Feng Shui for Real Life.* Available at http://fengshuiforreallife.com, accessed on 27 May 2014.

Pears P. (ed.) (2006) *Organic Gardening in Australia.* Camberwell, VIC, Australia: Dorling Kindersley.

Raffel, B. (ed.) (2005) *Macbeth (The Annotated Shakespeare).* New Haven, CT: Yale University Press.

Reichstein, G. (1998) *Wood Becomes Water.* New York, NY: Kodansha.

Reninger, E. (2012) *What is Qi?* Available at http://taoism.about.com/od/qi/a/Qi.htm, accessed on 29 December 2012.

Reninger, E. (2013) *Wu Wei the Action of Non-action.* Available at http://taoism.about.com, accessed on 4 August 2013.

Reston, J. (1971) 'Now about my operation in Peking.' *New York Times,* 26 July.

Scaer, R. (2005) *The Trauma Spectrum.* New York, NY: Norton.

Scherer, K. (2005) 'What are emotions and how can they be measured?' *Social Science Information.* New York, NY: Sage Publications.

Schwartz, J. (1997) *Brain Lock: Free Yourself from Obsessive-Compulsive Behaviour.* New York, NY: Harper Perennial.

Shah, I. (1967) *Tales of the Dervishes.* London: Penguin.

Simon, H. (2012) *Gallstones and Gall Bladder Disease.* Available at https://umm.edu/health/medical/reports/articles/gallstones-and-gallbladder-disease, accessed on 6 September 2013.

Solomon, R.C. (2003) *What Is an Emotion?* Oxford: Oxford University Press.

Sternberg, R.J. (1988) *The Triangle of Love.* New York, NY: Basic Books.

Stuart, J. (2007) 'What exactly is love?' *The Independent,* 13 February. Available at www.independent.co.uk/lifestyle/health-and-families/health-news/what-exactly-is-love-436234.htm, accessed on 10 December 2012.

Suttie, E. (2012) 'Dealing with grief: a TCM perspective.' *Points Newsletter,* October 2012. Available at www.acupuncture.com/newsletters/m_oct12/grief.htm, accessed on 19 October 2012.

Suzuki, S. (1970) *Zen Mind Beginner's Mind.* Berkeley, CA: Weatherhill.

Taylor, G. (ed.) (2008) *Henry V: The Oxford Shakespeare.* Oxford: Oxford Paperbacks.

Teeguarden, I.M. (1996) *A Complete Guide to Acupressure.* Tokyo: Japan.

Thompson, D. (2006) 'Seawater: A Safe Blood Plasma Substitute?' *Nexus,* 19–22.

Titan, S.M., Bingham, S., Welch, A., Luben, R. *et al.* (2001) 'Frequency of eating and concentrations of serum cholesterol in the Norfolk population of the European prospective investigation into cancer.' *British Medical Journal.* Available at www.bmj.com/content/323/7324/1286.1, accessed on 7 January 2016.

Tolle, E. (2004) *The Power of Now.* Novato, CA: New World Library.

Tortora, G.J. and Anagnostakos, N.P. (1990) *Principles of Anatomy and Physiology.* New York, NY: Harper Collins.

Unschuld, P.U. (1985) *Medicine in China.* Berkeley, CA: University of California Press.

Vines, T. (2005) 'An analysis of William Blake's Songs of Innocence and of Experience as a response to the collapse of values.' *Cross Sections 1,* 115–122.

Wetzler, S. (1992) *Living with the Passive-aggressive Man.* New York, NY: Touchstone.

Willmont, D. (1999) *Healing in the Winter.* Available at www.willmountain.com/v/Clinic/Winter.pdf, accessed on 6 August 2013.

Veith, I. (trans) (1949) *The Yellow Emperor's Classic of Internal Medicine.* Philadelphia, PA: Williams and Wilkins.

Waltz, R.D. (2012) *Cleansing and Supporting the Liver.* Available at www.naturalark.com/liverc.html, accessed 29 August 2012.

Waterfield, B. (2013) 'Sugar is addictive and the most dangerous drug of the times.' *Telegraph,* 17 September. Available at www.telegraph.co.uk/news/worldnews/europe/netherlands/10314705/Sugar-is-addictive-and-the-most-dangerous-drug-of-the-times.html, accessed on 3 September 2015.

White, E.B. (2012) *Wikiquote.* Available at https://en.wikiquote.org/wiki/E._B._White, accessed on 3 December 2012.

Wieger, L. (1965) *Chinese Characters.* New York, NY: Dover.

Wu, J.N. (1993) *Ling Shu or the Spiritual Pivot.* Honolulu, HI: University of Hawaii Press.

Zacks, D. (2006) 'Why does eyesight deteriorate with age?' *Scientific American 9.* Available at www.scientificamerican.com/article/why-does-eyesight-deterio, accessed on 7 January 2016.

Further Reading

Chia, M. and Winn, M. (1984) *Taoist Secrets of Love*. Santa Fe, NM: Aurora.

Cohen, K.S. (1997) *The Way of Qigong*. New York, NY: Ballantine.

Connelly, D.M. (1994) *Traditional Acupuncture: The Law of the Five Elements* (2nd ed.). Columbia, MD: Traditional Acupuncture Institute.

Cross, J.R. (2006) *Healing with the Chakra Energy System*. Berkeley, CA: North Atlantic.

Cross, J.R. (2008) *Acupuncture and the Chakra Energy System*. Berkeley, CA: North Atlantic.

Deadman, P. and Ali Khafaji, M., with Baker, K. (2005) *A Manual of Acupuncture* (revised ed.). Hove: Journal of Chinese Medicine.

Dolowich, G. (2003) *Archetypal Acupuncture: Healing with the Five Elements*. Aptos, CA: Jade Mountain.

Ellis, A., Wiseman, N. and Boss, K. (1989) *Grasping the Wind*. Brookline, MA: Paradigm.

Gach, M.R. (2004) *Acupressure for Emotional Healing*. New York, NY: Bantam.

Gerber, R. (2001) *Vibrational Medicine*. Rochester, VT: Bear.

Gerrard, D. (2001) *One Bowl: A Guide to Eating for Body and Spirit*. New York, NY: Marlowe.

Haas, E.M. (1981) *Staying Healthy with the Seasons*. Berkeley, CA: Celestial Arts.

Hicks, A. and Hicks, J. (1999) *Healing Your Emotions*. London: Thorsons.

Kaatz, D. (2005) *Characters of Wisdom*. Soudorgues: Petite Bergerie Press.

Larre, C. and Rochat de la Vallee, E. (1995) *Rooted in Spirit*. Barrytown, NY: Station Hill.

Marin, G. (2006) *Five Elements Six Conditions*. Berkeley, CA: North Atlantic.

Matsumoto, K. and Birch, S. (1986) *Extraordinary Vessels*. Brookline, MA: Paradigm.

Roth, G. (2010) *Women Food and God*. New York, NY: Scribner.

Teeguarden, I.M. (1978) *Acupressure Way of Health*. Tokyo: Japan Publications.

Teeguarden, I.M. (1987) *The Joy of Feeling*. Tokyo: Japan Publications.

Unschuld, P.U. (1986) *Nan-ching: The Classic of Difficulties*. Berkeley, CA: University of California Press.

Wong, L. and Knapsey, K. (2006) *Food for the Seasons*. Fitzroy, VIC, Australia: Red Dog.

Worsley, J.R. (1982) *Traditional Chinese Acupuncture. Meridians and Points* (volume 1). Tisbury: Element Books.

Index